Bio-Inspired Optimization for Medical Data Mining

Scrivener Publishing
100 Cummings Center, Suite 541J
Beverly, MA 01915-6106

Publishers at Scrivener
Martin Scrivener (martin@scrivenerpublishing.com)
Phillip Carmical (pcarmical@scrivenerpublishing.com)

Bio-Inspired Optimization for Medical Data Mining

Edited by

Sumit Srivastava

Department of Information Technology, Manipal University Jaipur, India

Abhineet Anand

Department of CSE, Bahra University, Shimla, Himachal Pradesh, India

Abhishek Kumar

Department of Computer Science & Engineering, Chandigarh University, Punjab, India

Bhavna Saini

Data Science and Analytics, Central University of Rajasthan, India

and

Pramod Singh Rathore

Department of Computer and Communication Engineering, Manipal University Jaipur, India

Scrivener Publishing

WILEY

This edition first published 2024 by John Wiley & Sons, Inc., 111 River Street, Hoboken, NJ 07030, USA and Scrivener Publishing LLC, 100 Cummings Center, Suite 541J, Beverly, MA 01915, USA

For more information about Scrivener publications please visit www.scrivenerpublishing.com.

Wiley Global Headquarters
111 River Street, Hoboken, NJ 07030, USA

For details of our global editorial offices, customer services, and more information about Wiley products visit us at www.wiley.com.

Library of Congress Cataloging-in-Publication Data

ISBN 978-1-394-21418-1

Cover image: Pixabay.Com
Cover design by Russell Richardson

Set in size of 11pt and Minion Pro by Manila Typesetting Company, Makati, Philippines

Printed in the USA

10 9 8 7 6 5 4 3 2 1

Contents

Preface

This book is organized into fourteen chapters. Chapter 1 begins by introducing the concept of bio-inspired algorithms and their underlying principles. It then explores the opportunities offered by these algorithms, such as their capacity to locate the best answers in very big and intricate search fields, their robustness in dealing with uncertainty and noise, and their potential for parallel and distributed computing. The chapter will also highlight the application areas where bio-inspired algorithms have shown promising results, including in optimization problems, pattern recognition, and swarm robotics.

In Chapter 2, the semipermeable membrane of an egg was separated and used to assess the Mace spice's *in vitro* antiurolithiatic efficacy. By performing *in vitro* urolithiasis on the chosen plant, Mace spice, and using the common medication Neeri, the percentage of kidney stone dissolving was discovered. The Mace spice's ethanol leaf extracts have the greatest medication dissolving rates. Thus, through our research, it has been established that the Mace spice plant contains antiurolithiatic properties.

In Chapter 3, Parkinson's disease (PD) is normally diagnosed in a person after a thorough physical examination by a doctor that considers the patient's medical past, neurological examination, evaluation of motor symptoms, and other supporting tests with precise diagnostic criteria. However, there is no surefire way to identify PD. Furthermore, other medical problems, including arthritis and stroke, should be evaluated on subsequent visits because they can show similarly to Parkinson's disease. Only 80.6% of PD diagnoses are correct overall. Machine learning techniques can be applied in a variety of ways to develop different methods to recognize the presence of PD in an individual, as well as identify it in the initial stages of the disease, to aid doctors in the diagnosis of PD.

Chapter 4 explains the importance of detecting the tumors immediately. Various mechanical methods exist for the detection of tumors, such as Magnetic Resonance Imaging (MRI), Computerized Tomography (CT) Scan, and Positron Emission Tomography (PET) Scan. These scans send the waves into the patient's body to obtain images of the organ or body part affected. Images obtained from these scans are of Digital Imaging and Communications in Medicine (DICOM) format. Different techniques are available for the classification of the tumor, such as segmentation, feature extraction, machine learning techniques, and deep learning models. These techniques are discussed and compared in this chapter, which will help researchers to find the optimal solution for their research in the detection and classification of different tumors and other deadly diseases. Finally, this chapter chronicles all the relevant and important literature related with tumor detection and how it can be classified using new age computer-based technology, such as deep learning and machine learning.

Chapter 5 addresses current developments in molecular subtyping and how they could enhance the precision of tumor categorization. The clinical ramifications of tumor detection and categorization, including diagnosis, prognosis, and treatment planning, are covered in the chapter's concluding section. In order to inform treatment choices, enhance patient outcomes, and save healthcare costs, this section emphasizes the significance of precise tumor diagnosis and classification. Healthcare workers, researchers, and students with an interest in tumor detection and treatment will find the chapter to be an invaluable resource.

In Chapter 6, researchers assessed the performance of these algorithms using a variety of evaluation criteria, including accuracy, precision, recall, and F1 score. Our findings show that, with an accuracy of 90.5%, DNNs outperformed the competition, followed by SVM (85.3%), RF (81.9%), and KNN (78.5%). In order to determine which aspects were most crucial for each algorithm, feature selection was also performed. Various algorithms were discovered that favored various feature sets. This research sheds light on the usefulness of various machine learning algorithms for classifying brain tumors, which will help in the creation of more precise and effective diagnostic equipment for this serious medical disease.

In Chapter 7, a series of mathematical equations simulate dingo behavior in the wild to find the best solutions to a variety of optimization challenges. The dingo optimizer has demonstrated promising results in several applications, including engineering design, financial forecasting, and bioinformatics. The algorithm is rather simple to implement and has the potential to be a useful tool for researchers and practitioners in a wide range of domains.

Chapter 8 discusses how genetic algorithms can be applied to the field of medicine. In addition to pharmacotherapy, other fields such as radiology, surgery, cardiology radiotherapy, pediatrics, endocrinology, obstetrics and gynaecology, pulmonary medicine, orthopaedics, rehabilitation medicine, neurology, infectious diseases, and health care administration have all found promising applications for the genetic algorithm. This chapter explains the genetic algorithm and how it may be used in healthcare administration, disease detection, treatment planning, drug safety monitoring, prognosis, and more. It also aids doctors in envisioning the future applications of this metaheuristic technique in healthcare.

Chapter 9 focuses on compounds that may comprise naturally occurring proteins or carbohydrates in our bodies. The immune system doesn't target these coated nanoparticles because it doesn't recognize them as being foreign when it sees them. Making the nanoparticles small enough to get past the body's natural defenses is another option. Small particles are harder for our immune system to find and recognize. The nanoparticles can therefore avoid detection and enter their target cells if we make them small enough. A computational method called an artificial immune system (AIS) algorithm can be used to create nanoparticles that bypass the immune system and deliver medications to specific cells. The AIS algorithm is inspired by the natural immune system. It is possible to create nanoparticles that can bypass the immune system and deliver medications to specific cells by using an artificial immune system algorithm.

In Chapter 10, the reader will learn about a novel ensemble approach that was developed for accurate blood vessel segmentation and classification. The retinal images had been accumulated from Digital Retinal Images for Vessel Extraction (DRIVE) and Structured Analysis of the Retina (STARE) datasets. The ensemble approach can segment the retinal blood vessels using bio-inspired algorithms and Cuttlefish Algorithm (CFA) for segmentation of the fundus image. The features are then extracted from the segmented pictures using the Enhanced Local Binary Pattern (ELBP) and Inverse Difference Moment Normalized (IDMN) algorithms.

Chapter 11 demonstrates how to predict behaviors and events thanks to data-driven linkages and patterns. Predictive analytics provides a look into the future by using past events. It is important to note that the predictive model was built using previous predictive approaches, even if it is not based on the production of a mathematical model or algorithms for the development of the forecast. Instead, it uses algorithms that are built into the identified tool. It is suggested that, via the usage of the model, the organizations that provide both public and private health services adopt it in a commercial setting, using the model's predictive capabilities for the client's diagnosis and the optimization of consultation procedures.

Chapter 12 focuses on neurological disease diagnosis, providing an overview of common diseases and current diagnostic techniques. It reviews traditional diagnostic methods and their limitations, highlighting the need for alternative approaches. The application of bio-inspired algorithms in neurological disease diagnosis is discussed in detail. Genetic algorithms can optimize feature selection and classification algorithms, as demonstrated through case studies and research findings. Neural networks are explored for their potential in improving disease diagnosis accuracy through bio-inspired optimization techniques. Other bio-inspired algorithms, such as ant colony optimization and particle swarm optimization, are also examined for their applications in feature selection, clustering analysis, and diagnostic model optimization. Finally, the chapter addresses the challenges and limitations associated with the use of bio-inspired algorithms in neurological disease diagnosis. It emphasizes the need for further research and development in this emerging field. Overall, bio-inspired algorithms hold great promise in advancing the field of neurological disease diagnosis, offering new opportunities for accuracy and efficiency.

As shown in Chapter 13, GA synergizes well with NNs to optimize models and approximate parameters, thereby enhancing the effectiveness of NNs. GA can be applied in various ways to design the best ANN for a given problem domain, including optimizing weights, selecting topology, choosing features, training, and improving interpretation. In the sections herein, several studies are presented that utilize different ANN optimization techniques through GA, depending on the research objectives.

Chapter 14 presents a modern idea that employs artificial intelligence and machine learning with a blend of bio-inspired methods. The biological inspiration behind this computing is Bio-Inspired Computing logics and can be applied in solving various applications. An organism's—or animal's—idea of fetching food, moving, and path formation are studied to determine how it can be best optimized and applied in the medical industry. The material in this chapter is based on the applications of bio-inspired systems in the medical therapy of the frontal and subsequent disorders. Furthermore, problems concerning the current challenges and future directions are also discussed.

We hope that you find this book to be informative and inspiring, and we extend our thanks to Martin Scrivener and his entire team for their dedicated support during publication.

Dr. Sumit Srivastava
Manipal University Jaipur (MUJ), India
Dr. Abhineet Anand
Department of CSE, Bahra University,
Shimla, Himachal Pradesh, India
Dr. Abhishek Kumar
Department of Computer Science & Engineering,
Chandigarh University, Punjab, India
Dr. Bhavna Saini
Department of Computer Science
Central University of Rajasthan, India
Pramod Singh Rathore
Department of Computer and Communication Engineering
Manipal University Jaipur (MUJ), India

1

Bioinspired Algorithms: Opportunities and Challenges

Shweta Agarwal*, Neetu Rani and Amit Vajpayee

Chandigarh University, Mohali, Punjab, India

Abstract

Bioinspired algorithms have received a lot of attention recently because of their potential to solve complex optimization problems by emulating the principles and behaviors found in nature. These algorithms, inspired by biological processes, such as evolution, swarm intelligence, and neural networks, have demonstrated promising results in various domains, including optimization, machine learning, robotics, and data mining. This chapter aims to give a brief summary of the opportunities and challenges associated with bioinspired algorithms. The chapter will begin by introducing the concept of bioinspired algorithms and their underlying principles. It will then explore the opportunities that these algorithms offer, such as their capacity to locate the best answers in very big and intricate search fields, their robustness in dealing with uncertainty and noise, and their potential for parallel and distributed computing. The chapter will also highlight the application areas where bioinspired algorithms have shown promising results, including in optimization problems, pattern recognition, and swarm robotics. However, along with the opportunities, bioinspired algorithms also present several challenges. The chapter will discuss these challenges, such as the need for parameter tuning, the lack of theoretical analysis and understanding, the risk of premature convergence, and the computational cost associated with large-scale problems. It will also address the ethical considerations and limitations of bioinspired algorithms, including concerns about fairness, transparency, and interpretability. To provide a comprehensive understanding, the chapter will discuss some of the prominent bioinspired algorithms, including artificial neural networks, ant colony optimization, particle swarm optimization and genetic algorithms. It will highlight their key features, advantages, and limitations, and provide examples of their applications in various domains. In conclusion, bioinspired algorithms offer exciting opportunities for solving complex problems in diverse

**Corresponding author*: ershweta.cs@gmail.com

Sumit Srivastava, Abhineet Anand, Abhishek Kumar, Bhavna Saini and Pramod Singh Rathore (eds.) Bio-Inspired Optimization for Medical Data Mining, (1–30) © 2024 Scrivener Publishing LLC

domains. However, their effective utilization requires addressing the associated challenges and considering ethical considerations.

Keywords: Bioinspired algorithms, ANN, ML, swarm intelligence, computational techniques, PSO, GA

1.1 Introduction

In this section, we explore the fascinating world of bioinspired algorithms and their significance in solving complex problems. Bioinspired algorithms draw inspiration from natural systems and processes, such as evolutionary principles, swarm behavior, and neural networks. We begin by defining bioinspired algorithms and discussing their importance in tackling challenging optimization problems. Furthermore, we provide an overview of the chapter, which includes an examination of different bioinspired principles and algorithms, an exploration of the opportunities they present, and an analysis of the challenges they entail. By delving into these topics, we aim to shed light on the exciting field of bioinspired algorithms and their potential for driving innovation.

1.1.1 Definition and Significance of Bioinspired Algorithms

Bioinspired algorithms, also known as nature-inspired algorithms or evolutionary computation, are computational techniques that draw inspiration from the principles, behaviors, and mechanisms observed in biological systems [1, 2]. These algorithms mimic the adaptive and problem-solving abilities found in nature to tackle complex optimization problems. By emulating the evolutionary processes, swarm behaviors, neural networks, or other biological phenomena, bioinspired algorithms offer innovative and efficient problem-solving approaches.

Bioinspired algorithms have gained significant importance in various fields due to their ability to handle complex and challenging problems. The application areas of these algorithms are optimization, machine learning, robotics, data mining, and pattern recognition. They offer a unique and alternative approach to problem-solving by leveraging the power of natural processes and behaviors.

1.1.2 Overview of the Chapter

This chapter aims to provide a comprehensive overview of bioinspired algorithms, their opportunities, and challenges. It will delve into various aspects of these algorithms, including their underlying principles, key algorithms, applications, and future research directions. The chapter will explore the significance of bioinspired algorithms in solving complex optimization problems and highlight their potential in different domains.

The chapter will discuss the opportunities offered by bioinspired algorithms. It will also explore their robustness in dealing with uncertainty and noise, as well as their potential for parallel and distributed computing. Furthermore, the chapter will highlight successful applications of bioinspired algorithms in areas such as optimization problems, pattern recognition, machine learning, and swarm robotics.

However, along with the opportunities, the chapter will address the challenges associated with bioinspired algorithms. It will discuss issues such as parameter tuning, the lack of theoretical analysis and understanding, the risk of premature convergence, and the computational cost for large-scale problems. The chapter will also touch upon ethical considerations and limitations related to fairness, transparency, and interpretability.

Overall, this chapter will provide readers with a comprehensive understanding of bioinspired algorithms, their opportunities, and the challenges they present. It will serve as a guide to explore the potential applications of these algorithms and inspire future research in this exciting and rapidly evolving field.

1.2 Bioinspired Principles and Algorithms

This section focuses on the exploration of bioinspired principles and algorithms. We delve into the fascinating world of evolutionary algorithms, which mimic the process of natural selection and genetics to solve optimization problems. Additionally, we examine swarm intelligence algorithms, inspired by collective behavior observed in social insects that simulate the behavior of a swarm or colony. Artificial neural networks, inspired by the functioning of the human brain, are also discussed for their applications in pattern recognition and machine learning. Lastly, we explore various other bioinspired algorithms that offer unique problem-solving mechanisms. Through this section, we aim to provide insights into the diverse range of bioinspired principles and algorithms driving innovation in various fields.

1.2.1 Evolutionary Algorithms

These are inspired by the process of natural evolution and genetics. These algorithms employ a population-based approach, where a set of potential solutions, known as individuals or chromosomes, undergoes selection, reproduction, and variation operations to evolve and improve over generations [3–5]. The fittest individuals are selected to form the next generation, while variation operations, such as mutation and crossover, introduce genetic diversity.

Genetic algorithms (GA), genetic programming (GP), and evolution strategies (ES) are examples of common evolutionary algorithms. These algorithms have been effectively used to address optimization issues such choosing the best setup, fine-tuning parameters, and selecting features [6, 7].

1.2.2 Swarm Intelligence Algorithms

The collective behaviors seen in social insect colonies and animal groupings serve as the inspiration for swarm intelligence systems [8]. These algorithms model the interactions and cooperation among simple agents, known as particles or agents, to solve complex problems. The agents communicate and exchange information locally to find globally optimal solutions through self-organization and emergent behaviors.

Popular swarm intelligence techniques include Particle Swarm Optimization (PSO) and Ant Colony Optimization (ACO). PSO simulates the behavior of particles in a search space to find the best solution, while ACO emulates the foraging behavior of ants to discover optimal paths in graph-based problems like the traveling salesman problem [9].

1.2.3 Artificial Neural Networks

The design and operation of biological neural networks in the brain serve as a model for artificial neural networks (ANNs). It consists of interconnected nodes, called artificial neurons or units, organized in layers. Each neuron processes input signals, applies activation functions, and propagates information through the network to produce output signals. ANNs can learn from examples and adjust their internal connections (weights) through a process known as training.

Different types of ANNs include feedforward neural networks, recurrent neural networks, and convolutional neural networks [9]. Machine learning applications, including classification, regression, pattern recognition, and natural language processing, have all seen extensive use of artificial neural networks (ANNs).

1.2.4 Other Bioinspired Algorithms

Apart from evolutionary algorithms, swarm intelligence algorithms, and artificial neural networks, there are various other bioinspired algorithms. Some notable examples include:

- Artificial immune systems: Inspired by the human immune system, these algorithms mimic immune mechanisms to solve optimization and pattern recognition problems.
- Bacterial forage optimization: This method simulates bacterial movement and interaction to solve optimization issues. It is inspired by bacterial foraging behavior.
- Firefly algorithm: Designed to optimize numerical operations, this algorithm replicates the attraction and movement of fireflies based on their flashing behavior.
- Grey wolf optimization: This algorithm emulates the leadership and teamwork among wolves to solve optimization issues. It was inspired by the social hierarchy and hunting behavior of grey wolves. These bioinspired principles and algorithms offer unique approaches to problem solving and optimization. They provide alternatives to traditional computational methods by leveraging the power of natural processes and behaviors observed in biological systems. A brief description of bioinspired principles and algorithms is mentioned in Table 1.1.

These bioinspired algorithms offer several advantages. They can effectively explore large and complex search spaces, making them suitable for problems with numerous possible solutions. They are robust and adaptable, capable of handling uncertainties, noisy data, and dynamic environments. Furthermore, bioinspired algorithms often exhibit parallel and distributed computing capabilities, enabling efficient solutions for computationally intensive tasks [10].

Despite their strengths, bioinspired algorithms also present challenges. Parameter tuning and algorithm configuration can be complex and require careful optimization. The lack of theoretical analysis and understanding of these algorithms limits their interpretability and hampers their adoption in certain domains. Additionally, there is a risk of premature convergence, where the algorithm settles on suboptimal solutions before reaching the global optimum. Furthermore, the computational cost associated with

Table 1.1 Bioinspired principles and algorithms.

Algorithm	Description
Evolutionary algorithms	Evolutionary algorithms, which are modelled after natural selection and genetics, iteratively create a population of potential solutions via mechanisms including mutation, crossover, and selection.
Swarm intelligence algorithms	Swarm intelligence algorithms replicate the behavior of a swarm or colony to solve optimization issues. These algorithms were inspired by the collective behavior seen in social insects. Ant colony optimization and particle swarm optimization are two examples.
Artificial neural networks	Artificial neural networks, which mimic the composition and operation of the human brain, are made up of linked nodes (neurons) that process and send information. They are frequently employed in tasks involving pattern recognition and machine learning.
Other bioinspired algorithms	This category can include a variety of algorithms such as artificial immune systems, cultural algorithms, firefly algorithms, and many others. Each algorithm has its own unique inspiration and mechanisms for problem-solving.

large-scale problems can be significant, requiring efficient implementation and computational resources [11].

To gain a comprehensive understanding of bioinspired algorithms, it is important to explore specific algorithms within each category. Genetic algorithms, particle swarm optimization, ant colony optimization, and artificial neural networks are among the most well-known and widely used bioinspired algorithms. Each algorithm has its own characteristics, advantages, and limitations, making them suitable for different problem domains and contexts [12].

Understanding the principles and applications of bioinspired algorithms opens up exciting opportunities for solving complex problems in various fields. Whether it is optimizing resource allocation, training neural networks, or simulating collective behaviors, bioinspired algorithms offer innovative approaches that can push the boundaries of traditional computational techniques. As research and development continue, these algorithms have the potential to drive advancements in optimization, machine learning, robotics, and other areas of science and engineering [13].

1.3 Opportunities of Bioinspired Algorithms

This section highlights the immense opportunities presented by bioinspired algorithms. We begin by exploring their ability to tackle complex optimization problems, where they demonstrate effectiveness in finding optimal solutions with diverse constraints and objectives [8]. Additionally, we delve into the robustness of bioinspired algorithms in handling uncertainty and noise, making them suitable for real-world applications. We also discuss the advantages of leveraging parallel and distributed computing to enhance the efficiency and scalability of these algorithms. Furthermore, we explore the wide range of application areas where bioinspired algorithms have been successfully implemented, accompanied by notable success stories. Through this section, we aim to showcase the promising opportunities that bioinspired algorithms offer in various domains are shown in Table 1.2.

1.3.1 Solving Complex Optimization Problems

Bioinspired algorithms offer opportunities for solving complex optimization problems that are challenging for traditional computational methods.

Table 1.2 Opportunities of bioinspired algorithms.

Opportunity	Description
Solving complex optimization problems	Bioinspired algorithms have shown effectiveness in tackling complex optimization problems with diverse constraints and objectives.
Robustness in dealing with uncertainty and noise	Bioinspired algorithms exhibit robustness and adaptability in handling noisy and uncertain environments, making them suitable for real-world applications.
Parallel and distributed computing	The inherent parallelism of many bioinspired algorithms enables efficient implementation on parallel and distributed computing platforms, accelerating optimization processes.
Application areas and success stories	Bioinspired algorithms have been successfully applied in various fields such as engineering design, scheduling, data mining, and image processing. Numerous success stories demonstrate their potential for solving practical problems.

These algorithms excel in exploring large solution spaces and finding near-optimal or optimal solutions. By leveraging principles inspired by biological systems, such as evolution, swarm behavior, or neural networks, bio-inspired algorithms can effectively handle problems with multiple variables, constraints, and objectives [14]. They can tackle optimization problems in diverse domains, including engineering, logistics, finance, and scheduling.

1.3.2 Robustness in Dealing With Uncertainty and Noise

One of the strengths of bioinspired algorithms is their robustness in dealing with uncertainty and noisy data. They are inspired by adaptive processes found in nature, allowing them to handle variations, uncertainties, and noisy input effectively. Bioinspired algorithms can adapt and adjust their strategies to optimize performance even in the presence of incomplete or noisy information. This makes them suitable for real-world applications where data may be imperfect or subject to fluctuations.

1.3.3 Parallel and Distributed Computing

Bioinspired algorithms lend themselves naturally to parallel and distributed computing paradigms. The population-based nature of these algorithms allows for parallel evaluation and exploration of multiple candidate solutions simultaneously. This parallelism can be effectively harnessed to speed up the optimization process and handle computationally intensive tasks. Distributed implementations of bioinspired algorithms enable efficient utilization of computational resources across multiple machines or nodes, making them scalable for large-scale problems.

1.3.4 Application Areas and Success Stories

These algorithms have been successfully applied in various domains, demonstrating their potential and effectiveness. Some notable application areas include:

- Optimization problems: Bioinspired algorithms have been used to optimize complex systems, such as supply chain management, network routing, resource allocation, and parameter optimization in engineering design.
- Pattern recognition and data mining: These algorithms have been employed for tasks, such as image and speech

recognition, classification, clustering, and anomaly detection in data mining.

- Machine learning: Bioinspired algorithms, particularly those based on artificial neural networks, have been applied in machine learning tasks such as regression, classification, and reinforcement learning.
- Robotics: Bioinspired algorithms have been used in swarm robotics, where multiple autonomous robots coordinate and collaborate to perform tasks, as well as in robot path planning and control.
- Bioinformatics: These algorithms have contributed to DNA sequence analysis, protein folding prediction, gene expression analysis, and biological network analysis.

Successful applications of bioinspired algorithms include the use of genetic algorithms in optimizing airline schedules, particle swarm optimization in image clustering, ant colony optimization in vehicle routing, and artificial neural networks in medical diagnosis.

These application areas and success stories demonstrate the versatility and effectiveness of bioinspired algorithms in solving real-world problems across various disciplines. They continue to inspire researchers and practitioners to explore new opportunities and push the boundaries of problem-solving approaches.

1.4 Challenges of Bioinspired Algorithms

This section explores the challenges associated with bioinspired algorithms. We discuss the importance of parameter tuning and algorithm configuration to achieve optimal performance. Additionally, we highlight the lack of rigorous theoretical analysis and understanding of these algorithms, which hinders their predictability and reliability. The risk of premature convergence, where suboptimal solutions are reached before the global optimum, is also examined. Furthermore, we address the computational cost involved in handling large-scale problems with high-dimensional search spaces. Lastly, we touch upon the ethical considerations and limitations that arise when employing bioinspired algorithms. Through this section, we shed light on the challenges that need to be addressed to harness the full potential of bioinspired algorithms.

1.4.1 Parameter Tuning and Algorithm Configuration

Bioinspired algorithms often rely on various parameters that need to be carefully tuned to achieve optimal performance. Selecting appropriate parameter values and configuring the algorithm can be challenging, as it requires a good understanding of the problem domain and the algorithm's behavior. The sensitivity of bioinspired algorithms to parameter settings makes parameter tuning a crucial and time-consuming task [10].

1.4.2 Lack of Theoretical Analysis and Understanding

Despite their wide use and empirical success, many bioinspired algorithms lack rigorous theoretical analysis and understanding. The behavior and convergence properties of these algorithms in different problem domains are not well understood [15]. This makes it difficult to predict their performance or provide theoretical guarantees of finding optimal or near-optimal solutions. The lack of theoretical foundation hampers the interpretability and reliability of these algorithms in certain applications.

1.4.3 Risk of Premature Convergence

Bioinspired algorithms are susceptible to premature convergence, where the algorithm settles on suboptimal solutions before reaching the global optimum. Premature convergence occurs when the algorithm converges too quickly or gets stuck in local optima. Balancing exploration and exploitation is a crucial challenge, as excessive exploration may lead to slow convergence, while excessive exploitation may limit the algorithm's ability to escape local optima [16, 17].

1.4.4 Computational Cost for Large-Scale Problems

Bioinspired algorithms can be computationally expensive, particularly for large-scale problems with high-dimensional search spaces. The evaluation and optimization of a large number of candidate solutions may require significant computational resources and time. As the problem size increases, the algorithm's scalability and efficiency become critical considerations [13, 18–24]. Developing efficient algorithms and leveraging parallel and distributed computing can help address these challenges.

1.4.5 Ethical Considerations and Limitations

Bioinspired algorithms, like any computational tool, have ethical considerations and limitations [17–19]. For example, the use of genetic algorithms in optimization may raise concerns about the potential for unintended consequences or biases in the generated solutions. Additionally, bioinspired algorithms may face limitations in handling certain problem types or may not be suitable for domains where interpretability and explainability are critical, such as legal or medical decision-making.

Addressing these challenges requires ongoing research and development. Efforts should focus on developing robust parameter tuning techniques, advancing the theoretical understanding of bioinspired algorithms, exploring methods to mitigate premature convergence, improving scalability for large-scale problems, and addressing ethical considerations and limitations. By overcoming these challenges, bioinspired algorithms can reach their full potential and provide effective solutions for complex problems across various domains.

The summary and comparison of these challenges are shown in Table 1.3 and Table 1.4.

Table 1.3 Challenges of bioinspired algorithms.

Challenge	Description
Parameter tuning and configuration	Selecting appropriate parameter values and configuring the algorithm for optimal performance.
Lack of theoretical analysis and understanding	Limited understanding of the algorithm's behavior and convergence properties in different problem domains.
Risk of premature convergence	Settling on suboptimal solutions before reaching the global optimum due to quick convergence or getting stuck in local optima.
Computational cost for large-scale problems	Increased computational resources and time required for evaluating and optimizing a large number of candidate solutions.
Ethical considerations and limitations	Potential ethical concerns and limitations in terms of unintended consequences, biases, and interpretability in certain applications.

Table 1.4 Opportunities and challenges comparison.

Opportunities	Challenges
Solving complex optimization problems	Parameter tuning and algorithm configuration
Robustness in dealing with uncertainty and noise	Lack of theoretical analysis and understanding
Parallel and distributed computing	Risk of premature convergence
Application areas and success stories	Computational cost for large-scale problems
	Ethical considerations and limitations

1.5 Prominent Bioinspired Algorithms

These algorithms, also recognized as nature-inspired procedures, are computational methods that draw inspiration from biological systems and natural processes to solve complex problems. These simulate the performance of biological entities, such as organisms, ecosystems, or cellular processes, to develop efficient and effective problem-solving techniques [25]. Figure 1.1 illustrates the various bioinspired optimization algorithms employed in the study. These algorithms serve as the foundation for exploring innovative solutions to complex optimization problems. Here are some prominent bioinspired algorithms:

1. **Genetic Algorithms (GAs):** These algorithms mimic the process of natural evolution via population of potential solutions to a problem and iteratively using genetic operators like selection, crossover, and mutation to evolve new generations of solutions. GAs are widely used for optimization problems, search tasks, and machine learning.
2. **Particle Swarm Optimization (PSO):** PSO is stimulated via collective bird behavior flocks or fish schools. It involves a population of particles that move through a multidimensional search space to find the optimal solution. The particles communicate and update their positions based on their own best-known position and the global best-known position found by the swarm. PSO is commonly used for optimization problems.

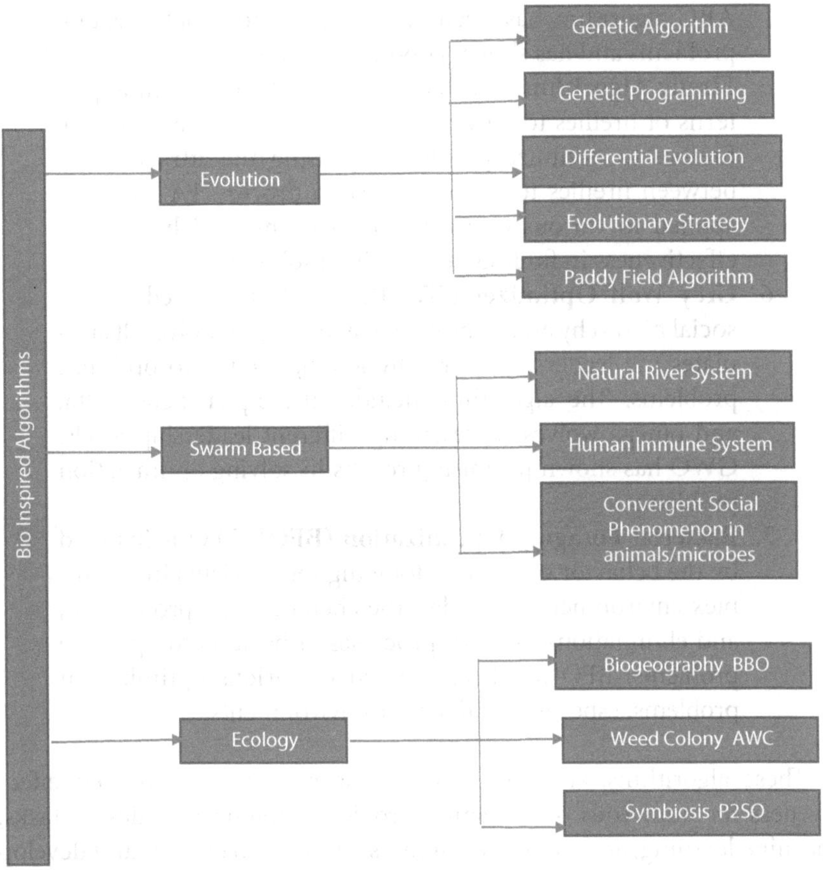

Figure 1.1 Bioinspired optimization algorithms.

3. **Ant Colony Optimization (ACO):** ACO is stimulated via foraging conduct of ants. It is used to solve optimization problems by simulating the behavior of ants depositing pheromone trails to communicate and find the shortest path between their nest and a food source. ACO has been successfully applied to problems like the traveling salesman problem and routing problems.
4. **Artificial Bee Colony (ABC) Algorithm:** This algorithm stirred via foraging activities of honeybees. It simulates the foraging, recruitment, and abandonment processes of a bee colony to optimize numerical and combinatorial problems.

ABC algorithm has been applied to various optimization problems and has shown good performance.

5. **Firefly Algorithm (FA):** FA is inspired by the flashing patterns of fireflies to attract mates. It models the behavior of fireflies to optimize problems by using the attractiveness between fireflies to guide the search process. FA has been applied to various optimization problems and has shown effectiveness in finding near-optimal solutions.
6. **Grey Wolf Optimizer (GWO):** GWO is inspired by the social hierarchy and hunting behavior of grey wolves. It simulates the leadership hierarchy among wolves to optimize problems. The algorithm includes the alpha, beta, delta, and omega wolves representing different leadership levels. GWO has shown promising results in solving optimization problems.
7. **Bacterial Foraging Optimization (BFO):** BFO is inspired by the behavior of bacteria foraging for nutrients in a complex environment. It models the chemotaxis, reproduction, and elimination-dispersal processes of bacteria to optimize problems. BFO has been applied to various optimization problems, especially in dynamic environments.

These algorithms, along with others, have demonstrated their effectiveness for numerous optimization problems, engineering design tasks, machine learning, and more. Researchers continue to explore and develop new bioinspired algorithms to tackle complex problems in different domains.

1.5.1 Genetic Algorithms

Genetic algorithms inspired from the process of natural selection and genetics to solve optimization problems. They belongs broader class of evolutionary algorithms, which simulate the mechanisms of natural evolution to find solutions for complex problems [26, 27].

In genetic algorithms, a population of potential solutions, represented as chromosomes or strings of genes, is evolved over multiple generations. Every chromosome encodes a possible solution to the problem at hand. The chromosomes are evaluated using a fitness function, which quantifies their quality or how well they solve the problem. The foremost steps of a genetic algorithm include:

1. Initialization: A population of random chromosomes is generated as an initial population.
2. Evaluation: Each chromosome is evaluated using a fitness function to determine its quality.
3. Selection: Chromosomes with higher fitness values have a higher probability of being selected for reproduction upon the principle of "survival of the fittest." Common selection techniques include tournament selection, roulette wheel selection, or rank-based selection.
4. Reproduction: Selected chromosomes are combined or modified to create new offspring for the next generation. Common reproduction techniques include crossover and mutation. Crossover use genetic information from two parent chromosomes to produce one or more offspring, and mutation presents small random variations for genetic information of a chromosome.
5. Replacement: The new offspring replace some of the existing chromosomes in the population, usually based on the principle of elitism, where the best individuals are preserved in each generation to ensure the overall quality of the population does not decrease.
6. Termination: The algorithm continues to iterate through the evaluation, selection, reproduction, and replacement steps till a termination condition is obtained.

Genetic algorithms explore the solution space by iteratively applying selection, reproduction, and replacement operations, gradually improving the quality of the population over time. By mimicking the process of natural evolution, genetic algorithms can effectively search for optimal solutions for complex problems, especially in cases where traditional optimization techniques may struggle. They have been successfully applied in various domains, including engineering, computer science, economics, and biology.

1.5.2 Particle Swarm Optimization

Particle Swarm Optimization (PSO) is a bioinspired algorithm that was initially proposed by Kennedy and Eberhart in 1995 [28]. It is stimulated via social behavior of bird flocking where individuals in a group cooperate and communicate with each other to achieve a common goal.

In PSO, a population of candidate solutions, called particles, move through a search space to discover the optimal solution [29].

The basic steps for PSO algorithm:

1. **Initialization:** Initialize a population of particles randomly within the search space. Each particle is assigned a random velocity.
2. **Evaluation:** Calculate the fitness of every particle depend upon objective function or fitness measure.
3. **Update pbest and gbest:** Update the personal best (pbest) position for every particle depend on its present fitness. Also, update the global best (gbest) position if a particle discovers a better solution than the current gbest.
4. **Update velocity and position:** Update the velocity and position of each particle based on its current velocity, its cognitive and social component, and random factors.
5. **Termination:** Repeat steps 2-4 until a termination condition is met. This condition could be extreme iterations, reaching a satisfactory fitness level, predefined threshold for improvement.

PSO widely applied in numerous optimization problems both single-objective and multiobjective problems. It has shown effectiveness in finding near-optimal solutions in continuous and discrete search spaces. The algorithm's ability to explore the search space and exploit promising regions makes it suitable for a wide range of applications.

PSO has also been extended and modified in several ways to address specific problem characteristics or improve its performance. Variants of PSO include adaptive PSO, chaotic PSO, hybrid PSO, and constrained PSO, among others.

1.5.3 Ant Colony Optimization

Ant colony optimization (ACO) based on the foraging behavior of ants [30]. ACO is inspired by the behavior of real ants when they search for food. Ants communicate with each other by depositing and following chemical pheromone trails. They leave pheromone trails to mark the paths they have explored, and the strength of the pheromone trail is directly proportional to the quality of the food source. Other ants can detect and follow these pheromone trails, and they tend to choose paths with stronger pheromone concentrations.

In the context of optimization problems, ACO uses a similar mechanism to find the optimal solution. It represents the problem as a graph, where each node represents a possible solution, and the edges represent the connections between the solutions. Initially, the pheromone concentration on each edge is set to a small positive value.

The ACO algorithm starts with a set of ants that independently explore the solution space by moving from one node to another through the graph. At each step, an ant chooses its next node based on a probabilistic decision rule, which takes into account the pheromone concentration on the edges and a heuristic information, which represents the desirability of moving from the current node to a neighboring node.

When an ant completes its tour and reaches the end, the pheromone trail is updated based on the quality of the solution found. Better solutions result in stronger pheromone concentrations. Over time, the pheromone trail is reinforced on the edges corresponding to good solutions, while weaker solutions lead to the evaporation of pheromone.

As ants continue to explore the solution space, the pheromone trail gradually converges towards the optimal solution. The exploration-exploitation trade-off is achieved through the combined effect of pheromone reinforcement and evaporation.

ACO successfully applied in numerous combinatorial problems such as the traveling salesman problem, vehicle routing problem, job scheduling, and many others. Its effectiveness lies in its ability to exploit the collective intelligence of the ant colony to find good solutions in complex and dynamic problem spaces.

1.5.4 Artificial Neural Networks

ANNs widely used in bioinspired algorithms due to their ability to simulate the behavior of biological neural networks. Bioinspired algorithms take inspiration from natural systems, such as the behavior of ants, bees, birds, and even the human brain, to solve complex optimization and learning problems. ANNs, as computational models of biological neural networks, can provide the foundation for these algorithms [31].

Bioinspired algorithms, also known as nature-inspired algorithms, aim to mimic the adaptive and evolutionary processes found in nature to solve various computational problems. These algorithms often exhibit robustness, scalability, and efficiency, making them suitable for a wide range of applications.

Here are a few examples of bioinspired algorithms that utilize artificial neural networks:

1. Artificial Bee Colony Algorithm (ABC): ABC is inspired by the foraging behavior of honey bees. It uses the concept of employed bees, onlooker bees, and scout bees to explore and optimize solutions. ANNs can be used in ABC to model the behavior of the bees, determine the quality of food sources, and guide the search process.
2. Particle Swarm Optimization (PSO): PSO is inspired by the collective behavior of bird flocking or fish schooling. It involves a swarm of particles moving through a search space to find the optimal solution. ANNs can be employed in PSO to model the movement and interactions of particles, and to evaluate fitness or objective functions.
3. Genetic Algorithms (GA): GA is inspired by the principles of natural selection and genetics. It uses the concepts of population, chromosomes, and genetic operators to evolve solutions over generations. ANNs can be integrated into GA as the individuals or chromosomes, allowing the genetic algorithm to search for optimal neural network architectures or learn the weights and connections of the network.
4. Ant Colony Optimization (ACO): ACO is inspired by the foraging behavior of ants, particularly the pheromone trails they use to communicate and find the shortest paths to food sources. ANNs can be used in ACO to simulate the pheromone trail updates and decision-making processes of ants, allowing for efficient exploration and exploitation of solution spaces.

By combining ANNs with these bioinspired algorithms, researchers and practitioners can harness the power of both biological systems and computational intelligence to solve complex optimization, prediction, and classification problems. ANNs provide the underlying learning and adaptive mechanisms, while the bioinspired algorithms offer efficient exploration and optimization strategies inspired by nature.

1.6 Applications of Bioinspired Algorithms

Bioinspired algorithms are computational methods that draw inspiration from biological systems and processes to solve complex problems

[22, 32, 33]. These algorithms mimic the behavior and mechanisms found in nature, such as the behavior of ants, the flight of birds, or the optimization of biological systems. Here are some applications of bioinspired algorithms:

1.6.1 Optimization Problems

Bioinspired algorithms have found wide applications in solving optimization problems. These algorithms take inspiration from biological systems, such as evolutionary processes, animal behavior, and natural selection, to develop efficient and robust optimization techniques [27]. Some popular bioinspired optimization algorithms include:

1. **Genetic Algorithms (GA):** Based on the principles of natural selection and genetics, GA mimics the process of evolution to search for optimal solutions to complex problems. It involves creating a population of candidate solutions and iteratively applying selection, crossover, and mutation operators to generate new generations.
2. **Particle Swarm Optimization (PSO):** Inspired by the behavior of bird flocking or fish schooling, PSO optimizes a problem by simulating the movement and interaction of a swarm of particles. Each particle represents a potential solution, and they update their positions based on their own best solution and the collective information obtained from other particles.
3. **Ant Colony Optimization (ACO):** ACO is inspired by the behavior of ants searching for food. It uses pheromone trails to guide the search process. Ants deposit pheromones on their paths, and other ants follow the paths with stronger pheromone concentrations. ACO has been successfully applied to problems such as the traveling salesman problem and vehicle routing.

1.6.2 Pattern Recognition and Machine Learning

Bioinspired algorithms have shown promise in the field of pattern recognition and machine learning. These algorithms leverage natural phenomena to design effective techniques for data analysis and classification [28]. Some notable bioinspired algorithms in this domain include:

1. **Artificial Neural Networks (ANN):** ANNs are inspired by the structure and function of biological neural networks. They consist of interconnected nodes, or "neurons," which process and transmit information. ANNs are used for tasks like image and speech recognition, natural language processing, and predictive modeling.
2. **Deep Learning:** Deep learning is a subset of machine learning that utilizes artificial neural networks with multiple hidden layers. Deep learning algorithms have achieved remarkable success in various tasks, including image and speech recognition, natural language processing, and autonomous driving.
3. **Support Vector Machines (SVM):** SVM is a machine learning algorithm that constructs a hyperplane or set of hyperplanes to separate different classes of data points. It is inspired by the structural risk minimization principle and has been widely applied in pattern recognition and classification tasks.

1.6.3 Swarm Robotics

Swarm robotics involves the coordination and cooperation of large groups of relatively simple robots to achieve complex tasks. Bioinspired algorithms are particularly well-suited for swarm robotics due to their ability to emulate the collective behavior observed in biological swarms [29]. Applications of bioinspired algorithms in swarm robotics include:

1. **Swarm Intelligence:** Swarm intelligence algorithms take inspiration from the behavior of social insect colonies, such as ants, bees, and termites. They enable a group of robots to work together, communicate, and self-organize to solve problems collectively. Swarm intelligence algorithms have been applied to tasks like exploration, mapping, and cooperative transport.
2. **Distributed Task Allocation:** Bioinspired algorithms can be used to develop efficient methods for task allocation in swarm robotics. These algorithms assign different tasks to individual robots based on their capabilities, proximity to the task, or local information exchange. This allows the swarm to optimize task allocation and achieve efficient collective behavior.

1.6.4 Other Domains

Bioinspired algorithms have also found applications in various other domains, including:

1. **Computational Biology:** Bioinspired algorithms are used to solve computational problems related to biological systems, such as protein folding, DNA sequencing, and gene expression analysis. These algorithms help researchers understand complex biological processes and develop new drugs or therapies [30].
2. **Smart Grid Optimization:** Bioinspired optimization algorithms are applied to optimize the operation and management of smart grids. These algorithms help in tasks like load balancing, demand response, energy scheduling, and power flow optimization [34].

Bioinspired algorithms are computational techniques that draw inspiration from biological systems and processes to solve complex problems. These algorithms have shown promising results in various domains, including optimization, machine learning, and data analysis. To further advance the field, researchers are focusing on several future research directions:

1.7 Future Research Directions

Bioinspired algorithms have been an exciting field of research, drawing inspiration from biological systems to solve complex problems. As we look into the future, several potential research directions emerge for bioinspired algorithms [35]:

1.7.1 Improving Efficiency and Scalability

Efficiency and scalability are crucial factors in the practical application of bioinspired algorithms. Researchers are exploring ways to enhance the efficiency of these algorithms by developing new search strategies, optimization techniques, and parallel computing approaches. This involves designing algorithms that can handle large-scale datasets and complex optimization problems more effectively. Additionally, advancements in hardware technology, such as the use of specialized architectures like GPUs and FPGAs, can significantly improve the efficiency and scalability of bioinspired algorithms.

1.7.2 Enhancing Interpretability and Explainability

Interpretability and explainability are important for building trust and understanding in the application of bioinspired algorithms. Researchers are working on developing methods to make these algorithms more interpretable, allowing users to understand how and why certain decisions are made. This involves investigating techniques such as feature selection, visualization, rule extraction, and model simplification to provide insights into the inner workings of the algorithms. By enhancing interpretability, bioinspired algorithms can be applied to critical domains, such as healthcare and finance, where transparency is essential.

1.7.3 Integration With Other Computational Techniques

Bioinspired algorithms can be joined with other computational techniques to leverage their strengths and overcome their limitations. Researchers are exploring ways to integrate bioinspired algorithms with machine learning approaches, such as deep learning, to create hybrid models that benefit from the complementary capabilities of both techniques. Additionally, the integration of bioinspired algorithms with statistical methods, fuzzy logic, swarm intelligence, and evolutionary computation can lead to more powerful and robust algorithms for solving complex problems.

1.7.4 Addressing Ethical Concerns

As bioinspired algorithms become more prevalent in various applications, ethical concerns arise regarding issues such as privacy, bias, fairness, and accountability. Future research aims to address these concerns by developing frameworks and guidelines for the ethical use of bioinspired algorithms. This involves considering the societal impact of these algorithms, ensuring transparency, fairness, and accountability in decision-making processes, and establishing regulations to govern their application. Additionally, research on the ethical implications of autonomous systems and artificial intelligence further contributes to addressing ethical concerns in the context of bioinspired algorithms.

Future research directions in bioinspired algorithms involve improving efficiency and scalability, enhancing interpretability and explainability, integrating with other computational techniques, and addressing ethical concerns. These advancements will contribute to the continued development and responsible application of bioinspired algorithms in solving real-world problems.

1.8 Conclusion

The field of bioinspired algorithms offers a promising avenue for solving complex problems by drawing inspiration from natural systems. These algorithms, inspired by the principles and behaviors observed in biological systems, have demonstrated their effectiveness in a wide range of applications. In this paper, we have explored the opportunities and challenges associated with bioinspired algorithms.

The opportunities presented by bioinspired algorithms are vast. By mimicking the processes and mechanisms found in nature, these algorithms provide a powerful framework for problem solving in various domains. They have shown remarkable success in optimization, machine learning, robotics, and other areas. Bioinspired algorithms offer the potential for developing innovative solutions that can outperform traditional approaches, especially in dealing with complex and dynamic environments.

Furthermore, bioinspired algorithms provide a means to tackle problems that are difficult to solve using traditional computational methods. They excel at handling nonlinear and multiobjective optimization problems, where conventional techniques may struggle. Additionally, bioinspired algorithms often offer robustness, adaptability, and scalability, enabling them to address real-world challenges effectively.

However, the field of bioinspired algorithms also faces several challenges. One of the primary concerns is the lack of a unified theoretical foundation. While biological systems serve as inspiration, translating their principles into algorithmic frameworks can be challenging. The complexity of biological systems often makes it difficult to understand and model their underlying mechanisms accurately.

Another challenge is the parameterization and fine-tuning of bioinspired algorithms. Many of these algorithms rely on numerous parameters, which must be carefully calibrated for optimal performance. Determining the appropriate parameter settings is often a trial-and-error process, requiring significant computational resources and expertise.

Additionally, the scalability of bioinspired algorithms remains a challenge. As problem sizes and data volumes increase, the computational demands of these algorithms can become prohibitive. Developing efficient and scalable implementations is crucial to unlock the full potential of bioinspired algorithms in solving real-world problems.

In conclusion, bioinspired algorithms offer exciting opportunities for addressing complex problems in various domains. Their ability to draw inspiration from natural systems and their robustness make them well-suited for tackling challenging optimization and machine learning tasks. However, several challenges, including the lack of a unified theoretical foundation, parameter tuning, and scalability, need to be addressed to fully exploit the potential of bioinspired algorithms. Overcoming these challenges will require interdisciplinary collaboration, theoretical advancements, and practical innovations. With continued research and development, bioinspired algorithms hold the promise of transforming problem-solving approaches and enabling breakthroughs in numerous fields.

1.8.1 Summary of Key Points

Bioinspired algorithms, also known as nature-inspired algorithms or evolutionary algorithms, are computational methods that draw inspiration from biological systems and processes to solve complex optimization problems. These algorithms mimic the behavior and principles observed in nature, such as natural selection, genetic variation, and swarm intelligence. Here are the key points summarizing the opportunities and challenges associated with bioinspired algorithms:

Opportunities:

1. Problem-solving versatility: Bio-inspired algorithms can be applied to a wide range of complex optimization problems in various fields, including engineering, finance, healthcare, and logistics.
2. Global optimization: These algorithms excel at finding global optima or near-optimal solutions, even in high-dimensional and multimodal search spaces.
3. Robustness: Bio-inspired algorithms exhibit robustness and adaptability, making them suitable for dynamic and uncertain environments.
4. Scalability: They can handle large-scale optimization problems with a large number of variables and constraints.
5. Exploration-exploitation tradeoff: Bio-inspired algorithms strike a balance between exploration (diversity) and exploitation (intensification) during the search process, allowing

them to efficiently explore the search space and converge to optimal solutions.

6. Inspiration from nature: Drawing inspiration from biological systems provides innovative and unconventional approaches to problem-solving, leading to potentially breakthrough solutions.

Challenges:

1. Algorithm design and parameter tuning: The performance of bio-inspired algorithms heavily depends on the choice and tuning of algorithmic parameters, which can be challenging and time-consuming.
2. Computational complexity: The computational requirements of bio-inspired algorithms can be high, especially for large-scale problems, which may limit their practicality in some cases.
3. Lack of theoretical guarantees: Unlike traditional optimization techniques, bio-inspired algorithms often lack strong theoretical guarantees, making it difficult to predict their convergence behavior or solution quality.
4. Premature convergence and local optima: Bio-inspired algorithms may suffer from premature convergence to suboptimal solutions or get trapped in local optima, especially in complex and deceptive problem landscapes.
5. Interpretability: Some bio-inspired algorithms, such as neural networks, are considered black boxes, making it challenging to understand and interpret their decision-making process.
6. Ethical considerations: As bio-inspired algorithms become more powerful and pervasive, ethical concerns, such as algorithmic bias, data privacy, and security, need to be carefully addressed.

Overall, bio-inspired algorithms offer promising opportunities for solving complex optimization problems, but they also present challenges that require careful consideration and further research to harness their full potential.

1.8.2 Implications and Future Prospects of Bioinspired Algorithms

Bio-inspired algorithms, also known as nature-inspired algorithms, are computational methods that draw inspiration from biological systems and processes to solve complex problems. These algorithms mimic the behavior, principles, and structures found in nature, such as evolutionary processes, swarm intelligence, neural networks, and immune systems. They have gained significant attention in various fields due to their ability to provide innovative and efficient solutions. Here are some implications and future prospects of bio-inspired algorithms:

1. **Optimization:** Bio-inspired algorithms have proven to be highly effective in solving optimization problems. They have been applied to various domains, including engineering design, logistics, finance, and data analysis. These algorithms can efficiently search large solution spaces, identify optimal solutions, and handle complex constraints. As computational power continues to increase, bio-inspired algorithms will play a crucial role in solving optimization challenges.
2. **Machine Learning:** Bio-inspired algorithms, particularly neural networks, have greatly influenced the field of machine learning. Neural networks, inspired by the structure and function of the human brain, have demonstrated remarkable performance in tasks such as pattern recognition, image processing, and natural language processing. The future prospects of bio-inspired algorithms in machine learning include developing more efficient and interpretable neural network architectures, improving transfer learning capabilities, and enhancing the ability to learn from limited labeled data.
3. **Robotics and Autonomous Systems:** Bio-inspired algorithms have immense potential in the field of robotics and autonomous systems. Nature-inspired techniques such as evolutionary algorithms, genetic algorithms, and swarm intelligence can be used to optimize robot behaviors, sensor networks, and control systems. These algorithms can enable robots to adapt to changing environments, exhibit collective intelligence, and perform complex tasks more effectively. As robotics continues to advance, bio-inspired algorithms will

contribute to the development of intelligent and versatile robotic systems.

4. **Data Science and Big Data Analytics:** With the increasing availability of large-scale datasets, bio-inspired algorithms are becoming crucial in the field of data science and big data analytics. They can be employed for clustering, classification, anomaly detection, feature selection, and data visualization. By integrating bio-inspired algorithms with traditional data analysis techniques, researchers can discover hidden patterns, extract meaningful insights, and make data-driven decisions in various domains such as healthcare, finance, and marketing.
5. **Cybersecurity:** Bio-inspired algorithms offer innovative solutions for addressing cybersecurity challenges. Techniques inspired by the immune system, such as artificial immune systems and intrusion detection systems, can detect and respond to threats in real-time. Additionally, evolutionary algorithms can be used to optimize cryptographic algorithms, intrusion detection systems, and malware detection mechanisms. Bio-inspired algorithms provide a unique approach to enhancing the security and resilience of computer systems.
6. **Sustainable and Green Computing:** Bio-inspired algorithms align well with the principles of sustainable and green computing. They often promote efficient resource utilization, adaptability, and fault tolerance. By leveraging the self-organization and self-adaptation found in natural systems, bio-inspired algorithms can contribute to energy-efficient computing, dynamic resource allocation, and optimization of renewable energy systems. They have the potential to shape the future of computing toward more sustainable practices.

In conclusion, bio-inspired algorithms have significant implications and promising future prospects across various domains. Their ability to solve complex optimization problems, contribute to machine learning advancements, improve robotics and autonomous systems, enhance data science capabilities, strengthen cybersecurity, and support sustainable computing makes them a valuable tool for tackling the challenges of the future. As research and technological advancements continue, bio-inspired algorithms will likely play an increasingly vital role in shaping our world.

References

1. Zang, H., Zhang, S., Hapeshi, K., A review of nature-inspired algorithms. *J. Bionic Eng.*, 7, 4, S232–S237, 2010.
2. Yang, X.S., *Nature-inspired metaheuristic algorithms*, Luniver Press, United Kingdom, 2010.
3. Bayer, P. and Finkel, M., Evolutionary algorithms for the optimization of advective control of contaminated aquifer zones. *Water Resour. Res.*, 40, 6, 1–19, 2004.
4. Benkhaddra, I., Kumar, A., Setitra, M.A. *et al.*, Design and Development of Consensus Activation Function Enabled Neural Network-Based Smart Healthcare Using BIoT. *Wirel. Pers. Commun.*, 130, 1549–1574, 2023. https://doi.org/10.1007/s11277-023-10344-0 Q2,Impact Factor -2.017.
5. Srivastav, A.L., Markandeya, Patel, N. *et al.*, Concepts of circular economy for sustainable management of electronic wastes: Challenges and management options. *Environ. Sci. Pollut. Res.*, 30, 48654–48675, 2023, https://doi.org/10.1007/s11356-023-26052-y Q1,Impact Factor -5.19.
6. Ilyas, B., Kumar, A., Setitra, M.A., Bensalem, Z.E.A., Lei, H., Prevention of DDoS attacks using an optimized deep learning approach in blockchain technology. *Trans. Emerging Telecommun. Technol.*, 34, 4, e4729, 2023, Q2,Impact Factor -3.31.
7. Kumar, A., Rathore, P.S., Dubey, A.K. *et al.*, LTE-NBP with holistic UWB-WBAN approach for the energy efficient biomedical application. *Multimed. Tools Appl.*, 82, 39797–39811, 2023, https://doi.org/10.1007/s11042-023-15604-6 Q1,Impact Factor -2.577.
8. Nicklow, J., Reed, P., Savic, D., Dessalegne, T., Harrell, L., Chan-Hilton, A., ASCE Task Committee on Evolutionary Computation in Environmental and Water Resources Engineering, State of the art for genetic algorithms and beyond in water resources planning and management. *J. Water Resour. Plann. Manage.*, 136, 4, 412–432, 2010.
9. Karaboga, D., An idea based on honey bee swarm for numerical optimization. Technical Report-tr06, vol. 200, pp. 1–10, Erciyes University, Engineering Faculty, Computer Engineering Department, Kayseri, 2005.
10. Zainal, N., Zain, A.M., Sharif, S., Overview of artificial fish swarm algorithm and its applications in industrial problems. *Appl. Mech. Mater.*, 815, 253–257, 2015.
11. Krizhevsky, A., Sutskever, I., Hinton, G.E., Imagenet classification with deep convolutional neural networks. *Commun. ACM*, 60, 6, 84–90, 2017.
12. Fong, S., Opportunities and challenges of integrating bio-inspired optimization and data mining algorithms, in: *Swarm Intelligence and Bio-Inspired Computation*, pp. 385–402, 2013.
13. Binitha, S. and Sathya, S.S., A survey of bio inspired optimization algorithms. *Int. J. Soft Comput.*, 2, 2, 137–151, 2012.

14. Eiben, A.E. and Smith, J.E., *Introduction to evolutionary computing*, Springer-Verlag, Berlin Heidelberg, 2015.
15. Mitchell, M., *An introduction to genetic algorithms*, Penguin Random House LLC, United Kingdom, 1998.
16. Cloete, T., Engelbrecht, A.P., Pampara, G., Cilib: A collaborative framework for computational intelligence algorithms-part II, in: *2008 IEEE International Joint Conference on Neural Networks (IEEE World Congress on Computational Intelligence)*, pp. 1764–1773, IEEE, 2008, June.
17. Jakšić, Z., Devi, S., Jakšić, O., Guha, K., A comprehensive review of bio-inspired optimization algorithms including applications in microelectronics and nanophotonics. *Biomimetics*, 8, 3, 278, 2023. https://doi.org/10.3390/biomimetics8030278.
18. Colomer, M. À., Margalida, A., Pérez-Jiménez, M.J., Population dynamics P system (PDP) models: A standardized protocol for describing and applying novel bio-inspired computing tools. *PloS One*, 8, 4, e60698, 2013.
19. Lipson, H. and Pollack, J.B., Automatic design and manufacture of robotic lifeforms. *Nature*, 406, 6799, 974–978, 2000.
20. Beyer, H.G. and Arnold, D.V., Theory of evolution strategies — A tutorial. In: *Theoretical Aspects of Evolutionary Computing*, L. Kallel, B. Naudts, A. Rogers (eds.), Natural Computing Series, Springer, Berlin, Heidelberg, 2001, https://doi.org/10.1007/978-3-662-04448-3_6.
21. Caruana, R., Lou, Y., Gehrke, J., Koch, P., Sturm, M., Elhadad, N., Intelligible models for healthcare: Predicting pneumonia risk and hospital 30-day readmission, in: *Proceedings of the 21th ACM SIGKDD international conference on knowledge discovery and data mining*, pp. 1721–1730, 2015, August.
22. Gandomi, A.H., Yang, X.S., Alavi, A.H., Mixed variable structural optimization using firefly algorithm. *Comput. Struct.*, 89, 23–24, 2325–2336, 2011.
23. Wang, S., Li, Y., Yang, H., Liu, H., Self-adaptive differential evolution algorithm with improved mutation strategy. *Soft Comput.*, 22, 3433–3447, 2018.
24. Holland, J.H., Genetic algorithms and the optimal allocation of trials. *SIAM J. Comput.*, 2, 2, 88–105, 1973.
25. Wang, D., Tan, D., Liu, L., Particle swarm optimization algorithm: an overview. *Soft Comput.*, 22, 387–408, 2018.
26. Bonabeau, E., Dorigo, M., Theraulaz, G., *Swarm intelligence*, Oxford University Press, New York, 1999.
27. Dorigo, M., Maniezzo, V., Colorni, A., Ant system: optimization by a colony of cooperating agents. *IEEE Trans. Syst. Man Cybern. Part B Cybern.*, 26, 1, 29–41, 1996.
28. Conforth, M. and Y., Toward Evolving Neural Networks using Bio-Inspired Algorithms, in: *IC-AI*, pp. 413–419, Meng, 2008, July.
29. Selvaraj, C., Kumar, R.S., Karnan, M., A survey on application of bio-inspired algorithms. *Int. J. Comput. Sci. Inf. Technol.*, 5, 1, 366–70, 2014.

30. Fan, X., Sayers, W., Zhang, S., Han, Z., Ren, L., Chizari, H., Review and classification of bio-inspired algorithms and their applications. *J. Bionic Eng.*, 17, 611–631, 2020.
31. Kar, A.K., Bio inspired computing–a review of algorithms and scope of applications. *Expert Syst. Appl.*, 59, 20–32, 2016.
32. Far, A.B., Flitti, F., Guo, B., Bermak, A., A bio-inspired pattern recognition system for tin-oxide gas sensor applications. *IEEE Sens. J.*, 9, 6, 713–722, 2009.
33. Bhargava, N., Rathore, P.S., Bhowmick, A., Study of X Ray Detection Using CNN in Machine Learning, in: *International Conference on Advancements in Smart Computing and Information Security*, pp. 295–303, Cham: Springer Nature, Switzerland, 2022, November.
34. Fadel, E., Faheem, M., Gungor, V.C., Nassef, L., Akkari, N., Malik, M.G.A., Akyildiz, I.F., Spectrum-aware bio-inspired routing in cognitive radio sensor networks for smart grid applications. *Comput. Commun.*, 101, 106–120, 2017.
35. Gill, S.S. and Buyya, R., Bio-inspired algorithms for big data analytics: a survey, taxonomy, and open challenges, in: *Big Data Analytics for Intelligent Healthcare Management*, pp. 1–17, Academic Press, Elsevier Inc., 2019.

2

Evaluation of Phytochemical Screening and *In Vitro* Antiurolithiatic Activity of *Myristica fragrans* by Titrimetry Method Using Machine Learning

G. Lalitha[1], S. Surya[1] and M.P. Karthikeyan[2*]

[1]*Department of Biochemistry, Dr. NGP Arts & Science College, Coimbatore, Tamil Nadu, India*
[2]*School of CS & IT, Jain (Deemed-to-be University), Bengaluru, Karnataka, India*

Abstract
Medicinal plants play a great role in human health and diseases they are considered as backbone of all the traditional medicine. *Myristica fragrans* (mace spice) is traditionally used as antibacterial, antifungal, analgesic, antidepressant, sedative, hypnotic, antidiarrhea, chemoprotective, neuropharmacologic, and antidiabetic. Hence, our study showed interest *in vitro* antiurolithiatic activity. Presence of alkaloids, flavonoids, glycosides, tannins and phenolics, saponins, protein and amino acids, phytosterols, and terpenoids were all found in the extract after a phytoconstituent analysis. Evaluation of antiurolithiatic activity using titrimetry method showed *Myristica fragrans* had the highest calcium oxalate dissolution as 82% compared with standard drug neeri was used. The ethanolic and aqueous extracts of mace spice exhibited the maximum calcium oxalate dissolution, according to this investigation.

Keywords: *Myristica fragrans*, phytochemical analysis, antiurolithiatic activity

**Corresponding author*: karthi.karthis@gmail.com

Sumit Srivastava, Abhineet Anand, Abhishek Kumar, Bhavna Saini and Pramod Singh Rathore (eds.) Bio-Inspired Optimization for Medical Data Mining, (31–40) © 2024 Scrivener Publishing LLC

2.1 Introduction

Plants have provided us food, raw materials, and a variety of other necessities for the existence of life since the beginning of time. Even today's conventional medicine employs many plant-derived substances used as medicines. The increased incidence adverse drug reactions caused by the overuse of synthetic drugs has prompted people should turn to nature for secure cures. Due to their effects that have been professionally verified, herbs and herbal medications have drawn people's curiosity.

Urolithiasis refers to stone originating anywhere in the urinary tract, such as the kidneys and bladder. Urinary stones play an important role in daily urological practise [1]. Urinary saturation is a very rare condition, and it affects only a small number of individuals. The most common urologic condition today, stone production is also the oldest and most painful. This is because to dietary and lifestyle changes. The most common urologic condition today, stone production is also the oldest and most painful. This is because to dietary and lifestyle changes. According to reports, the average lifetime risk of developing stones is in the region of 5% to 10%, with men more likely than women to get stones and an incidence peak between the fourth and fifth decades of life. One frequent element of treating stone illness is preventing the production of new stones [2].

Renal calculus is a complex condition can be caused by the interaction of various contagious, pathological, and genetic factors. The third most typical cystitis infection is urolithiasis. The non-metallic solid minerals that are present in the urinary system are referred as. Lithogenesis inhibitors found in urine, such as magnesium, citrate as well as an imbalance of promoter and inhibitors in the kidney, causes this complex process [3]. As a result, lithogenesis may be influenced by an imbalance among promoters such low urine volume, oxalate, uric acid, and phosphate. Nearly eighty percentage all stones examined were found to be calcium oxalate 50% or 5% calcium phosphate or in combination found to be 45%, 15% to 20% magnesium phosphate, 10% uric acid, 1% cystine can all be found in calcium-containing stones. Stone sickness is two to three times more common in men than in women. It has a 70% to 81% male recurrence rate and a 47% to 60% female recurrence rate.

The selected plant, *Myristica fragrans* (mace spice), has a significant role in Indian culture and folk medicines. Mace has pharmacological functions such as antibacterial, antifungal, anti-inflammatory, anti-ulcer, analgesic, antidepressant, sedative, hypnotic, antioxidant, antidiarrhea, chemoprotective, neuropharmacologic, and antidiabetic [4]. The objective of the current review is to evaluate the medicinal plant *Myristica fragrans* (mace spice's) *in vitro* antiurolithiatic activity.

2.2 Methodology

2.2.1 Collection of Plant Material

The mace spice was purchased from the local market, Coimbatore, Tamil Nadu, India. With tap water, the plant material was cleaned, then dried in the shade.

The basic plant extract was created using the Soxhlet extraction technique. A rotary evaporator was used to filter and evaporate the 15 g of powdered plant material (mace spice) with 150 ml of aqueous and ethanol extracts until they were completely dry. Additionally, it was stored at 4°C in a refrigerator to maintain its antiurolithiatic properties.

2.2.2 Qualitative Analysis of Phytochemicals

Using a conventional technique, preliminary phytochemical screening was conducted for a variety of phytoconstituents, including alkaloids, flavonoids, carbohydrates and reducing sugar, steroids, proteins, tannins, glycosides, saponins, and triterpenoids were used as standard protocol [5]. Figure 2.1 shows the Powder formation of mace spice.

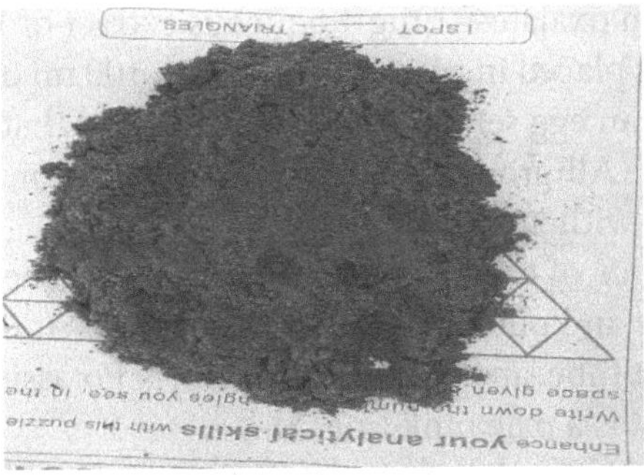

Figure 2.1 Powder formation of mace spice.

2.2.3 Study of *In Vitro* Antiurolithiatic Activity Using Titrimetry Method

2.2.3.1 *Preparation of Calcium Oxalate*

Experimental kidney stones were prepared using sodium oxalate in 10 ml of 2N H_2SO_4 and calcium chloride dehydrate with distilled water. They were then allowed to react in a beaker with enough distilled water to produce calcium oxalate as a precipitate. The precipitate was cleaned of any remaining sulphuric acid using an ammonia solution before being rinsed with double distilled H_2O and dried at 60°C [6].

2.2.3.2 *Preparation of Semipermeable Membrane From Eggs*

Before being put in a beaker with 700 ml of 10% acetic acid, the eggs were thoroughly washed in distilled water. The semipermeable membrane had completely decalcified after being soaked overnight. On next day, semipermeable membrane was carefully removed from decalcified egg using syringe to remove the entire content of the egg, washed thoroughly with double distilled water and kept in ammonia solution has to neutralize acid traces found in solution and again washed with distilled water, then it was stored in the refrigerator, pH 7 to 7.4 has to be maintained for further process.

2.2.3.3 *In Vitro Antiurolithiatic Test Using Titrimetry Method*

Group I: calcium oxalate—1 mg serve as blank;
Group II: calcium oxalate—1 mg + neeri - 10 mg serve as positive control;
Group III: calcium oxalate—1 mg + Ethanol extract of 10 ml was taken
Group IV: Calcium oxalate—1 mg + aqueous extract of 10 ml was taken.

Each group was placed in a beaker filled with 100 ml of Tris buffer 0.1 M and suspended in an egg semipermeable membrane that was secured with thread at one end. All groups are kept in an incubator, and it was maintained for 2 hours with 40°C.

The full substance of each group was taken out of the sutured semipermeable membrane and put into a different test tube. Add 2 ml of 1N sulfuric acid to each test tube, and then titrate with 1N Potassium permanganate until the end point is a pale pink tint [7].

The total amount of calcium oxalate was calculated by the quantity of undissolved calcium oxalate that is still present is deducted from the total amount utilized in the experiment in order to calculate the total amount of calcium oxalate that has been dissolved by different solvent extracts.

2.3 Result and Discussion

Alkaloids, flavonoids, glycosides, tannins and phenolics, saponins, protein and amino acids, phytosterols, and terpenoids were all found in the extract after a phytoconstituent analysis. The phenolic compounds usually exhibit ubiquitous in plant metabolites. Flavonoids, alkaloids possess antioxidant, antimicrobial, and anticancer property, several reports were shown the importance of phytoconstituents [8–11]. Table 2.1 shows the Phytoconstituents of *Myristica fragrans*.

Table 2.1 Phytoconstituents of *Myristica fragrans*.

Phytochemical Screening	Test	Ethanol extract of *Myristica fragrans*
Dragendorff's Hager's Mayer	Alkaloids	+ + +
General test	Glucoside	+
Ferric chloride	Tannins and phenolics	+
Foam	Saponins	+ +
Shinoda Lead acetate	Flavanoids	+ +
Fehling's test Molisch test	Carbohydrates	+ +
Million's Biuret	Proteins and Amino acids	+ +
Salkowaski	Phytosterols	+ +
Ruthenium red test	Gum and mucilage	-
Libermann-Buchardt Test	Terpenoids	+

**+, presence; –, absence.*

2.3.1 *In Vitro* Antiurolithiatic Activity Test

Each group was placed in a beaker filled with 0.1 M Tris buffer of 100 ml and suspended in an egg semipermeable membrane that was secured with thread at one end.

Each group's whole material was taken out of the sutured semipermeable membrane and put into a separate test tube. Until a light pink end point was reached, substance from each test tube was independently titrated. All the groups spent 2 hours in an incubator that was heated to 37°C.

2.3.2 Analysis of Dissolved Calcium Oxalate

Drug therapy changed as a result of the demands of population health. Numerous serious medical conditions, including liver disorders, arthritis, age-related issues, certain viral infections, and cancer, cannot be adequately treated by traditional therapy. These are some of the most exciting areas of study and development for plant-based medicines. Additionally, plant sources used efficient, innovative, used as a treatment medicine for kidney procumbens [12, 13].

Many phytotherapies has been used for several phases of pathophysiology, in contrast to allopathic medications, which focus on just one element of urolithiatic pathophysiology. Approximately 80% of people rely on traditional medicine, which is primarily made up of ingredients from plants. Plant-based drug development activities are still a significant source of fresh therapeutic candidates. Nephrolithiasis and urolithiasis both are example of lithiasis, which is a major cause of acute and chronic failure. When it comes to the numerous types of stones that have been found, calcium stones mostly affect males, whereas phosphate stones mostly affect women [10]. As opposed to allopathic medicine, which focuses on several aspects of when it comes to the numerous types of stones that have been found, calcium stones mostly affect males, whereas phosphate stones mostly affect women [10]. Unlike allopathic treatment, urolithiatic medications that exclusively focus on one element. Most plant-based treatments have been demonstrated to enhance pathophysiology and to be efficient at different stages of stone pathology [14–16].

Plant-based drug development activities still have a significant impact. An origin of fresh drug leads Stone formation, or lithiasis, is a medical problem [17–19]. It comprises nephrolithiasis and urolithiasis found in the ureter, bladder, or both [20]. This condition is a substantial cause of both acute and chronic renal failure [22]. There are several different varieties of calcium stones, and they are often found in. Phosphate stones are more prone to form in women

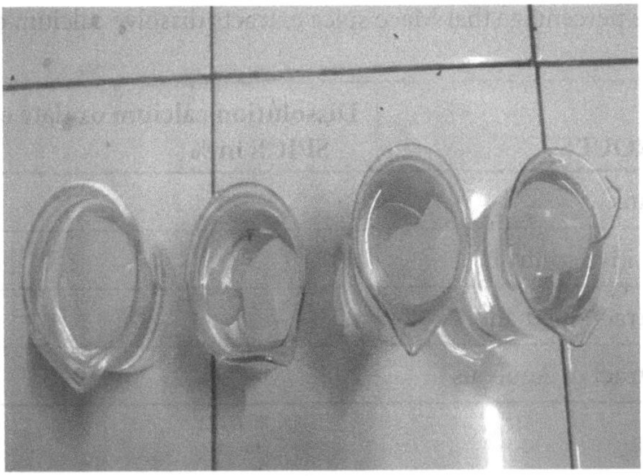

Figure 2.2 Egg semipermeable membrane in 0.1 M Tris buffer.

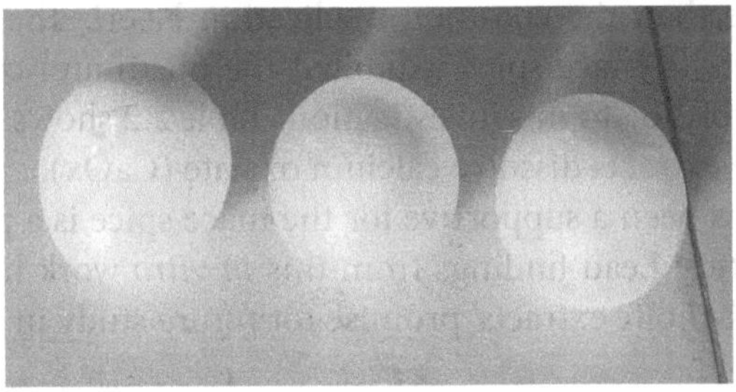

Figure 2.3 Decalcified eggs.

[21]. Figure 2.2 shows the egg semipermeable membrane in 0.1M Tris Buffer. Figure 2.3 shows the decalcified eggs.

GROUP I: Undissolved calcium oxalate—10 mg, total calcium oxalate—10 mg. There is no dissolution process occurs.

GROUP II: Undissolved calcium oxalate—1.9 mg, total calcium oxalate—10 mg. 8.1 mg of calcium oxalate was dissolved by neeri.

GROUP III: Undissolved calcium oxalate—1.8 mg, total calcium oxalate—10 mg. The remaining 8.2 mg of calcium oxalate was dissolved by ethanol extract of mace spice.

GROUP IV: Undissolved calcium oxalate—2.6 mg, Total calcium oxalate—10 mg. The remaining 7.4 mg of calcium oxalate was dissolved by aqueous extract of mace spice.

The ethanolic and aqueous extracts of mace spice are examined in this study for their antiurolithiatic properties. Aqueous extract has calcium

Table 2.2 The percentage that Mace spice extracts dissolve calcium oxalate (CaOx).

S. no	GROUPS	Dissolution calcium oxalate of MACE SPICE in %
1	Blank	0
2	Positive control	80
3	Extract of ethanol	82
4	Extract of Aqueous	74

oxalate dissolution of 74%, whereas the ethanolic extract had the greatest percentage of calcium oxalate (CaOx) dissolution, 82%. Both ethanolic extracts from the mace spice were shown to be more potent at reducing calcium oxalate than the common medication Neeri. The ethanolic and aqueous extracts of mace spice exhibited the maximum calcium oxalate dissolution, according to this investigation. Table 2.2 shows the percentage that Mace spice extracts dissolve calcium oxalate (CaOx).

This work has been a supportive for the mace spice is a plant with lithotriptic properties. Lead findings from this *in vitro* work have shown the aqueous and ethanolic extracts' promise for future study in this field.

2.4 Conclusion

Semipermeable membrane of egg was separated and used to assess the Mace spice's *in vitro* antiurolithiatic efficacy. By performing *in vitro* urolithiasis on the chosen plant, Mace spice, and using the common medication Neeri, the percentage of kidney stone dissolving was discovered. The Mace spice's ethanol leaf extracts have the greatest medication dissolving rates. Thus, through our research, it has been established that the mace spice plant contains antiurolithiatic properties.

References

1. Sumayyasikandari, P.M., *In vitro* antiurolithiatic activity of uteamonosperma Lam. and Nigella Sativa Linn. seeds. *Ann. Phytomed.*, 4, 105–7, 2015.
2. Gupta, S.K., Baghel, M., Bhuyan, C., Ravi Shankar, B., Ashok, B.K., Patil, P.D., Evaluation of the anti-urolithiatic activity of Pashanabhedadi Ghrita against

experimentally induced renal calculi in rats. *AYU Int. Q. J. Res. Ayurveda*, 33, 429–34, 2012.
3. Makasana, A., Ranpariya, V., Desai, D., Mendpara, J., Parekh, V., Evaluation for the anti-urolithiatic activity of Launaeaprocumbens against ethylene glycol-induced renal calculi in rats. *Toxicol. Rep.*, 1, 46–52, 2014.
4. Nifras, M.M.M., Fasmila, M.F.F., Fatheena, J.F., Muthalib, A.M., A comprehensive review on therapeutic uses of *Myristica fragrans* in traditional systems of medicine. *Int. J. Unani Integr. Med.*, 5, 2, 111–117, 2021.
5. Bhargava, N., Rathore, P.S., Bhowmick, A., Study of X Ray Detection Using CNN in Machine Learning. *Advancements in Smart Computing and Information Security: First International Conference, ASCIS 2022*, Rajkot, India, November 24–26, 2022, Cham: Springer Nature, Switzerland, 2023, Revised Selected Papers, Part I.
6. Benkhaddra, I., Kumar, A., Setitra, M.A. *et al.*, Design and Development of Consensus Activation Function Enabled Neural Network-Based Smart Healthcare Using BIoT. *Wirel. Pers. Commun.*, 130, 1549–1574, 2023, https://doi.org/10.1007/s11277-023-10344-0 Q2,Impact Factor -2.017.
7. Ilyas, B., Kumar, A., Mo., A., Setitra, Z., Bensalem, E.A., Lei, H., Prevention of DDoS attacks using an optimized deep learning approach in blockchain technology. *Trans. Emerging Telecommun. Technol.*, 34, 4, e4729, 2023. Q2,Impact Factor -3.31.
8. Kumar, A., Rathore, P.S., Dubey, A.K., Agrawal, R., Sharma, K.P., LTE-NBP with holistic UWB-WBAN approach for the energy efficient biomedical application. *Multimed. Tools Appl.*, 82, 39797–39811, 2023.
9. Kumar, A.,Kumar, S.A., Dutt, V., Shitharth, S., Tripathi, E., IoT based arrhythmia classification using the enhanced hunt optimization based deep learning. *Expert Sys.*, 40, 7, 1–10, 2023.
10. Bhargava, N., Rathore, P.S., Bhowmick, A., Study of X Ray Detection Using CNN in Machine Learning, in: *International Conference on Advancements in Smart Computing and Information Security*, pp. 295–303, Cham: Springer Nature, Switzerland, 2022, November.
11. Lalitha, G., Dr.Nazeema, T.H., Sharmila, L., Phytochemical screening and evaluation of Antimicrobial activity, Antioxidant activity, Anticoagulant activity and Fibrinolytic activity of leaves of Andrographis paniculata (leaf). *Int. J. Pharma Bio Sci.*, 6, 2, 475–484, 2015.
12. Jagannath N., Chikkannasetty, S.S., Govindadas, D., Devasankaraiah, G., Study of anti urolithiatic activity of Asparagus racemosus on albino rats. *Indian J. Pharmacol.*, 44, 576–9, 2012.
13. Ramu, R., Doraiswamy, R., Yadav, H.M., Antiurolithiatic activity of Aqueous bark extract of Crateva Magna Lour. (DC). *Int. J. Res. Ayurveda Pharm.*, 8, 271–8, 2017.
14. Subramoniam, Present scenario, challenges and future perspectives in plant-based medicine development. *Ukaaz Ann. Phytomed.*, 3, 31–6, 2014.

15. Kumar, A.S., Kavimani, S., Jayaveera, K.N., Anti-diabetic and antihyperlipidemic effects of methanol extracts of Chloris barbata (SW.) in Streptozotocin-induced diabetic rats. *Eur. J. Exp. Biol.*, 2, 1346–53, 2012.
16. Atodriya, U., Baard, R., Upadhya, S., Upadhyay, U., Antiurolithiatic activity of Dolichosbiflorus seeds. *J. Pharmacogn Phytochem.*, 2, 209–13, 2013.
17. Moses, R., Pais, V.M., Jr, Ursiny, M., Prien, E.L., Jr, Miller, N., Eisner, B.H., Changes in stone composition over two decades: evaluation of over 10,000 stone analyses. *Urolithiasis*, 43, 135–9, 2015.
18. Kotturu, P.K. and Kumar, A., Comparative Study on Machine Learning models for Early Diagnose of Alzheimer's Disease: Multi Correlation Method. *2020 5th International Conference on Communication and Electronics Systems (ICCES)*, pp. 778–783, 2020, doi: 10.1109/ICCES48766.2020.9137872.
19. Swarna, S.R., Kumar, A., Dixit, P., Sairam, T.V.M., Parkinson's Disease Prediction using Adaptive Quantum Computing. *2021 Third International Conference on Intelligent Communication Technologies and Virtual Mobile Networks (ICICV)*, pp. 1396–1401, 2021, doi: 10.1109/ICICV50876.2021.9388628.
20. Dhole, A.R., Dhole, V.R., Magdum, C.S., Mohite, S., Herbal Therapy for Urolithiasis: A Brief Review. *Res. J. Pharmacol. Pharmacodyn.*, 5, 1, 06–12, 2013.
21. Subramoniam, A. and Pushpangadan, P., Development of Phytomedicines for liver diseases. *Indian J. Pharmacol.*, 31, 166–175, 1999.
22. Yang, D., Tiselius, H.G., Lan, C., Chen, D., Chen, K., Ou, L. *et al.*, Metabolic disturbances in Chinese children with urolithiasis: A single center report. *Urolithiasis*, 45, 285–290, 2017.

3

Parkinson's Disease Detection Using Voice and Speech—Systematic Literature Review

Ronak Khatwad[1], Suyash Tiwari[1], Yash Tripathi[1], Ajay Nehra[1] and Ashish Sharma[2]*

[1]Dept. of CSE, IIIT Kota, MNIT Jaipur, Jaipur, India
[2]Dept. of CSE, Manipal University Jaipur, Jaipur, India

Abstract
Parkinson's disease (PD) is normally diagnosed in a person after a thorough physical examination by a doctor that considers the patient's medical history, neurological examination, evaluation of motor symptoms, and other supporting tests with precise diagnostic criteria. However, there is no surefire way to identify PD. Furthermore, other medical problems, including arthritis and stroke, should be evaluated on subsequent visits because they can show similarly to Parkinson's disease. Only 80.6% of PD diagnoses are correct overall. Machine learning techniques can be applied in a variety of ways to develop different methods to recognize the presence of PD in an individual, as well as identify it in the initial stages of the disease, to aid doctors in the diagnosis of PD. The primary objective of this SLR is to explore the different methods in which features and machine learning systems can be combined to detect individuals with Parkinson's disease (PD). We gathered, summarized, and analyzed research publications on PD detection using voice and speech datasets (and closely related topics) published between the years 2016 and 2022 for this SLR. To search for all the publications related to the issue, articles were gathered by executing a keyword-based automated search using ScienceDirect and PubMed.

Keywords: Parkinson's disease, Bradykinesia, Ysphonia, gait, sleep disturbance, dementia, constipation, Braak model

**Corresponding author*: ashish@iiitkota.ac.in

Sumit Srivastava, Abhineet Anand, Abhishek Kumar, Bhavna Saini and Pramod Singh Rathore (eds.) Bio-Inspired Optimization for Medical Data Mining, (41–74) © 2024 Scrivener Publishing LLC

3.1 Introduction

A neurodegenerative condition called Parkinson's disease [1] is characterized by a progressive depletion of dopamine in the brain. The substantia nigra region of the brain is affected by this age-related illness. This region has a midbrain dopaminergic nucleus, plays a vital role in regulating motor activity and reward functions. It is a crucial brain region for the generation of dopamine. The manifestation of PD symptoms occurs when there is a significant loss of dopaminergic neurons or an alteration in the amount of dopamine in the brain.

As one ages, the number of connections between brain cells decreases, and the neurons shrink in size. Unlike cells found in muscles, skin, and bones, nerve cells lack the ability to regenerate themselves. As we age, our neurons deteriorate or die. Parkinson's disease is linked to both motor and non-motor characteristics, including the ability to plan, initiate, and complete movements. Motor symptoms, which include Bradykinesia (slowness in walking), Ysphonia (changes in speech), gait (short steps), and stiff muscles, are those that affect how the body moves. Sleep disturbance, loss of smell, dementia, constipation, hallucinations, and other nonmotor symptoms are a few examples.

Parkinson's disease cannot be prevented because the cause of the death of dopamine-producing neurons is still unclear, but the condition can be caught early and treated appropriately to decrease the disease's course. Parkinson's disease patients receive treatment with drugs like syndopa and levodopa, the dosage of which depends on how severe the condition is.

Parkinson's disease affects over 1% of individuals who are 65 years or older [1]. Ninety percent of persons with PD report speech impairment [2, 3], and A significant number of individuals exhibit speech-related symptoms during the initial stages of the condition [4]. Symptoms of PD include reduced inflection in pitch or loudness for expressing emotion or meaning, decreased intensity, altered voice quality, and a limited range of articulatory movements. Repeated syllables can cause a decline in volume and articulation. Rush (words that are spoken quickly) and dysfluency (caused by hesitations or a loss of rhythm) make comprehension even more difficult. This collection of flaws is often referred to as hypokinetic dysarthria [5]. Its manifestation is somewhat dependent on internal cues and sensory processing, similar to bradykinesia [6, 7]. Although PD patients talk softly, they mistakenly think their speech is louder than it actually is [8]. Most aspects of parkinsonian dysarthria improve in response to outside signals [9].

Apart from the aforementioned conditions, voice patterns can also be affected by autism, dyslexia, heart disease, and Alzheimer's disease [10–12].

As per the Braak model that describes the progression of a PD in a pathological manner, Lewy (alpha-synuclein) pathology first affects the medulla oblongata and pons [13]. In Braak stages 1 and 2 of PD, speech impairment may manifest before the appearance of additional motor symptoms [14, 15]. The prosody of speech was recently shown to be impacted in people with solitary REM sleep behavior disorder and decreased olfaction, which are premonitory nonmotor deficits [16]. Perceptual speech analysis contributes significantly to our present understanding of parkinsonian speech problems. The subjective approach suffers from several drawbacks, such as inherent variations in people's voices, external cues effects, and context-related variations in verbal communication. In order to address these challenges, computerized speech or voice analysis has been suggested as a potential method for the diagnosis and monitoring of PD.

This review seeks to fill the gaps between these several fields, advance technological knowledge, and specify clinical needs. Our literature review began in the year 2016 as the starting point since our preliminary reading indicated that the pace of research in this area has increased since that year [17, 18]. The aim of our literature review was to establish connections among different studies on speech and voice in PD and determine the acoustic features and phonemes that best indicate the disease's seriousness.

3.2 Research Questions

Research questions serve the purpose of clarifying the objectives of a systematic review, enabling the readers to comprehend what the review aims to achieve. The questions are devised to encompass all the essential concepts and significant aspects relevant to detecting PD. The aim is to explore the literature, analyze and consolidate the accessible data on research topics, types, methodologies, contributions, and gaps, from the viewpoint of scholars and practitioners, in the context of PD detection. The research questions that were given priority include:

1. What are the individual stages that make up the process of detecting PD?
2. What are the different datasets based on the voice that can be utilized to train models for the identification of PD?

3. What are the different voice recording characteristics that can be extracted and utilized for training models to detect PD in individuals?
4. What ML/Non-ML algorithms have been used for PD detection?
5. What are the accuracy metrics used?

3.3 Method

The systematic review followed the PRISMA guidelines. All papers were collectively evaluated to identify those that were not suitable for further assessment based on three criteria:

(i) insufficient statistical analysis;
(ii) poor data analysis; and
(iii) inadequate methodological details.

The selected publications were analyzed to assess both the technical and medical aspects, as well as the quality of the methodology and the reliability of the results. Additionally, papers that did not meet the criteria for statistical analysis, data analysis, or methodological detail were excluded from further assessment.

3.3.1 Search Strategy

The study utilized the combination of search terms "Parkinson's disease," "speech," "voice," and "machine learning" to search two databases, ScienceDirect and PubMed, for publications between 2016 and 2022. A total of 220 papers were screened based on the title and abstract, and 60 papers were selected for full-text reading.

3.3.2 Inclusion Criteria

Several studies have been selected or rejected for this systematic literature review (SLR) based on specific parameters. Inclusion and exclusion criteria were used to determine which studies met the requirements for this review. The inclusion criteria for a study refer to the specific characteristics that it must possess to be considered for the review and this is shown below in Figure 3.1 that represent the flow diagram of PRISMA. The following inclusion criteria were considered for this SLR:

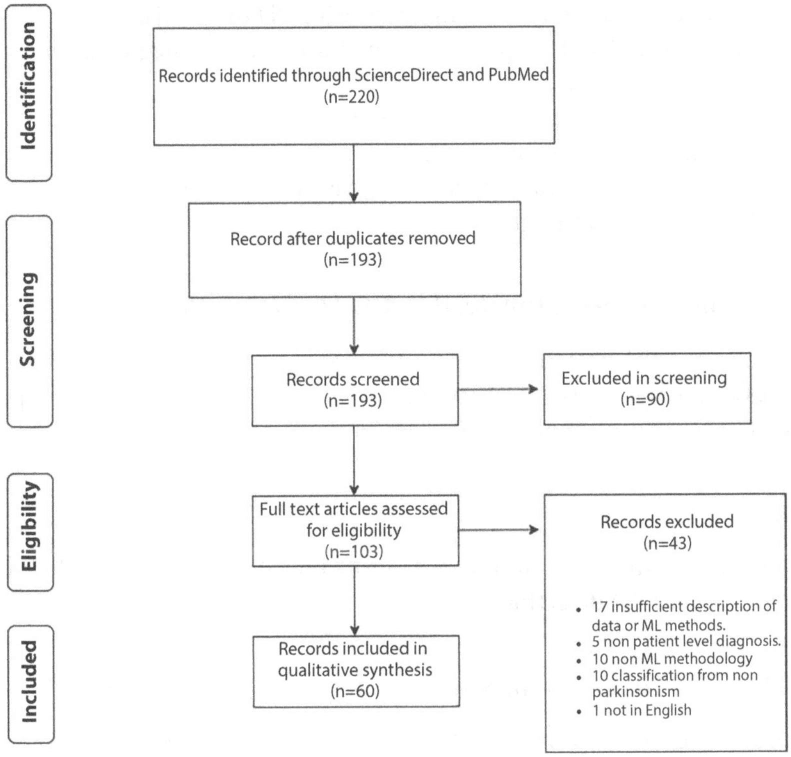

Figure 3.1 The flow diagram of PRISMA for literature search and selection process illustrates the number of research papers that were found, filtered, and included in the SLR.

1. Research papers published between 2016 and 2022 that explored the application of speech and/or voice in detection or monitoring PD were included in this study.
2. Differentiating between individuals with PD and healthy controls (HC) based on classification.
3. Differentiating PD from other syndromes of parkinsonism.

Studies that fell into one or more of the following groups were not included:

1. studies on Parkinsonism or associated illnesses that did not involve PD classification or detection;
2. studies which involved PD detection using other datasets other than voice and speech datasets were excluded;

3. studies that have nothing to do with PD diagnosis;
4. study did not employ any metrics to assess categorization performance;
5. study's descriptions of the machine learning techniques, data sets, and subjects used were insufficient or inaccurate;
6. not original documents for a journal article or a conference; and
7. article not in English.

3.3.3 Subprocesses Involved in PD Detection Process

Typically, the PD detection process encompasses the subprocesses of pre-processing of the dataset, feature extraction process, feature selection process, and classification of selected features.

3.3.4 Data Sets

Following are the voice and speech recording datasets used by different researchers for PD detection:

3.3.4.1 Parkinson's Data Set—UCI Machine Learning Dataset

Max Little, in association with the National Center for Speech and Speech in Denver, Colorado, recorded speech signals to create this dataset [22]. It comprises biomedical voice measurements from 31 individuals, of which 23 have PD. Each row of the table represents one of these individuals' 195 audio recordings, and each column is a specific audio measurement [22]. The dataset aims to distinguish healthy people from those with PD, with the "status" column setting healthy individuals to 0 and PD patients to 1. Of the 23 attributes in the dataset, 21 are acoustic features.

3.3.4.2 PC-GITA Dataset

The dataset comprises voice recordings of 50 individuals diagnosed with PD and their age and gender-matched HC who are all Spanish native speakers [23]. The recordings were taken using a rule that adhered to technical requirements and recommendations from experts in the fields of linguistics, phonetics, and neurology. The tasks included in this dataset cover various aspects of speech, such as sustained vowel vocalization, diadocokinetic assessment, 45 words, 10 sentences, reading texts, and monologs.

3.3.4.3 mPower Dataset

The mPower project, which aimed to evaluate innovative metrics to complement traditional behavioral symptom assessments for tracking Parkinson's disease progression and diagnosis, generated this dataset through a mobile application-based study [23]. This study seeks to comprehend the sources of, frequency of, and degree of variation in patient symptoms, as well as any potential moderators of such differences. This dataset contains data from seven different modules:

1. *Demographics:* Participants in this survey replied to inquiries about their health history and general demographic information [21].
2. *MDS-UPDRS:* Selected questions from the UPDRS scale of the Movement Disorder Society were answered by survey respondents [21].
3. *PDQ-8:* The PD questionnaire short form was used for participants to respond to in this survey.
4. *Memory:* Participants engage in a brief visuospatial game associated with the Corsi block-tapping test in this module [21].
5. *Tapping:* In this module, participants perform multiple taps on their mobile's screen.
6. *Voice:* In this module, participants initially capture the surrounding noise level for 5 seconds, and upon its acceptability, they proceed to record their voice saying "aaah" for 10 seconds [21].
7. *Walking:* Participants are instructed to walk back and forth for a duration of 20 to 30 seconds while keeping their mobile in their pocket in this module [21]. They are subsequently asked to stand still for another 20 to 30 seconds.

3.3.4.4 Mobile Device Voice Recordings (MDVR-KCL) Dataset

The dataset was captured at the KCL Hospital in Denmark Hill, Brixton, London, where a standard examination room measuring approximately ten square meters with a typical reverberation time of 500 milliseconds was employed for speech recordings [19]. Motorola Moto G4 smartphones were used to record the data. The dataset includes voice recordings collected from 16 individuals diagnosed with PD and 21 healthy individuals [19]. The first task involved reading a paragraph of text, and the second task involved engaging in spontaneous conversation, both of which were completed by all 37 participants. The recordings are approximately 150 seconds long and are saved in the WAV format.

3.3.4.5 *Italian Parkinson's Voice and Speech (IPVS) Dataset*

The Italian Parkinson's Voice and Speech dataset is a collection of audio recordings of individuals with Parkinson's disease speaking in Italian [20]. The dataset was created to support research in the area of voice and speech analysis for the early detection and monitoring of Parkinson's disease.

The dataset contains audio recordings from 28 individuals with Parkinson's disease and 20 healthy individuals serving as controls. Each participant was asked to read a set of standardized sentences in Italian, resulting in a total of 2,000 utterances in the dataset. The recordings were made in a soundproof room using a high-quality microphone and were stored in WAV format.

The dataset also includes various measures of speech quality and voice characteristics, such as the fundamental frequency, jitter, shimmer, and harmonics-to-noise ratio. These measures can be used to evaluate the severity of Parkinson's disease and track changes in speech quality over time.

3.3.4.6 *Parkinson Speech Dataset With Multiple Types of Sound Recordings Dataset*

The Parkinson Speech Dataset with Multiple Types of Sound Recordings is a collection of audio recordings of individuals with Parkinson's disease and healthy controls [24]. The dataset was created to support research in the area of speech analysis for the detection and monitoring of Parkinson's disease. The dataset contains several types of sound recordings, including sustained phonation, vowel prolongation, and reading tasks. The recordings were made using several devices, including smartphones, tablets, and professional microphones. The dataset includes a total of 756 recordings from 42 individuals, including 23 individuals with Parkinson's disease and 19 healthy controls.

In addition to the audio recordings, the dataset also includes various measures of speech quality and voice characteristics, such as jitter, shimmer, fundamental frequency, and harmonics-to-noise ratio. These measures can be used to evaluate the severity of Parkinson's disease and track changes in speech quality over time and below Table 3.1 shows the Comparison of Parkinson's voice datasets. The Table 3.2 shows the Comparison of various techniques used for PD detection

Table 3.1 Comparison of Parkinson's voice datasets.

Name	Total participants	Number of recordings	Dataset availability	Recording availability	Task
Mobile Device Voice Recordings at King's College London (MDVR KCL) [19]	37 (PD=16, HC=21) -	73	Public	Yes	Spontaneous Dialogue Read text
Italian Parkinson's Voice and Speech Dataset [20]	65 (PD=28, HC=37)	495	Public	Yes	Reading Exercise, Pronunciation of vowels
mPower Database [21]	5826	65022	Public	Yes (requires synapse account)	say 'Aaaaah' into the microphone at a steady volume for up to 10 s.
Parkinson's Disease Dataset [22]	31 (PD=23, HC=8)	197	Public	No	Vowel Phonations
PC-GITA Dataset [23]	100(PD=50, HC=50)	Not Available	Private	No	Vowel Phonation, Word Phonation, Sentence Phonation, Dialogue, Spontaneous Speech
Parkinsons Telemonitoring Dataset [22]	42 (PD=42, HC=0)	5875	Public	No	Sustained Phonations, Running Speech
Parkinson Speech Dataset with Multiple Types of Sound Recordings [24]	Training: 40(PD=20, HC=20, Testing: 28(PD=28, HC=0)	Training: 872, Testing: 168	Public	No	Training: Vowel, word and sentence phonation, Testing: Vowel Phonation

Table 3.2 Comparison of various techniques used for PD detection.

Authors	Source of data	Number of HC	Number of PD	Classifiers	Results
Maryam [26]	UCI Dataset	20 HC	20 PD	EWNN	Accuracy = 92.9%
Qiang Li, Huiling Chen [25]	UCI Dataset	8 HC	23 PD	IGWOKELM	Accuracy = 97.45% Sensitivity = 99.38%
Chao Ma, Hui-Ling Chen [27]	UCI Dataset	8 HC	23 PD	Kernel Extreme Learning Machine with feature weighting using Subtractive Clustering	Accuracy = 97.40% Sensitivity = 99.38%.
Samiappan, Dhanalakshmi, Masunda, Sam [31]	UCI Dataset	20 HC	20 PD	SVM, HMM	Accuracy = 95.16%, Specificity = 91.67%.
Pawalai Kraipeerapun and Somkid Amornsamankul [30]	UCI Dataset	20 HC	20 PD	CMTNN	Accuracy = 70%
Hongpeng Zhou, Tianyi Gao [28]	UCI Dataset	8 HC	23 PD	SVm-RBF	Accuracy = 96.29%
N. Sairam, Indrajit [29]	UCI Dataset	8 HC	23 PD	Pegasos, SMO, SVM and AdaBoost	Accuracy = 98.24%

(Continued)

Table 3.2 Comparison of various techniques used for PD detection. (*Continued*)

Authors	Source of data	Number of HC	Number of PD	Classifiers	Results
Harshul Garg, Zaid [33]	UCI Dataset	8 HC	23 PD	KNN	Accuracy = 90%
Shreerag, Swain [32]	UCI Dataset	8 HC	23 PD	KNN, random forest, ANN, LR	Accuracy = 94.87%
Arif, Akin [34]	UCI Dataset	8 HC	23 PD	rotation forest	Accuracy = 87%
Akin [35]	UCI Dataset	8 HC	23 PD	rotation forest	Accuracy = 96.9%
Musa [36]	UCI Dataset	8 HC	23 PD	radial basis function-support vector machine	Accuracy = 98.9%
Hasan, Marziye [37]	UCI Dataset	8 HC	23 PD	extreme learning machine	Accuracy = 88.72%
Alavi, Nikookar [38]	UCI Dataset	8 HC	23 PD	ensemble learning	Accuracy = 90.6%
Yunfeng Wu, Yao [39]	UCI Dataset	8 HC	23 PD	generalized logistic regression	Sensitivity = 0.9796
Kumar, Yadav, Sahoo [40]	UCI Dataset	8 HC	23 PD	decision tree classifier	Accuracy = 0.76
Ertam, Tuncer [41]	UCI Dataset	40 HC	40 PD	KNN and SVM	Accuracy = 91.25%

(*Continued*)

Table 3.2 Comparison of various techniques used for PD detection. (*Continued*)

Authors	Source of data	Number of HC	Number of PD	Classifiers	Results
Luo, Cai [42]	UCI Dataset	8 HC	23 PD	Mean average precision, SVM-Radial basis function, fisher linear discriminant analysis	Accuracy = 91.8%
Safra, Frid [43]	Participants	9 HC	43 PD	SVM-RBF	Accuracy = 81.8%
Perez, Montana [44]	Participants	27 HC	27 PD	SVM	Accuracy = 94.4%
Isenkul [45]	Participants	20 HC	20 PD	KNN, SVM, SVMRBF	Accuracy = 77.5%
Vicsi, Tulics [46]	Participants	27 HC	51 PD	ANN, SVM, KNN	Accuracy = 84.62%
Saurabhchand [47]	Participants	56 HC	52 PD	Siamese LSTM-based NN	EER = 1.9%
Atkins, John, Reza [48]	Participants	2023 HC	246 PD	gradient boosted decision tree, LR	F1 score = 0.836
Skalski, Hemmerling [49]	PC-GITA	50 HC	50 PD	ResNet	Accuracy = 91.7%
Abiyev and Abizade [50]	UCI Dataset	8 HC	23 PD	Fuzzy neural system	Testing accuracy = 100%

(*Continued*)

Table 3.2 Comparison of various techniques used for PD detection. (*Continued*)

Authors	Source of data	Number of HC	Number of PD	Classifiers	Results
Aich, Kim, Younga, Hui, Al-Absi, and Sain [51]	UCI Dataset	8 HC	23 PD	Some examples of machine learning algorithms are RPART, C4.5, PART, Boosted C5.0, Bagging CART, SVM, and random forest	NPV = 0.9995 Accuracy = 97.57% Specificity = 99.87% Sensitivity = 97.56%
Al-Fatlawi, Jabardi, and Ling [52]	UCI Dataset	8 HC	23 PD	DBN of 2 RBMs	Testing Testing accuracy = 94%
Sayaydeha and Mohammad, M. F. [53]	UCI Dataset	8 HC	23 PD	EFMM-OneR	Accuracy = 94.21%
Ali, Khan, Arshad, Ali, and Anwar [33]	UCI Dataset	20 HC	20 PD	Linear regression, LDA, KNN, Gaussian Na¨ıve Bayes, SVM-RBF decision tree, SVM-linear, validation	Accuracy = 70%

(*Continued*)

Table 3.2 Comparison of various techniques used for PD detection. (*Continued*)

Authors	Source of data	Number of HC	Number of PD	Classifiers	Results
Ali, Zhu, Zhang, and Liu [54]	UCI Dataset	20 HC	20 PD	LDA-NN-GA validation	Training: Sensitivity = 95%, Accuracy = 95% Test: Sensitivity = 100%, Accuracy = 100%
Alqahtani, Alshamrani, Syed, and Olatunji [55]	UCI Dataset	8 HC	23 PD	NNge with AdaBoost	Testing accuracy = 96.30%
Anand, Haque, Alex, and Venkatesan [56]	UCI Dataset	8 HC	23 PD	Logistic regression, random forest, SVM, KNN, na¨ıv Bayes, decision tree, DNN	Accuracy = 95.513%
Bakar, Ispawi, Ibrahim, and Tahir [57]	UCI Dataset	8 HC	23 PD	MLP	MSE = 0.03552, Training accuracy = 97.86%, Test accuracy = 92.96%
Cai, Gu, Wen, Zhao, Huang, Huang [58]	UCI Dataset	8 HC	23 PD	FKNN, SVM, KELM	Accuracy = 97.89%

(*Continued*)

Table 3.2 Comparison of various techniques used for PD detection. (*Continued*)

Authors	Source of data	Number of HC	Number of PD	Classifiers	Results
Celik, and Omurca [59]	UCI Dataset	20 HC	20 PD	D SVM, Logistic Regression, ET, Gradient boosting, Random Forest	Accuracy = 76.03%
C, imen, and Bolat [60]	UCI Dataset	20 HC	20 PD	MLP, GRNN	Spread parameter = 195.1189, GRNN: Error rate = 0.0995
Dash, Thulasiram, And Thulasiraman [61]	UCI Dataset	8 HC	23 PD	ECFA-SVM	Accuracy = 97.95%, Precision = 97.90%, F-measure = 97.90%, Sensitivity = 97.90%, Specificity = 96.50%, AUC = 97.20%
Dastjerd, Sert, Ozyer, and Alhajj [62]	UCI Dataset	20 HC	20 PD	Fuzzy Classifier	Testing Accuracy = 100%

(*Continued*)

Table 3.2 Comparison of various techniques used for PD detection. (*Continued*)

Authors	Source of data	Number of HC	Number of PD	Classifiers	Results
Dinesh, and He [63]	UCI Dataset	8 HC	23 PD	BPM, Boosted Decision Tree, Decision Forests, Decision Jungle, Averaged Perceptron, Locally Deep SVM, Logistic Regression, NN, SVM	Accuracy = 91.2105% Precision = 93.5714% F-score = 94.2368% AUC = 96.6293% %
Erdogdu Sakar, Serbes, and Sakar [64]	UCI Dataset	8 HC	42 PD	KNN, SVM, ELM	Accuracy = 96.43%., MCC = 0.77
Gunduz H. [66]	UCI Dataset	64 HC	188 PD	CNN	Accuracy = 86.9%, F-measure = 91.7% MCC = 63.2 %
Haq, Li, Memon, Khan, Din, Ahad [67]	UCI Dataset	8 HC	23 PD	DNN, SVM, KNN, Logistic Regression	Accuracy = 98%, Sensitivity = 99%, Specificity = 95%
Haq, Li, Memon, khan, Malik, Ahmad [68]	UCI Dataset	8 HC	23 PD	SVM-RBF, SVM-linea	Accuracy = 99% Specificity = 99% Sensitivity = 100%

(*Continued*)

Table 3.2 Comparison of various techniques used for PD detection. (*Continued*)

Authors	**Source of data**	**Number of HC**	**Number of PD**	**Classifiers**	**Results**
Hariharan, Polat, and Sindhu [69]	UCI Dataset	8 HC	23 PD	LS-SVM, PNN, GRNN with conventional	AUC = 100, Accuracy = 100%, Sensitivity = 100%, Precision = 100%, Specificity = 100%
Islam, Parvez, Hai, and Goswami [70]	UCI Dataset	8 HC	23 PD	FBANN, SVM-linear, Random tree	MSE = 0.027, Accuracy = 97.37%, Precision = 0.979, Sensitivity = 98.60%, FPR = 6.38%, Specificity = 93.62%
Ji, and Li [71]	UCI Dataset	8 HC	23 PD	SVM-linea	Error rate 0.13
Junior, Costa, Chen, and Guido [72]	UCI Dataset	20 HC	20 PD	GBM, Decision tree, XGBoost, random forest, SVM	FNR = 10 Accuracy = 72.5%
Karapinar Senturk [73]	UCI Dataset	8 HC	23 PD	CART, SVM, ANN	Accuracy = 93.84%
Goyal *et al.* [33]	MDVR-KCL	21 HC	16 PD	CNN	Validation accuracy of 99.37%

(*Continued*)

Table 3.2 Comparison of various techniques used for PD detection. (*Continued*)

Authors	Source of data	Number of HC	Number of PD	Classifiers	Results
Chetan *et al.* [75]	MDVR-KCL	21 HC	16 PD	KNN	Accuracy upto 98%
Adedolapo *et al.* [76]	MDVR-KCL	21 HC	16 PD	KNN, Decision Trees, (SVM), Naïve Bayes, Logistic Regression (LR), Random Forest, Gradient Boosting	Accuracy upto 90.9%
Lamba *et al.* [74]	MDVR-KCL	21 HC	16 PD	KNN, XGBoost, Random Forest, Logistic Regression	Accuracy = 90%
Adedolapo *et al.* [76]	IPVS	37 HC	28 PD	KNN, Decision Trees, (SVM), Naïve Bayes, Gradient Boosting, Logistic Regression and Random Forest	Accuracy up 99%
Lamba *et al.* [74]	IPVS	37 HC	28 PD	KNN, XGBoost, Random Forest, Logistic Regression	Accuracy = 100%

(*Continued*)

Table 3.2 Comparison of various techniques used for PD detection. *(Continued)*

Authors	Source of data	Number of HC	Number of PD	Classifiers	Results
Hires *et al.* [77]	PC-GITA	50 HC	50 PD	CNN	Accuracy = 99%
Karan *et al.* [78]	PC-GITA	50 HC	50 PD	SVM, SVR	Vowels: accuracy: 92% Words: accuracy: 97%
Er *et al.* [79]	PC-GITA	50 HC	50 PD	ResNet-LSTM	Accuracy = 98.61%
Amato *et al.* [80]	PC-GITA	50 HC	50 PD	SVM, DT, NB, kNN	Accuracy = 94.3%
Sechidis *et al.* [81]	PC-GITA	50 HC	50 PD	SVM, RF, MLP	Vowels: accuracy: 96%

3.3.4.7 Parkinson's Telemonitoring Dataset

The Parkinson's Telemonitoring dataset is a collection of data that was collected from individuals with Parkinson's disease using a telemonitoring system [22]. The dataset was created to support research in the area of remote monitoring of Parkinson's disease symptoms. The dataset contains data from 42 individuals with Parkinson's disease who were monitored remotely for up to 6 months. The data include various measures of motor symptoms, such as tremors, bradykinesia, and dyskinesia, as well as medication usage and side effects. The telemonitoring system used to collect the data included a smartphone application and a wearable device that recorded accelerometer and gyroscope data. The data were collected in real time and transmitted to a secure server for analysis.

The Parkinson's telemonitoring dataset is a valuable resource for researchers and clinicians working in the area of remote monitoring of Parkinson's disease symptoms. It is publicly available for research purposes and can be downloaded from the Parkinson's Disease Digital Biomarker DREAM Challenge website.

3.4 Algorithms

Good volume of relevant work had been done in relation to Parkinson Disease detection and diagnosis. The field is increasingly adopting Machine Learning due to its ability to recognize patterns.

Author—Anurag Jain, Rohit Lamba, Tarun Gulati, and Pooja Rani
Paper—"A Speech-Based Hybrid Decision Support System for Early Detection of Parkinson's Disease" [74]
In this study, two different speech datasets were utilized—the IPVS dataset consisting of 28 individuals with PD and 20 healthy peoples (HC), and the MDVR-KCL dataset comprising of 16 PD and 21 healthy individuals HC. Both datasets contain voice recordings in ".wav" file format. Feature extraction was performed using the Parselmouth Python library, resulting in the extraction of 17 acoustic features. The resultant table matrix comprises of 19 columns, including a voice ID column, 17 feature columns, and a status column. To identify the most distinguishing features, two different techniques genetic algorithm and extra tree were utilized. The extra tree technique identified 10 features from the 17 available, while the genetic algorithm method identified 8 features. The extra tree method utilized 10 estimators, while the genetic algorithm method utilized 18 generations

with a population size of 100 in each individual generation. The next generation was created by combining 20 randomly selected chromosomes and 20 best chromosomes, with 0.5 as crossover rate. A mutation rate of 0.05 was used to bring diversity in the population. To detect PD, four different classifiers were used: (i) K-NN, (ii) XGBoost, (iii) RF, and (iv) LR.

Author—Chethan C R, Divitha D, Abhishek M S, Aditya C R, Nagaraju T R, Paper—"Diagnosis of Parkinson Disorder through Speech Data" [75]

In this study 13 different acoustic features were obtained from each captured voice signal. In this study, a function was developed that takes multiple intricate measurements on an input audio file. These measurements were then transferred to the Parselmouth library, which implements Praat within the Python code. They have used MDVR-KCL dataset. They have used K Nearest Neighbour classifier to classify PD from healthy individuals and has reached the accuracy of 85% considering all features and in case only optimized features were used the accuracy were 98%, 94%, and 93%.

Author—Mehmet Bilal Er , Ibrahim Isik, Esme Isik
Paper—"Parkinson's detection based on combined CNN and LSTM using enhanced speech signals with Variational mode decomposition" [79]

This study has proposed a speech signals based model, which was based on deep learning to identify PD. They have used PC-GITA dataset. They have applied noise reduction using the variational mode decomposition method to produce images from voice samples. Three networks, ResNet-18, 50, and 101, were put to use to extract different features, and to classify these features LSTM model is used. The parameters used to measure performance were precision, accuracy and sensitivity, and 98.61% accuracy was obtained.

Author—Sruthi Kurada, Abhinav Kurada
Paper—"VGGish Embeddings Based Audio Classifiers to Improve Parkinson's Disease Diagnosis" [65]

The outcomes of five distinct feature extraction techniques are compared in this study. King's College London's Mobile Device Voice Recordings dataset provided the audio data for this study (MDVR-KCL). The five feature extraction techniques used in our study are: VG—Gish embeddings, ResNet50-based extraction, mel-frequency cepstral coefficient (MFCC)-based filter banks, a dysphonia-specific handpicked feature set extracted through PRAAT, and a larger handpicked set extracted through the DisVoice framework. The YouTube 8M dataset's substantial number of audio samples served as the pre-training data for the 11-layer CNN VGGish model. This model is modified from the VGG16 architecture to accommodate log mel spectrogram-based inputs for feature extraction. An evenly dispersed training set that contained 80% of the voice clips was used to train each model. The hyperparameters were adjusted using fivefold cross-validation process on the training set. The clips in the training set for each patient belonged to only one fold in order to prevent the revealing of patient-specific information. A held-out set comprising 20% of the data was used to evaluate performance.

Author—Hakan Gunduz
Paper—"Deep Learning-Based Parkinson's Disease Classification Using Vocal Feature Sets" [66]
By applying filters of various sizes to layer-wise inputs of CNN, the Convolution is performed. The activation function is applied to the results of the convolution layers. The quantity of connections between the successive layers is the primary distinction between ANN and CNN. Additionally, CNN filters transform the receptive field data to a high-level feature representation on deeper layers.

Here authors have created multiple categorization frameworks with various input layers in accordance with feature combination strategies. One input layer, six convolution layers, one fully linked (dense) layer, and one output layer make up our first framework, a nine-layered CNN. In this framework, before sending various feature sets to input layer of network they are combined. Parallel layers are used in the second framework. Two convolutional layers make up each branch of the parallel layer, which is utilized to sort out the deep features from each feature set independently. Using the KERAS software and predefined hyperparameters, they have train their CNN classifiers. The first method to stop overfitting in training is the L2 regularizer. Another method for addressing the issue of overfitting is dropout. Given that CNN takes into account the spatial link between nearby features, we must rearrange the features in the input data for a better prediction of relationships between the features.

SVM Support Vector Machines is a ML model that comes under the category of supervised learning and is used for classification and regression problems. When dealing with dichotomous classification tasks, if the data exhibit linearity, discrimination can be achieved using numerous hyperplanes. SVM, through kernel techniques, can effectively perform nonlinear categorization. For example, the fitted model complexity can be defined by taking C as the regularization parameter.

Author—Arif Gulten, Akin Ozcift
Paper—"Classifier ensemble construction with rotation forest to improve medical diagnosis performance of machine learning algorithms" [34]
In this particular study, an evaluation is provided that can aid in the CFS algorithm's ability to minimize the feature dimensions of three datasets used for benchmarking purposes. To measure the accuracy of algorithms employed in the diagnosis of Parkinson's, diabetes, and heart disorders, 30 base and ensembles of RF classifiers are used. Leave-one-out is used to validate every experiment (10-fold cross validation). with enhanced precision. The goodness of features in a classification issue can be described as follows from the perspective of correlation: A feature is typically considered to be good if it associates strongly to the class but not correlated with any other features. In order to lower the risk of Parkinson's, heart, and diabetes datasets, they have employed the best-first search strategy in the WEKA machine learning tool to implement the CFS algorithm.

Single base classifier is less accurate than Classifier ensembles. Like Random Forest, RF consists of independent decision trees. When building an algorithm, classifiers employ hyperplanes that are parallel to the axis of features, and slight rotations of these axis leads to different trees. Finding the principle components of each K-subset using principal component analysis (PCA) is supposed to prevent the variability of information in the data. For the base classifier, new features are produced using K axis rotations. This method's rotation strategy provides the ensemble with precision and variety. Decision trees are used for the rotation job in the classic Rotation Forest algorithm because of their sensitivity to feature axes rotation.

3.5 Features

This section briefly describes several features that are employed for voice-based Parkinson's diagnosis.

3.5.1 Acoustic Features

3.5.1.1 Jitter (Local, Absolute)

This feature also goes by the name of jitta, the value is determined by computing the mean of the absolute (i.e, nonrelative) difference between consecutive intervals. The benchmark value of jitta in detection of pathologies in adults is evaluated as 83.2 μs.

$$jitta = \frac{1}{N-1}\sum_{i=1}^{N-1} |T_i - T_{i-1}| \tag{3.1}$$

3.5.1.2 *Jitter (Local)*

Also known as jitt, it is the average of the absolute (i.e., nonrelative) difference between consecutive intervals which is then divided according to the average interval. In order to identify pathologies, a threshold value of 1.04% is used for jitt.

$$jitt = \frac{jitta}{\frac{1}{N}\sum_{i=1}^{N} T_i} \times 100 \tag{3.2}$$

3.5.1.3 *Jitter (rap)*

It shows the mean disturbance, i.e., the mean absolute difference between one interval and the mean of the interval and its two neighbors, divided according to the average interval. In order to identify pathologies, a threshold value of 0.68% is used for jitter.

$$rap = \frac{\frac{1}{N-1}\sum_{i=1}^{N-1} \left| T_i - \frac{1}{3}\sum_{n=i-1}^{i+1} T_n \right|}{\frac{1}{N-1}\sum_{i=1}^{N} T_i} \times 100 \tag{3.3}$$

3.5.1.4 *Jitter (ppq5)*

The disturbance ratio is shown by this feature within 5 intervals, i.e, it is estimated by taking the mean (average) absolute difference between the chosen period and its 4 closest neighbors.

$$ppq5 = \frac{\frac{1}{N-1}\sum_{i=2}^{N-2} \left| T_i - \frac{1}{5}\sum_{n=i-2}^{i+2} T_n \right|}{\frac{1}{N}\sum_{i=1}^{N} T_i} \times 100 \tag{3.4}$$

3.5.1.5 *Shimmer (Local)*

The value obtained by dividing the mean amplitude difference between consecutive periods by mean amplitude is called Shim. In order to identify pathologies, a threshold value of 3.81% is used for Shim.

$$Shim = \frac{\frac{1}{N-1}\sum_{i=1}^{N-1} |A_i - A_{i+1}|}{\frac{1}{N}\sum_{i=1}^{N} A_i} \times 100 \tag{3.5}$$

3.5.1.6 *Shimmer (local, dB)*

ShdB is the mean of the absolute variation in the base 10 logarithm of the disparity between successive periods. To identify pathologies, ShdB has a threshold value of 0.350 dB.

$$ShdB = \frac{1}{N-1}\sum_{i=1}^{N-1} \left| 20 * \log \frac{A_{i+1}}{A_i} \right| \tag{3.6}$$

3.5.1.7 *Shimmer (apq3)*

A metric can be obtained by dividing the average variation in amplitude between a period and the mean amplitude of its adjacent periods by the mean amplitude. This metric represents the average of the absolute difference.

$$apq3 = \frac{\frac{1}{N-1}\sum_{i=1}^{N-1} \left| A_i - \frac{1}{3}\sum_{n=i-1}^{i+1} A_n \right|}{\frac{1}{N}\sum_{i=1}^{N} A_i} \times 100 \tag{3.7}$$

3.5.1.8 *Shimmer (apq5)*

The value is obtained by dividing the mean absolute deviation between the amplitude of a period and the average amplitude of its four closest neighbors by the mean amplitude.

$$apq5 = \frac{\frac{1}{N-1}\sum_{i=2}^{N-2}\left|A_i - \frac{1}{5}\sum_{n=i-2}^{i+2} A_n\right|}{\frac{1}{N}\sum_{i=1}^{N} A_i} \times 100 \tag{3.8}$$

3.5.2 Spectogram-Based Methods

3.5.2.1 MFCC

MFCC are cepstral coefficients derived on a the mel scale, which is a twisted frequency scale that focuses on human auditory perception. To calculate MFCC from audio the following steps are employeed:

- Perform a Fourier transform on a signal (a windowed segment of the signal may be used).
- Use triangular overlapping windows or cosine overlapping windows to map the spectrum powers onto the mel scale.
- Logarithmically transform the powers at each mel frequency.
- Treat the mel log power list as a signal and apply a discrete cosine transform.
- The amplitudes of the resulting spectrum are referred to as MFCCs.

The procedure for calculating MFCCs from a continuous speech signal is illustrated in Figure 3.2.

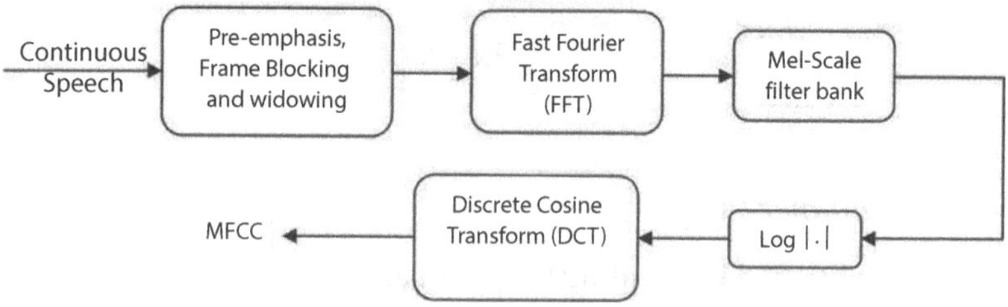

Figure 3.2 Block diagram of the MFCC computation process.

3.6 Conclusion

There is still much work to be done in order to detect Parkinson's disease early and accurately. Different methods of evaluation are being used in order to try to perfect the system. These methods include coherence, relevance, feedback, and knowledge-based. Our SLR is based on the idea that a systematic review of previous work in this domain is necessary. Several different PD detection techniques have been analyzed, and Machine Learning techniques including Logistic Regression (LR), KNN algorithm, SVM, Random Forest, and Gradient Boost are found to be the most implemented detection technique.

We have come to the following conclusions based on our systematic literature review:

- As many machine learning techniques are used in different research, we will be focusing on Neural Network for PD detection as it is observed that neural networks are more effective than generic machine learning techniques.
- One issue is that there are very few research which focused on early-stage PD detection, so we are focusing for early-stage PD detection.
- We will be using MDVR-KCL dataset, which is a voice recording dataset. This data set is recorded using mobile phone in normal room conditions; hence, we can use it for different real application, and it is also cost effective than other dataset as it does not require any special devices for recording,
- Most of the research have used common features, such as acoustic features, MFCC, AWT, etc. We will be using BARC Wavelet Feature, which is a wavelet-based feature.

References

1. Brakedal, B., Toker, L., Haugarvoll, K., Tzoulis, C., A nationwide study of the incidence, prevalence and mortality of Parkinson's disease in the Norwegian population. *NPJ Parkinsons Dis.*, 8, 1, 19, 2022.
2. Fabbri, M., Guimarães, I., Cardoso, R., Coelho, M., Guedes, L.C., Rosa, M.M., Godinho, C., Abreu, D., Gon¸calves, N., Antonini, A., Ferreira, J.J., Speech and voice response to a levodopa challenge in late-stage Parkinson's disease. *Front. Neurol.*, 8, 432, 2017.

3. Rusz, J., Tykalová, T., Novotný, M., Ružicka, E., Dušek, P., Distinct patterns of speech disorder in early-onset and late-onset de-novo Parkinson's disease. *NPJ Parkinsons Dis.*, 7, 1, 98, 2021.
4. Rusz, J., Cmejla, R., Ruzickova, H., Ruzicka, E., Quantitative acoustic measurements for characterization of speech and voice disorders in early untreated Parkinson's disease. *J. Acoust. Soc. Am.*, 129, 1, 350–367, 2011.
5. Sapir, S., Ramig, L., Fox, C., Speech and swallowing disorders in Parkinson disease. *Curr. Opin. Otolaryngol. Head Neck Surg.*, 16, 3, 205–210, 2008.
6. Ramig, L.O., Fox, C., Sapir, S., Speech treatment for Parkinson's disease. *Expert Rev. Neurother.*, 8, 2, 297–309, 2008.
7. Hammer, M.J. and Barlow, S.M., Laryngeal somatosensory deficits in Parkinson's disease: implications for speech respiratory and phonatory control. *Exp. Brain Res.*, 201, 3, 401–409, 2010.
8. Ho, A.K., Bradshaw, J.L., Iansek, T., Volume perception in parkinsonian speech. *Mov. Disord.*, 15, 6, 1125–1131, 2000.
9. Sadagopan, N. and Huber, J.E., Effects of loudness cues on respiration in individuals with Parkinson's disease. *Mov. Disord.*, 22, 5, 651–659, 2007.
10. Levanon, Y. and Lossos-Shifrin, L., Method and system for diagnosing pathological phenomenon using a voice signal. *Acoust. Soc. Am. J.*, 128, 2, 963, 2010.
11. Bonneh, Y.S., Levanon, Y., Dean-Pardo, O., Lossos, L., Adini, Y., Abnormal speech spectrum and increased pitch variability in young autistic children. *Front. Hum. Neurosci.*, 4, 237, 2011.
12. López-de-Ipinã, K., Alonso, J.-B., Travieso, C.M., Solé-Casals, J., Egiraun, H., Faundez-Zanuy, M., Ezeiza, A., Barroso, N., Ecay-Torres, M., Martinez-Lage, P., Lizardui, U.M., On the selection of non-invasive methods based on speech analysis oriented to automatic Alzheimer disease diagnosis. *Sensors*, 13, 5, 6730–6745, 2013.
13. Braak, H., Bohl, J.R., Müller, C.M., Rüb, U., de Vos, R.A., Del Tredici, K., Stanley Fahn lecture 2005: The staging procedure for the inclusion body pathology associated with sporadic Parkinson's disease reconsidered. *Mov. Disord.*, 21, 12, 2042–2051, 2006.
14. Harel, B.T., Cannizzaro, M.S., Cohen, H., Reilly, N., Snyder, P.J., Acoustic characteristics of Parkinsonian speech: A potential biomarker of early disease progression and treatment. *J. Neurolinguistics*, 17, 6, 439–453, 2004.
15. Ma, A., Lau, K.K., Thyagarajan, D., Voice changes in Parkinson's disease: what are they telling us? *J. Clin. Neurosci.*, 72, 1–7, 2020.
16. Rusz, J., Janzen, A., Tykalová, T., Novotný, M., Zogala, D., Timmermann, L., Růžička, E., Sônka, K., Dušek, P., Oertel, W., Dysprosody in isolated REM sleep behavior disorder with impaired olfaction but intact nigrostriatal pathway. *Mov. Disord.*, 37, 3, 619–623, 2022.
17. Moro-Velazquez, L., Gomez-Garcia, J.A., Arias-Londonõ, J.D., Dehak, N., Godino Llorente, J.I., Advances in Parkinson's disease detection and

assessment using voice and speech: a review of the articulatory and phonatory aspects. *Biomed. Signal Process. Control*, 66, 102418, 2021.
18. Mei, J., Desrosiers, C., Frasnelli, J., Machine learning for the diagnosis of Parkinson's disease: A systematic review. arXiv preprint arXiv:2010.06101, 10, 2020.
19. Jaeger, H., Trivedi, D., Stadtschnitzer, M., Mobile device voice recordings at King's College London (MDVR-KCL) from both early and advanced Parkinson's disease patients and healthy controls. Zenodo, 2019.
20. Dimauro, G. and Girardi, F., Italian parkinson's voice and speech, 2019.
21. Bot, B., Suver, C., Chaibub Neto, E., Kellen, M., Klein, A., Bare, J.C., Doerr, M., Pratap, A., Wilbanks, J., Dorsey, E., Friend, S., A., The mpower study, parkinson disease mobile data collected using researchkit. *Sci. Data*, 3, 03, 160011, 2016.
22. Little, M.A., McSharry, P.E., Roberts, S.J., Costello, D.A., Moroz, I.M., Exploiting nonlinear recurrence and fractal scaling properties for voice disorder detection. *Biomed. Eng. Online*, 6, 1, 23, Jun 2007.
23. Orozco-Arroyave, J.R., Arias-Londo no, J.D., Vargas-Bonilla, J.F., Gonz alez-R ativa, M.C., N oth, E., New Spanish speech corpus database for the analysis of people suffering from Parkinson's disease, in: *Proceedings of the Ninth International Conference on Language Resources and Evaluation (LREC'14)*, Reykjavik, Iceland, May 2014, European Language Resources Association (ELRA), pp. 342–347.
24. Tsanas, A., Little, M., Mcsharry, P., Ramig, L., Accurate telemonitoring of parkinson's disease progression by noninvasive speech tests. *IEEE Trans. Biomed. Eng.*, 57, 11, 884–93, 2009.
25. Li, Q., Chen, H., Huang, H., Zhao, X., Cai, Z.N., Tong, C., ... Tian, X., An enhanced grey wolf optimization based feature selection wrapped kernel extreme learning machine for medical diagnosis. *Comput. Math. Methods Med.*, 2017, 9512741-1, 2017.
26. Khan, M.M., Mendes, A., Chalup, S.K., Evolutionary Wavelet Neural Network ensembles for breast cancer and Parkinson's disease prediction. *PloS One*, 13, e0192192, 2018, doi: 10.1371/journal.pone.0192192.
27. Ma, C., Ouyang, J., Chen, H.-L., Zhao, X.-H., An efficient diagnosis system for Parkinson's disease using kernel-based extreme learning machine with subtractive clustering features weighting approach. *Computat. Math. Methods Med.*, 2014, 985789, 2014, doi: 10.1155/2014/985789.
28. Ma, H., Tan, T., Zhou, H., Gao, T., Support Vector Machinerecursive feature elimination for the diagnosis of Parkinson disease based on speech analysis, in: *2016 Seventh International Conference on Intelligent Control and Information Processing (ICICIP) (Siem Reap)*, pp. 34–40, 2016.
29. Mandal, I. and Sairam, N., Accurate telemonitoring of Parkinson's disease diagnosis using robust inference system. *Int. J. Med. Inf.*, 82, 359–377, 2013, doi: 10.1016/j.ijmedinf.2012.10.006.

30. Kraipeerapun, P. and Amornsamankul, S., Using stacked generalization and complementary neural networks to predict Parkinson's disease, in: *2015 11th International Conference on Natural Computation (ICNC)*, Zhangjiajie, pp. 1290–1294, 2015, doi: 10.1109/ICNC.2015.7378178.
31. Kuresan, H., Samiappan, D., Masunda, S., Fusion of WPT and MFCC feature extraction in Parkinson's disease diagnosis. *Technol. Health Care*, 27, 363–372, 2019, doi: 10.3233/THC-181306.
32. Marar, S., Swain, D., Hiwarkar, V., Motwani, N., Awari, A., Predicting the occurrence of Parkinson's disease using various classification models). *2018 International Conference on Advanced Computation and Telecommunication (ICACAT)*, Bhopal, pp. 1–5, 2018, doi: 10.1109/ICACAT.2018.8933579.
33. Moharkan, Z.A., Garg, H., Chodhury, T., Kumar, P., A classification based Parkinson detection system, in: *2017 International Conference On Smart Technologies For Smart Nation (SmartTechCon)*, Bengaluru, pp. 1509–1513, 2017, doi: 10.1109/SmartTech- Con.2017.8358616.
34. Ozcift, A. and Gulten, A., Classifier ensemble construction with rotation forest to improve medical diagnosis performance of machine learning algorithms. *Comp. Methods Progr. Biomed.*, 104, 443–451, 2011, doi: 10.1016/j.cmpb.2011.03.018.
35. Ozcift, A., SVM feature selection based rotation forest ensemble classifiers to improve computer-aided diagnosis of Parkinson disease. *J. Med. Syst.*, 36, 2141–2147, 2012, doi: 10.1007/s10916-011-9678-1.
36. Peker, M., A decision support system to improve medical diagnosis using a combination of k-medoids clustering based attribute weighting and SVM. *J. Med. Syst.*, 40, 116, 2016, doi: 10.1007/s10916-016-0477-6.
37. Shahsavari, M.K., Rashidi, H., Bakhsh, H.R., Efficient classification of Parkinson's disease using extreme learning machine and hybrid particle swarm optimization, in: *2016 4th International Conference on Control, Instrumentation, and Automation (ICCIA)*, Qazvin, pp. 148–154, 2016, doi: 10.1109/ICCIAutom.2016.7483152.
38. Sheibani, R., Nikookar, E., Alavi, S.E., An ensemble method for diagnosis of Parkinson's disease based on voice measurements. *J. Med. Signals Sens.*, 9, 221–226, 2019.
39. Wu, Y., Chen, P., Yao, Y., Ye, X., Xiao, Y., Liao, L. *et al.*, Dysphonic voice pattern analysis of patients in Parkinson's disease using minimum interclass probability risk feature selection and bagging ensemble learning methods. *Comput. Math. Methods Med.*, 2017, 4201984, 2017, doi: 10.1155/2017/4201984.
40. Yadav, G., Kumar, Y., Sahoo, G., Predication of Parkinson's disease using data mining methods: a comparative analysis of tree, statistical, and support vector machine classifiers. *Ind. J. Med. Sci.*, 65, 231–242, 2011, doi: 10.4103/0019-5359.107023.
41. Yaman, O., Ertam, F., Tuncer, T., Automated Parkinson's disease recognition based on statistical pooling method using acoustic features. *Med. Hypoth.*, 135, 109483, 2020, doi: 10.1016/j.mehy.2019.109483.

42. Yang, S., Zheng, F., Luo, X., Cai, S., Wu, Y., Liu, K. *et al.*, Effective dysphonia detection using feature dimension reduction and kernel density estimation for patients with Parkinson's disease. *PloS One*, 9, e88825, 2014, doi: 10.1371/journal.pone.0088825.
43. Frid, A., Safra, E.J., Hazan, H., Lokey, L.L., Hilu, D., Manevitz, L. *et al.*, Computational diagnosis of Parkinson's disease directly from natural speech using machine learning techniques, in: *2014 IEEE International Conference on Software Science, Technology and Engineering*, Ramat Gan, pp. 50–53, 2014, doi: 10.1109/SWSTE.2014.17.
44. Montanã, D., Campos-Roca, Y., Pérez, C.J., A Diadochokinesis-based expert system considering articulatory features of plosive consonants for early detection of Parkinson's disease. *Comp. Methods Programs Biomed.*, 154, 89–97, 2018, doi: 10.1016/j.cmpb.2017.11.010.
45. Sakar, B.E., Isenkul, M.E., Sakar, C.O., Sertbas, A., Gurgen, F., Delil, S. *et al.*, Collection and analysis of a Parkinson speech dataset with multiple types of sound recordings. *IEEE J. Biomed. Health Inform.*, 17, 828–834, 2013, doi: 10.1109/JBHI.2013.2245674.
46. Sztahó, D., Tulics, M.G., Vicsi, K., Valálik, I., Automatic estimation of severity of Parkinson's disease based on speech rhythm related features, in: *2017 8th IEEE International Conference on Cognitive Infocommunications (CogInfoCom)*, Debrecen, pp. 000011–000016, 2017, doi: 10.1109/CogInfoCom.2017.8268208.
47. Bhati, S., Velazquez, L.M., Villalba, J., Dehak, N., LSTM siamese network for Parkinson's disease detection from speech, in: *2019 IEEE Global Conference on Signal and Information Processing (GlobalSIP)*, Ottawa, ON, pp. 1–5, 2019, doi: 10.1109/GlobalSIP45357.2019.8969430.
48. Tracy, J.M., Özkanca, Y., Atkins, D.C., Hosseini Ghomi, R., Investigating voice as a biomarker: deep phenotyping methods for early detection of Parkinson's disease. *J. Biomed. Inform.*, 104, 103362, 2019, doi: 10.1016/j.jbi.2019.103362.
49. Wodzinski, M., Skalski, A., Hemmerling, D., Orozco-Arroyave, J.R., N¨oth, E., Deep learning approach to Parkinson's disease detection using voice recordings and convolutional neural network dedicated to image classification, in: *2019 41st Annual International Conference of the IEEE Engineering in Medicine and Biology Society (EMBC)*, Berlin, pp. 717–720, 2019, doi: 10.1109/EMBC.2019.8856972.
50. Abiyev, R.H. and Abizade, S., Diagnosing Parkinson's diseases using fuzzy neural system. *Comput. Mathe. Methods Med.*, 2016, 1267919, 2016, doi: 10.1155/2016/1267919.
51. Aich, S., Kim, H., Younga, K., Hui, K.L., Al-Absi, A.A., Sain, M., A supervised machine learning approach using different feature selection techniques on voice datasets for prediction of Parkinson's disease, in: *2019 21st*

International Conference on Advanced Communication Technology (ICACT), PyeongChang, pp. 1116–1121, 2019, doi: 10.23919/ICACT.2019.8701961.

52. Al-Fatlawi, A.H., Jabardi, M.H., Ling, S.H., Efficient diagnosis system for Parkinson's disease using deep belief network, in: *2016 IEEE Congress on Evolutionary Computation (CEC)*, Vancouver, BC, pp. 1324–1330, 2016, doi: 10.1109/CEC.2016.7743941.
53. Sayaydeha, O.N.A. and Mohammad, M.F., Diagnosis of the Parkinson disease using enhanced fuzzy min-max neural network and OneR attribute evaluation method, in: *2019 International Conference on Advanced Science and Engineering (ICOASE)*, Zakho-Duhok, pp. 64–69, 2019, doi: 10.1109/ICOASE.2019.8723870.
54. Ali, L., Zhu, C., Zhang, Z., Liu, Y., Automated detection of Parkinson's disease based on multiple types of sustained phonations using linear discriminant analysis and genetically optimized neural network. *IEEE J. Transl. Eng. Health Med.*, 7, 1–10, 2019c, doi: 10.1109/JTEHM.2019.2940900.
55. Alqahtani, E.J., Alshamrani, F.H., Syed, H.F., Olatunji, S.O., Classification of Parkinson's disease using NNge classification algorithm, in: *2018 21st Saudi Computer Society National Computer Conference (NCC)*, Riyadh, pp. 1–7, 2018, doi: 10.1109/NCG.2018.8592989.
56. Anand, A., Haque, M.A., Alex, J.S.R., Venkatesan, N., Evaluation of machine learning and deep learning algorithms combined with dimentionality reduction techniques for classification of Parkinson's disease, in: *2018 IEEE International Symposium on Signal Processing and Information Technology (ISSPIT)*, Louisville, KY, pp. 342–347, 2018, doi: 10.1109/ISSPIT.2018.8642776.
57. Bakar, Z.A., Ispawi, D., II, Ibrahim, N.F., Tahir, N.M., Classification of Parkinson's disease based on Multilayer Perceptrons (MLPs) neural network and ANOVA as a feature extraction, in: *2012 IEEE 8th International Colloquium on Signal Processing and its Applications*, Malacca, pp. 63–67, 2012, doi: 10.1109/CSPA.2012.6194692.
58. Cai, Z., Gu, J., Wen, C., Zhao, D., Huang, C., Huang, H., ... Chen, H., An intelligent Parkinson's disease diagnostic system based on a chaotic bacterial foraging optimization enhanced fuzzy KNN approach. *Comp. Math. Methods Med.*, 2018, 2396952, 2018, doi: 10.1155/2018/2396952.
59. Celik, E. and Omurca, S., II, Improving Parkinson's disease diagnosis with machine learning methods, in: *2019 Scientific Meeting on Electrical Electronics Biomedical Engineering and Computer Science (EBBT)*, Istanbul, pp. 1–4, 2019, doi: 10.1109/EBBT.2019.8742057.
60. Çimen, S. and Bolat, B., Diagnosis of Parkinson's disease by using ANN, in: *2016 International Conference on Global Trends in Signal Processing, Information Computing and Communication (ICGTSPICC)*, Jalgaon, pp. 119–121, 2016, doi: 10.1109/ICGT-SPICC.2016.7955281.
61. Dash, S., Thulasiram, R., Thulasiraman, P., An enhanced chaosbased firefly model for Parkinson's disease diagnosis and classification, in: *2017*

International Conference on Information Technology (ICIT), Bhubaneswar, pp. 159–164, 2017, doi: 10.1109/ICIT.2017.43.
62. Dastjerd, N.K., Sert, O.C., Ozyer, T., Alhajj, R., Fuzzy classification methods based diagnosis of Parkinson's disease from speech test cases. *Curr. Aging Sci.*, 12, 100–120, 2019, doi: 10.2174/1874609812666190625140311.
63. Dinesh, A. and He, J., Using machine learning to diagnose Parkinson's disease from voice recordings, in: *2017 IEEE MIT Undergraduate Research Technology Conference (URTC)*, Cambridge, MA, pp. 1–4, 2017, doi: 10.1109/URTC.2017.8284216.
64. Erdogdu Sakar, B., Serbes, G., Sakar, C.O., Analyzing the effectiveness of vocal features in early telediagnosis of Parkinson's disease. *PloS One*, 12, e0182428, 2017, doi: 10.1371/journal.pone.0182428.
65. Kurada, S. and Kurada, A., Poster: VGGish Embeddings Based Audio Classifiers to Improve Parkinson's Disease Diagnosis, in: *2020 IEEE/ACM International Conference on Connected Health: Applications, Systems and Engineering Technologies (CHASE)*, Crystal City, VA, USA, pp. 9–11, 2020, doi: 10.1145/3384420.3431775.
66. Gunduz, H., Deep learning-based Parkinson's disease classification using vocal feature sets. *IEEE Access*, 7, 115540–115551, 2019, doi: 10.1109/ACCESS.2019.2936564.
67. Haq, A.U., Li, J., Memon, M.H., Khan, J., Din, S.U., Ahad, I. *et al.*, Comparative analysis of the classification performance of machine learning classifiers and deep neural network classifier for prediction of Parkinson disease, in: *2018 15th International Computer Conference on Wavelet Active Media Technology and Information Processing (ICCWAMTIP)*, Chengdu, pp. 101–106, 2018.
68. Haq, A.U., Li, J.P., Memon, M.H., Khan, J., Malik, A., Ahmad, T. *et al.*, Feature selection based on L1-Norm support vector machine and effective recognition system for Parkinson's disease using voice recordings. *IEEE Access*, 7, 37718–37734, 2019, doi: 10.1109/ACCESS.2019.2906350.
69. Hariharan, M., Polat, K., Sindhu, R., A new hybrid intelligent system for accurate detection of Parkinson's disease. *Comput. Methods Programs Biomed.*, 113, 904–913, 2014, doi: 10.1016/j.cmpb.2014.01.004.
70. Islam, M.S., Parvez, I., Hai, D., Goswami, P., Performance comparison of heterogeneous classifiers for detection of Parkinson's disease using voice disorder (dysphonia), in: *2014 International Conference on Informatics, Electronics Vision (ICIEV)*, Dhaka, pp. 1–7, 2014, doi: 10.1109/ICIEV.2014.6850849.
71. Ji, W. and Li, Y., Energy-based feature ranking for assessing the dysphonia measurements in Parkinson detection. *IET Signal Proc.*, 6, 300–305, 2012, doi: 10.1049/iet-spr.2011.0186.
72. Junior, S.B., Costa, V.G.T., Chen, S., Guido, R.C., U-healthcare system for pre-diagnosis of Parkinson's disease from voice signal, in: *2018 IEEE International Symposium on Multimedia (ISM)*, Taichung, pp. 271–274, 2018.

73. Karapinar Senturk, Z., Early diagnosis of Parkinson's disease using machine learning algorithms. *Med. Hypoth.*, 138, 109603, 2020, doi: 10.1016/j.mehy.2020.109603.
74. Lamba, R., Gulati, T., Jain, A., Rani, P., A speech-based hybrid decision support system for early detection of Parkinson's disease. *Arab. J. Sci. Eng.*, 48, 2, 2247–2260, 2023.
75. Diagnosis of Parkinson's Disorder through Speech Data using Machine Learning Algorithms. *IJITEE*, 9, 69–72, 2020. 10.35940/ijitee.C8060.019320.
76. Toye, A.A. and Kompalli, S., Comparative study of speech analysis methods to predict parkinson's disease, arXiv preprint arXiv:2111.10207, 2021, November 15. arXiv.org. Retrieved December 10, 2022, from https://arxiv.org/abs/2111.10207.
77. Hires, M., Gazda, M., Drotár, P., Pah, N.D., Motin, M.A., Kumar, D.K., Convolutional neural network ensemble for Parkinson's disease detection from voice recordings. *Comput. Biol. Med.*, 141, 105021, 2022. ISSN 0010-4825, https://doi.org/10.1016/j.compbiomed.2021.105021.
78. Karan, B., Sahu, S.S., Orozco-Arroyave, J.R., Mahto, K., Non-negative matrix factorization-based time-frequency feature extraction of voice signal for Parkinson's disease prediction. *Comput. Speech. Lang.*, 69, 101216, 2021. ISSN 0885-2308, https://doi.org/10.1016/j.csl.2021.101216.
79. Er, M.B., Isik, E., Isik, I., Parkinson's detection based on combined CNN and LSTM using enhanced speech signals with Variational mode decomposition. *Biomed. Signal Process. Control*, 70, 103006, 2021. ISSN 1746-8094, https://doi.org/10.1016/j.bspc.2021.103006.
80. Amato, F., Borzí, L., Olmo, G., Orozco, J.R., An algorithm for Parkinson's disease speech classification based on isolated words analysis. *Health Inf. Sci. Syst.*, 9, 1–15, 2021.
81. Sechidis, K., Fusaroli, R., Orozco-Arroyave, J.R., Wolf, D., Zhang, Y.-P., A machine learning perspective on the emotional content of Parkinsonian speech. *Artif. Intell. Med.*, 115, 102061, 2021. ISSN 0933-3657, https://doi.org/10.1016/j.artmed.2021.102061.

4

Tumor Detection and Classification

Hermehar P.S. Bedi*, Sukhpreet Kaur and Saumya Rajvanshi

Department of Computer Science and Engineering, Chandigarh Engineering College - CGC, Mohali, Punjab, India

Abstract

Uncontrolled growth of abnormal tissues in the body is referred to as the tumor. Broadly, tumors can be classified into two types: benign and malignant. The World Health Organization (WHO) claims that in the year 2020, cancer alone contributed 10 million deaths, making it the leading death causing disease. National Cancer Registry Programme of Indian Council of Medical Research (ICMR), estimated cases of cancer in India have seen a rise from 1,392,179 in 2020 to 14,61,427 in 2022 and reported a mortality of 7,70,230 and 8,08,558 in 2020 and 2022, respectively, which is a significant increase. Till date, more than 120 types of brain tumors have been found, which have different shapes and sizes. Due to these factors, it is important to detect the tumors immediately. Various mechanical methods exist for the detection of tumors, such as magnetic resonance imaging (MRI), computed tomography (CT) scan, and positron emission tomography (PET) scan. All these scans send the waves into the patient's body to obtain the images of the organ or body part affected. Images obtained from these scans are of Digital Imaging and Communications in Medicine (DICOM) format. Different techniques available for classification of the tumor, such as aegmentation, feature extraction, machine learning techniques, and deep learning models, have been discussed and compared in this chapter, which can help researchers in finding the optimal solution for their research in the detection and classification of different tumors and other deadly diseases. Finally, this chapter comes up with all the relevant and important literature related with tumor detection and how it can be classified using the new age computer-based technology, such as deep learning and machine learning.

***Keywords*:** Tumors, machine learning models, deep learning models, segmentation, feature extraction, region of interest

**Corresponding author*: hermeharbedi@gmail.com

Sumit Srivastava, Abhineet Anand, Abhishek Kumar, Bhavna Saini and Pramod Singh Rathore (eds.) Bio-Inspired Optimization for Medical Data Mining, (75–102) © 2024 Scrivener Publishing LLC

4.1 Introduction

Cancer is the uncontrolled growth of cells, which spread over the other organs and parts of the body. Cancer can be caused almost everywhere in the body and till now there is no well-known cause of cancer. Cancers can generally be divided into two categories:

1) Hematologic: This is a type of cancer, which starts in the blood forming tissues such as bone marrow or in the cells of the immune systems. Examples of such cancers are leukemia, lymphoma, and multiple myeloma.
2) Solid tumors: This is a type of cancer of the body organs or tissues. These generally do not contain the cysts or liquid areas. Examples of such cancers are brain, breast, prostate, and lung.

According to the World Health Organization (WHO), in 2020, cancer contributed 10 million deaths, making it the leading death causing disease of 2020 [1]. National Cancer Registry Programme of Indian Council of Medical Research (ICMR), estimated cases of cancer in India have seen a rise from 1,392,179 in 2020 to 14,61,427 in 2022 and reported a mortality of 7,70,230 and 8,08,558 in 2020 and 2022, respectively, which is a significant increase [2].

Tumors are also like cancer, i.e., these are also the uncontrolled growth of abnormal tissues in the body. Tumors can be classified into two categories:

1) Benign: these are tumors, which are not cancerous in nature.
2) Malignant: these are tumors, which are cancerous in nature. So, malignant tumors fall under the solid tumors category of cancer. This is the most dangerous form of tumors. Malignant tumors alone contribute 14,000 deaths in a year.

Based on the severity level, tumors are classified into three different grades:

1) Grade 1: It is the least dangerous grade, where the tumor cells resemble the normal cells and these cells do not grow much rapidly.

2) Grade 2: It is the grade of tumors, where the tumor cells do not resemble the normal cells and the growing is also fast as compared to the normal cells.
3) Grade 3: It is the grade of tumors, where the tumor cells look abnormal and starts spreading or replicating at very fast pace.

According to a report "Cancer Statistics 2020," which is published by American Cancer Society, approximately 24,000 people would have been affected by only one kind of tumor, the brain tumor, and it will contribute 19,000 deaths in USA alone [3].

Till today, there are more or less 120 types of brain tumors found in different shapes and sizes, which, due to the complex structure of brain, is difficult to detect [4].

Imaging plays a very crucial role in the detection and treatment of brain tumors and the factor, which has emerged as an indicator in the planning of treatment and the outcome assessment is the size of the tumor [5].

4.2 Methods Used for Detection of Tumors

There are several radiological techniques available for detecting different tumors. Radiological techniques, such as magnetic resonance imaging (MRI), computed tomography (CT), positron emission tomography (PET) scans along with the combination of these techniques, such as PET-MRI and PET-CT scans, are also used to detect the tumors. The main principle behind these scans is sending different kinds of waves (depending on the type of scan) into the patient's body, gathering the images, and identifying the abnormalities in those images.

Most common scans used for the detection of tumors are discussed below:

1) MRI: The term MRI, which stands for magnetic resonance imaging, is an advanced image-based diagnosing technique used for the detection of different diseases in the body based on the frequency and intensity of the protons and their resonance. MRI works on the principal of nuclear magnetic resonance (NMR), which produces the high-quality images of the parts, instead of using uniform field, a varying magnetic field is applied across the body part. Protons of different regions come to the resonance at non-identical frequencies.

Intensity of signals is proportional to the number of protons at each magnetic field. Images and data obtained from this are then used by doctors to detect the tumors. For easy and detailed reading, these images are broken into slices or small segments by the process named segmentation, which is discussed later in this chapter [6].

2) CT: The term CT, which stands for computed tomography, is an image-based diagnosing technique used for the different diseases in the body using a beam of X-rays. In CT scan, a narrow beam of X-Rays is aimed at a patient and then it is revolved around the body of the patient, which produces the signals that are processed and the cross-sectional images known as slices are generated by the machine [7].
3) PET: The term PET, which stands for positron emission tomography, is a noninvasive functional imaging method, which works at the molecular level. It gives a detailed quantitative information about the disease and is many times used to find out the cancer, infection, and inflammation by perceiving the emitted photons from a radiotracer dye, which is localized to abnormal cells. In PET scan, the patient is injected with a radioactive dye, which is referred to as the tracer or radiotracer dye, which helps in identifying the disease by highlighting the part affected [6, 8].

Presently, the process of anomaly detection through the above stated imaging techniques is performed manually in most of the cases, and the doctors spend a lot of time detecting and segmenting it. The manual techniques are prone to human error, which can sometimes cost the life of patient. To overcome this problem and save the lives of patient, researchers have shifted their focus on various machine learning (ML)– and deep learning (DL)–based techniques for automatic detection and segmentation [4], which are further discussed as we delve deeper in this chapter. In order to reduce the errors, early detection of tumors and high accuracy of the ML and DL models to predict and detect the tumors, following points are made in context to the chapter: 1) Data capturing 2) Image Pre-processing 3) Segmentation 4) Feature Extraction 5) Training the ML or DL models using suitable classification algorithms [9].

1. Data Capturing: The first step to detect and classify the tumor is the collection of data, in this case, the images using

which the tumor could be found out. The dataset can contain different types of images, such as axial, sagittal, and coronal.

2. Image Pre-processing: This is the step, in which the unwanted data known as noise is removed from the image using different methods, such as mean filter, median filter, and hybrid filters. Filters are used to alter the size, shade, color and also to subdue the inflated frequencies of the image. Many times, during the pre-processing stage only the image reconstruction also takes place.
3. Segmentation: After the images have been processed and the noise has been removed, now the next step is to divide/slice/split the images into smaller parts. All the pixels are assigned a tag. This slicing of the image creates a number of sets of pixels within an image. Every set of the pixels contain pixels having same tag. Similar tags of pixels denote a distinct feature [6]. There are different segmentation techniques used for segmenting the images, which are further discussed in the chapter. Figure 4.1 shows the steps for classifying the tumors.

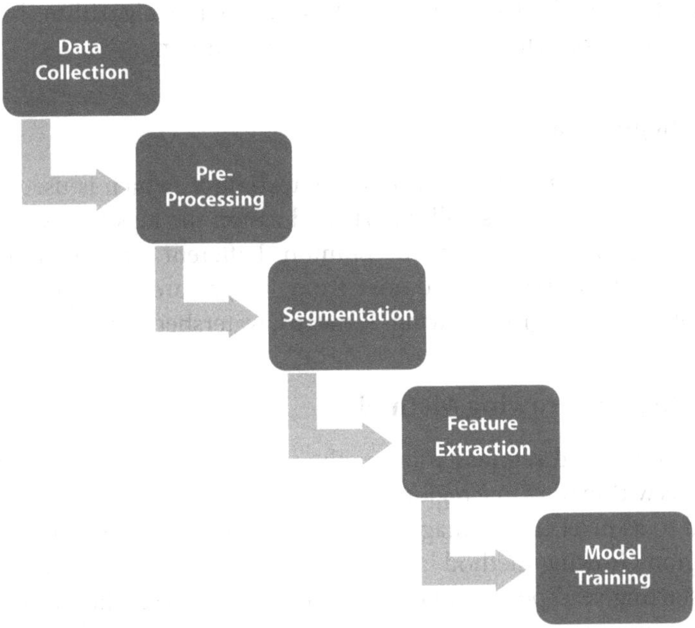

Figure 4.1 Steps for classifying the tumors.

4. Feature Extraction: Extracting the features from the images is a tedious, time consuming and one of the most important tasks. Features that have been used to probe the images help people differentiate between the tumors and other tissues. Different features, such as standard deviation, kutosis, variance, etc., are extracted during this stage [6, 9].
5. Training the model using suitable classification algorithms: This is the step, where the model is trained using the different classification algorithms. After model training, the trained model is validated or tested. Different ML and DL algorithms are used to train the model, which are discussed and compared further in the next topics as we delve deeper into the models.

4.3 Methods Used for Classification of Tumors

For classification of tumors, different classification techniques are used such as the Segmentation, Machine Learning and Deep Learning models. To classify the tumors, the models are trained using different classification algorithms such as KNN, SVM, DT, Random Forest, XGBoost Classifier, ResNet 18, DenseNet 169, DenseNet 201 etc. Different algorithms have different accuracy of detecting and classifying the tumors.

4.3.1 Segmentation

As discussed earlier, segmentation is the technique, which is used to split the image into different smaller parts and assign the tags to pixels. Pixels having same tag have feature in common. Different segmentation techniques used to classify the tumors from images are Histogram Based, Threshold based, Region growing, K means, watershed etc.

4.3.2 Region Growing Method

It is a region-based segmentation method, which rely on the assumption that pixels within the same region have same values. Region Growing is also referred to as pixel-based image segmentation technique shown in Figure 4.2. Region Growing method inspects the adjacent or the bordering pixels of the starting seed point and decides whether the pixel should be added to the region or not. Region Growing Method comprises of three different methods, which include Seeded Region Growing Method, Unseeded Region

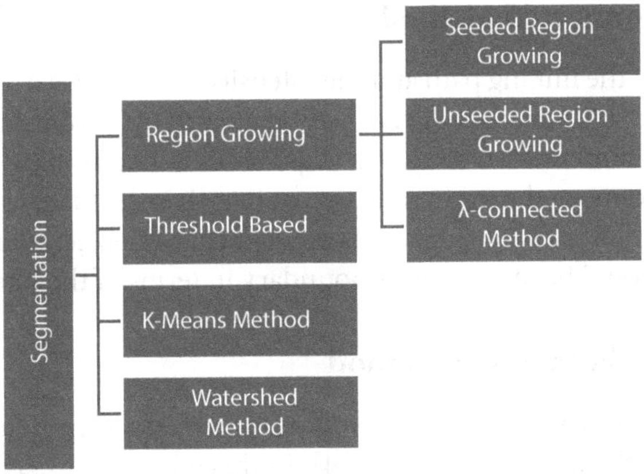

Figure 4.2 Different types of segmentation.

Growing Method and λ Region Growing Method. This method correctly separates the region based on the properties of similar pixels [10].

4.3.3 Seeded Region Growing Method

It is one of the simplest and very alluring for semantic image segmentation. Since, it is fast and free from the tuning points, it is most frequently used or it is given the preference to be used [11]. To check whether a pixel belongs to the region or not, the difference between the intensity of the pixel and region mean is used [12]. This method performs the segmentation in the respect of a set of a point, which is known as seed. It is the choice of seeds which decides what is Region of Interest (ROI) and what is irrelevant. In this, the number of seeds are grouped into n sets let us assume them to be $A_1, A_2, A_3, \ldots, A_n$. Individual sets may consist of single point. From the seeds, the algorithm then finds the tessellation of the image into regions with the property all the components of the region meets with one of the A_i and based on this, the region is chosen to be homogenous. This process develops synthetically from the seeds. Each step of seeded region growing method includes the addition of one pixel to one of the above sets [13]. According to the study of Praveen Gamage, the seeded region growing method shows the highest accuracy of 92% [14].

4.3.4 Unseeded Region Growing Method

It is the upgraded variant of the Seeded Region Growing method, in which the explicit seeds are not required [6].

4.3.5 λ-Connected Method

It is drawn on the linking path and the intensity of the pixels of images under consideration. It is related to fuzzy method created by Rosenfeld who treated image as a 2 dimensional fuzzy set. A pixel set is said to be λ connected if there is a λ connected path for any two points (λ is the fuzzy value between 0 and 1). The main key on which it is based is that an object must be smooth inside and should have a gap at its boundary in terms of the intensity [15].

4.3.6 Threshold Based Method

It is one of the best and the simplest segmentation techniques available, which shows the accuracy of 91% [14]. In this type of segmentation, firstly the image is converted to binary form from the already existing greyscale image. In this, the intensity of pixels is compared to threshold intensity or the intensity, which has already been defined [6], threshold values are obtained from the histogram of the edges of the original images [16]. The value of histogram is calculated on the basis of the edge detection, which means that the value of threshold is precise only if the edge detection is errorless [17]. This technique takes as a hypothesis that all the pixels, which lies in the same range belongs to one class [18].

4.3.7 K-Means Method

This type of segmentation technique uses the raw image, that is the image, which has not been pre-processed as a point having a location in the k-space. It is an unsupervised technique, due to which it requires less human interaction. It is useful for the large images having bad or poor contrast. It is susceptible to sample selection and setting up the fuzzy sets might be difficult [19].

4.3.8 Watershed Method

This method has the ability to classify the intensities with very less differences, which is not possible by other methods such as snake and level set method [6]. This method only works on the pre- processed image. If the image is not already processed, then it will lead to over segmentation of the image. According to the study of [14], this method shows the accuracy of 85.5%, which is one of the least as compared to other segmentation techniques used by him. Table 4.1 shows the advantages and disadvantages of different segmentation techniques and Table 4.2 shows the different segmentation technique and the Table 4.3 shows the Comparison of region based and threshold based segmentation techniques.

4.3.9 Comparison of Different Segmentation Techniques Based on the Advantages and Disadvantages

Table 4.1 Advantages and disadvantages of different segmentation techniques [20, 21].

Technique	Advantages	Disadvantages
Thresholding Method	1. No pre-requisites are required. 2. It is the simplest method.	1. It is sensitive to noise. 2. It is largely dependent on peaks 3. Difficult to set the threshold value. 4. No spatial details are considered.
Region Growing Method	1. It is more immune to noise. 2. More useful if similarity criteria can be defined easily.	1. Takes more time and consumes more memory.
Watershed Method	1. This is a more stable method. 2. Boundaries detected are more continuous results are more stable, detected boundaries are continuous	1. Difficult to calculate the gradients.
Edge Based Method	1. It is easy and simple to implement. 2. Edges are recognized along with their edges.	1. Sensitive to noise. 2. Edge detection can be shaky at times. 3. It can be inconsistent at times.

4.3.10 Comparison of Different Segmentation Techniques Based on Accuracy

Table 4.2 Comparison of different segmentation techniques based on accuracy.

Reference	Author	Technique used	Accuracy
[14]	Praveen Gamage	Seeded Region Growing	92%
[22]	Astina Minz *et al.*	Threshold Based	89.90%
[14]	Praveen Gamage	Threshold Based	91%
[23]	Veenu Nookala *et al.*	K- Mean	87.5%

4.3.11 Comparison of Region Based and Threshold Based Segmentation Techniques Based on Different Parameters

Table 4.3 Comparison of region based and threshold based segmentation techniques [24].

Parameters	Region based	Threshold based
Speed	Slow	Fast
Accuracy	Exceptional	Moderate
Multiple Object Detection	Fair	Poor
Computational Complexity	Rapid	Less

4.4 Machine Learning

Machine learning (ML) is a process of feeding machine with sufficient data to train and predict the possible outcome using different techniques. Efficiency of the technique or algorithm depends upon the quality and usefulness of the data. There are different types of Machine learning available,

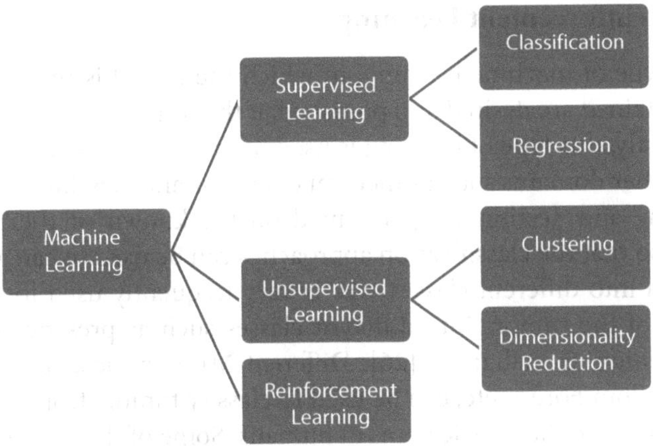

Figure 4.3 Types of machine learning techniques.

which are supervised learning, unsupervised learning and reinforcement learning shown in Figure 4.3.

4.4.1 Supervised Learning

Supervised machine learning is the type of machine learning, in which the machine is supervised for learning. The most common example of this supervised learning is the classification. For supervised learning, the data provided is the labelled. Supervised learning is further divided into two categories: Classification and Regression. In the supervised learning, generally, a set of n features X_1, X_2,...,X_n is provided, which is measured on n observations, and a response Y also measured on those same n observations. The goal is then to predict Y using X_1, X_2,...,X_n.

4.4.2 Unsupervised Learning

It is the type of machine learning, in which the data is neither labelled nor classified and algorithms are used to find the pattern in such datasets. The algorithms are hence required to classify and label the data in the dataset without having any external guidance or human interference to perform the task [25]. Unsupervised learning is further divided into two sub groups, which are: Clustering and Dimensionality Reduction.

4.4.3 Reinforcement Learning

It is the type of machine learning, in which the model is rewarded if the results obtained are desired and punished, if the results obtained are undesired. Mostly, this type of learning is used in the games and very less often used in other domains such as medical diagnosis and classification.

Training and Testing are performed on the known or the unknown datasets, so that the classification approaches can be used to categorize the input data into different classes. ML is very frequently used for the classification of the tumors into different classes such as presence of tumor or not, benign or malignant [26]. Different ML methods, such as KNN, SVM, Random Forest, etc, can be used to classify tumors from the images of different radio diagnostic scans of humans. Some of the ML techniques, which are actively been used to detect and classify the tumors into the one of the above stated types are discussed below.

4.4.4 K-Nearest Neighbour (KNN)

It is one of the easiest classification algorithms, which provide the results with high accuracy. Most of the times, KNN is used for the pattern recognition. In KNN, all the available cases are stockpiled and the new cases are classified based on the similarity measure. The instance is classified on the basis of the votes received for its nearest neighbour class shown in Figure 4.4. Generally, the Euclidean formula is used to find the distance between the instance and its nearest neighbour. Sometimes, Manhattan and Minkowski formulas are also used to calculate the same.

Euclidean Formula:

$$\sqrt{\sum_{i=1}^{k}(x_i - y_i)^2}$$

Manhattan Formula:

$$\sum_{i=1}^{k}|x_i - y_i|$$

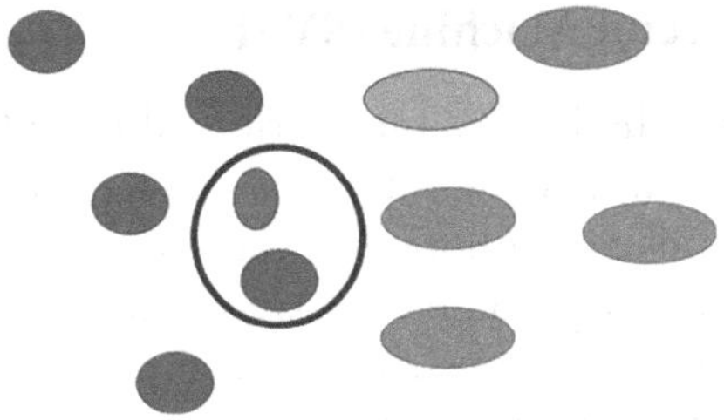

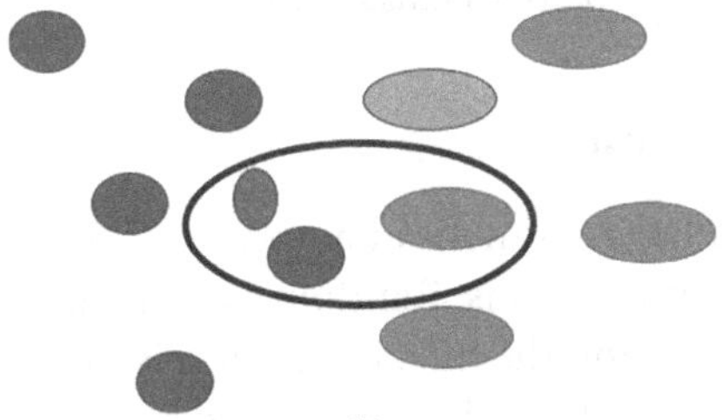

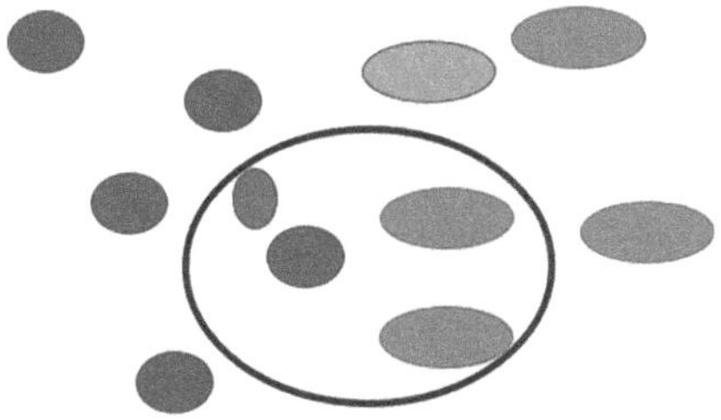

Figure 4.4 (a) 1 nearest neighbour. (b) 2 nearest neighbours. (c) 3 nearest neighbours.

Minkowski Formula:

$$\left(\sum_{i=1}^{k}\left(|x_i - y_i|\right)^q\right)^{1/q}$$

4.4.5 Support Vector Machine (SVM)

SVM is used to split the images into various different classes as is done by the KNN algorithm. It is also a type of classification algorithm, which classifies the given image into different classes. It uses a hyperplane that differentiates between the two given classes and then classifies the given the instance into the class. It constructs a hyperplane based out of a kernel function as shown in the graph 4.1 below, where feature vectors on the left side belong to the -1 (negative) class and the feature vectors on the right side belongs to the +1 (positive) class [27].

4.4.6 Random Forest

Random Forest is a bagging method algorithm, which uses the bootstrap average to make the predictions. Random Forest algorithm creates several different decision trees and the final prediction is made by taking into consideration the majority vote, which is finalized by analysing the predictions of all the decision trees [28].

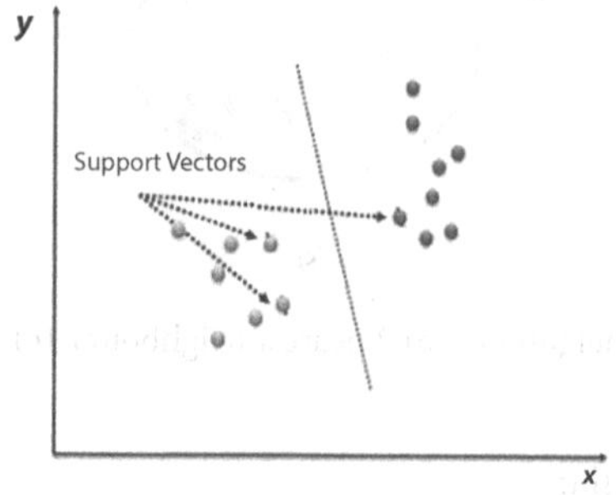

Graph 4.1 Classification using SVM [27].

4.5 Deep Learning (DL)

Deep Learning is a very active area of research in the Machine Leaning and Artificial Intelligence communities. The key basis or the foundation of Deep learning is the Neural Networks. Neural Networks caught more fame in the late 1980's and early 1990's. there are different types of neural networks such as Convolutional Neural Networks for image classification and Recurrent Neural Networks for time series and other sequences [29]. Different DL methodologies are used to cram the medical data. These methodologies include CNN, encoded CNN, 3D CNN, U-Net, LSTM, RNN, which are discussed further in the chapter [26].

4.5.1 Convolutional Neural Networks (CNN)

CNN is a multi-layered neural network, which focuses to process the grid structured data. CNN basically works by combining the two specialized layers, which are the Convolution layer and the Pooling layers.

4.5.1.1 Convolution Layer

This layer performs an operation, known as convolution, which is based on the linear algebra operation, which multiplies matrix of the filter in the image to be processed [30]. The main work of this layer is to find out whether a particular feature is present in an image or not. The convolution layer is made up of large number of filters, known as convolution filters. These filters work on a simple operation, which is already described as convolution, which works by recursively multiplying matrix elements followed by the addition of the results [29]. Working of convolution filter can be understood by taking an example of two matrices one of an image and the other of the filter. Consider the image matrix of 4x3 and the convolution filter matrix of 2×2.

$$\text{Image matrix} = \begin{bmatrix} a\,b\,c \\ d\,e\,f \\ g\,h\,i \\ j\,k\,l \end{bmatrix}$$

$$\text{Convolution filter matrix} = \begin{bmatrix} w\;x \\ y\;z \end{bmatrix}$$

Resultant matrix obtained will be the convolved image, which will be smaller than the original image because its dimension is given by the number of 2×2 submatrix in the original image. The convolved image can have same dimensions as that of the original image, if we use padding.

$$\text{Resultant matrix} = \begin{bmatrix} aw+bx+dy+ez & bw+cx+ey+fz \\ dw+ex+gy+hz & ew+fx+hy+iz \\ gw+hx+jy+kz & hw+ix+ky+lz \end{bmatrix}$$

The convolved image spotlights the region of an original image, that matches with the convolution filter.

4.5.1.2 *Pooling Layer*

It is the layer which takes the maximum or the average value of the pixel proportions of an image [30]. This layer provides a method to concise a larger image into smaller image. The max-pooling operation summarizes each non-duplicating 2x2 block of pixels in an image using the maximum value in the block. This reduces the size of an image and also, it provides the location invariance [29].

$$\textbf{max pooling} \quad \begin{bmatrix} 1234 \\ 1301 \\ 0521 \\ 1204 \end{bmatrix} \rightarrow \begin{bmatrix} 3\;4 \\ 5\;4 \end{bmatrix}$$

The max pooling matrix is obtained by collecting the maximum values of the 2x2 sub matrix.

4.5.1.3 *Architecture of CNN*

The convolution layer is surrounded by the kernel around the input sample to calculate different feature maps. Features identified from the input samples are represented by the small boxes on the feature map. These feature maps are then sent to the maximum collection layer. The maximum collection layer stores the relevant features and rejects the other. The features of the max-pooling layer are converted to a single dimensional (1D) vector of features in the fully connected layer, which is used to calculate the probability of the output. The architecture of the CNN is represented in Figure 4.5 [31].

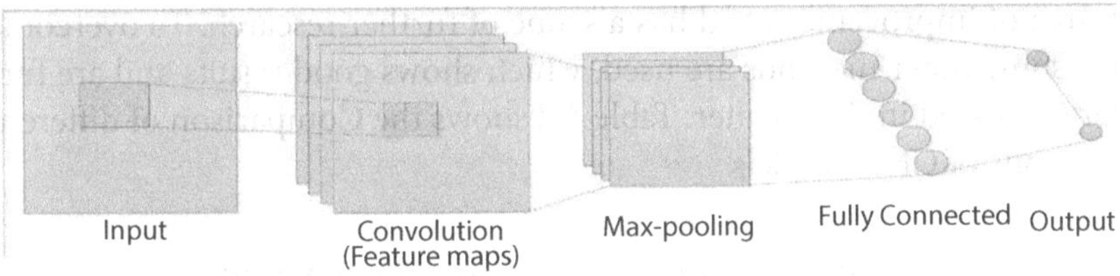

Figure 4.5 Architecture of CNN [31].

4.5.1.3.1 Convolution Layer

As discussed above, it is the layer, which focuses on extracting the features by recursively multiplying matrix elements followed by the addition of the results.

4.5.1.3.2 Subsampling Layer

The main work of this layer is to reduce the size of the image data and increase the invariance of feature positions. The max pooling as discussed above divides the image into different smaller grids and then take the value which is maximum from each grid to produce the smaller image matrix, which makes it easy for the next convolution layer to process.

4.5.1.3.3 Fully Connected Layer

This layer basically changes the dimensions of the image so that it can is easy to classify it linearly. In the convolution layer, each neuron shall be converted into 1D data before assigning it to another layer, which is connected as a whole [32].

The typical architecture of the CNN for the classification of an image is shown in Figure 4.6 [29].

The main drawback of CNN is that it is inefficient for the classification of 3D MRI images. It shows less accuracy, when it comes to the classification of tumors from the 3 dimensional images of the MRI, which is still

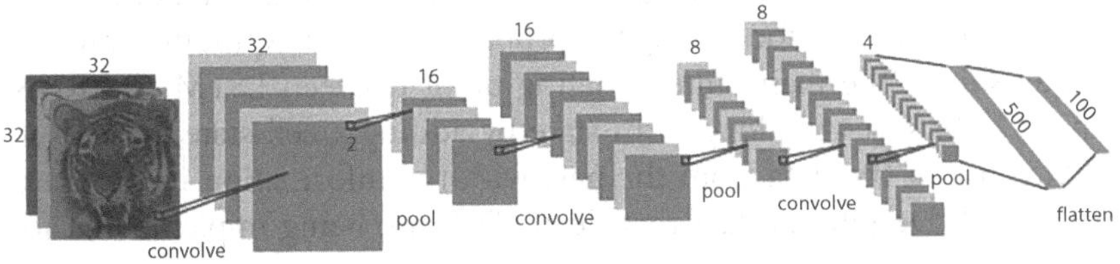

Figure 4.6 CNN architecture for the classification of an image showing convolution and pooling layers [29].

an area of improvement and has a scope of further research. To overcome this, some other methods are used, which shows good results and are further discussed in the chapter. Table 4.4 shows the Comparison of different variations of CNN models.

4.5.1.4 Comparison of Different Variations of CNN Techniques

Table 4.4 Comparison of different variations of CNN models [28].

Sr. no.	Author	Variation	Results
[33]	Pan Y. *et al.*	Traditional CNN	18% improvement as compared to the baseline neural networks.
[34]	Moeskops P. *et al.*	Transfer Learning	Mean classification accuracy of 98% achieved
[35]	Sajjad M. *et al.*	U-Net Architecture	Dice score – 0.89353 and sensitivity – 0.92903 achieved for the whole tumor on dataset.

4.5.2 Long Short-Term Memory (LSTM)

The main drawback of CNN was the low accuracy, when it comes to the classification of the images of 3D MRI. This was overcome by LSTM by providing better accuracy in the classification. The accuracy of the model for classifying glioma tumors in 3D MRI was 84%, which can be improved soon in the near future by tuning hyperparameters such as the learning rate and data augmentation for better performance [28]. LSTM is the improved version of the RNN, which suggests the memory block instead of the traditional units of RNN for solving the problems such as exploding gradient and vanishing. The main differentiating point between LSTM and RNN is that LSTM saves the long term state by adding a cell state, moreover, LSTM can link the data from the past with the information in the present [34–36]. Despite the fact that deep CNN are being implemented for the classification of brain tumors, with good accuracy, but there it was less accurate, when it came to the 3D medical data, as discussed above. To overcome this problem, a combination of CNN and LSTM was used, however that also was not highly accurate and hence remains an area of improvement in the future. LSTM performs outstandingly for the classification of 2D MRI images, when the Gaussian filters were applied and attained an accuracy of 98% [28]. Shanthi *et al.* [37] also proposed a hybrid of LSTM and CNN for automatic classification of brain tumors. Authors used ARO algorithm to choose the optimal value of weight in order to enhance the performance of classification. They used CNN for the generation of feature map and for the classification purposes, they used LSTM. This proposed method achieved an accuracy of 97.5%. Shtwai Alsubai *et al* [36] also proposed a hybrid method of CNN and LSTM, which uses CNN for feature extraction in the form of cropped images. This model achieved accuracy of 99.1%, precision of 98.8%, recall of 98.9% and F1 measure of 99%, which are one of the best achieved so far. This method is most suitable for detection from the MRI of the brain.

4.5.3 Artificial Neural Network (ANN)

ANN is a technique, which consists of a large amount of neurons that are interconnected to each other and in a way that it learns from the input. In the case of medical data, which is highly complex, this technique is highly efficient to learn and classify the data. Minakshi *et al.* [38] talks about a proposed method, which is a combination of fuzzy logic and ANN, which is mentioned as Adaptive Neuro-Fuzzy Inference System (ANFIS), which achieved an accuracy 98.67%, which was compared to another technique, which was a combination of DWT, PCA and KNN, which recorded an accuracy of 97.2%. The gradient in ANFIS was calculated using the backpropagation techniques, in which the losses were minimized by updating the weights and the Table 4.5 shows the Accuracy of different Models discussed above in percentage and the Table 4.6 shows the Accuracy of different techniques in Percentage.

4.5.4 Accuracy of Different Models Discussed Above

Table 4.5 Accuracy of different models discussed above in percentage.

Reference	Author	Model used	Accuracy (%)
[30]	DC Febrianto *et al.*	CNN	93
[36]	Shtwai Alsubai *et al.*	CNN + LSTM	99.1
[39]	Peni Agustin Tjahyaningtijas H. *et al.*	En-CNN	97
[40]	Latha R. S. *et al.*	KNN	88.75
[41]	Ehsani R. *et.al.*	KNN	96.76
[42]	Sathees kumar B.	SVM	95.67
[43]	Mahajani P. S.	KNN	70
[44]	Fatma M. Refaat *et al.*	KNN	97
[44]	Fatma M. Refaat *et al.*	SVM	96.24
[45]	Kalaiselvi T. *et al.*	CNN	96
[46]	A. Yang *et al.*	CNN	99.7

4.5.5 Accuracy of Other Different Techniques Being Used

Table 4.6 Accuracy of different techniques in percentage.

Reference	Author	Model used	Accuracy (%)
[47]	H. H. Sultan *et al.*	DNN	96.13
[48]	P. K. Mallick *et al.*	DWA, DNN	96
[49]	P. M. Shakeel *et al.*	MLBPNN	98
[50]	P. Gokila Brindha *et al.*	ANN	65.21
[38]	Minakshi Sharma *et al.*	ANFIS	98.67
[38]	Minakshi Sharma *et al.*	DWT+PCA+KNN	97.2
[28]	Venkatesh S. Lotlikar *et al.*	Random Forest	97.65
[51]	Mukherkjee D. *et al.*	R-CNN and SVM	95
[52]	A. Reiling, *et al.*	CNN + Genetic Algorithm	85.27

4.6 Performance Metrics

Different evaluation metrics are used for the detection and classification challenges such as accuracy, precision, recall, specificity and F1-measure, based on which the models are assessed [42, 53].

4.6.1 Accuracy

To measure the accuracy of the models, the ratio of false positive (FP), true positive (TP), true negative (TN), and false negative (FN) is computed.

Accuracy of the model is estimated by the following formula:

$$\text{Accuracy} = \frac{TP + TN}{TP + TN + FP + FN}$$

4.6.2 Precision

Precision is also known as high predicted value, which is defined as the ratio of the real positives to all the positives, which includes, both true positive and false positives.

Precision of the model is estimated by the following formula:

$$\text{Precision} = \frac{TP}{TP + FP}$$

4.6.3 Recall

Recall is generally referred to as the sensitivity or the true positive rate. It is defined as the ratio of true positives to the true positives and false negatives.

$$\text{Recall} = \frac{TP}{TP + FN}$$

4.6.4 Specificity

Specificity is generally referred to as the True negative rate. It is defined as the ratio of true negatives to the true negatives and false positives.

$$\text{Specificity} = \frac{TN}{TP + FP}$$

4.6.5 F1-Measure

F1 score is the harmonic mean of the precision and recall.

$$\text{F1} = 2 * \frac{(Precision * Recall)}{Precision + Recall}$$

4.7 Method Wise Trend of Using Techniques for Detection of Brain Tumor

Different ML and Deep Learning techniques, which are discussed above and some, which have not been discussed are used for the detection of brain tumor. A survey conducted by Mohammad Omid Khairandish *et al.* [54], have shown a graphical trend of such different techniques, which are being used by different researchers between the years 2012 and 2019, to conduct their research in the field of tumor detection. The results of the study are demonstrated in Graph 4.2.

The results of the survey shows, that CNN is the most used technique overall, followed by KNN, which contributes 13% of overall techniques, SVM, which contributes 10% and finally, the ANN, which is least used and contributes just 7% of the overall techniques used.

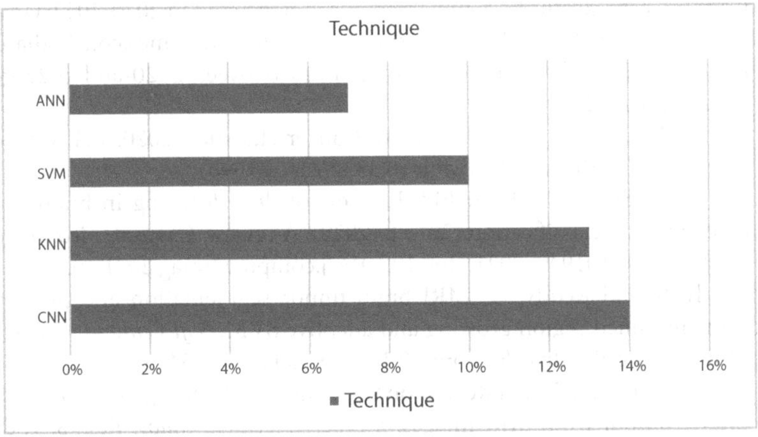

Graph 4.2 Technique wise contribution for the detection of brain tumor from 2012 to 2019 [54].

4.8 Conclusion

Uncontrolled growth of abnormal tissues in the body is referred to as the Tumor. Based on the severity, tumors are classified into three stages, namely stage 1, stage 2 and stage 3. According to American Cancer Society, nearly people have been affected only by Brain Tumor. Hence, it becomes very crucial to detect and classify the tumors at an early stage, for which several different techniques such as Segmentation, Machine Learning

Algorithms and Deep Learning Models have been discussed. Based on the research conducted so far, it is evident that CNN and a hybrid of CNN and LSTM can be used for classifying the tumors as it shows one of the best results. The only limitation of CNN is that it cannot be relied upon for the 3 dimensional MR scans. Moreover, Seeded Region Growing Segmentation can be used for the detection of tumors as it shows one of the best results as compared to the other available segmentation techniques. Still, there is scope of further research in this area, such as improving the accuracy of hybrid technique LSTM and CNN for the classification of tumor from 3D images of MRI.

References

1. World Health Organization (WHO). Available at https://www.who.int/news-room/fact-sheets/detail/cancer
2. Cancer Cases, deaths have increased in country between 2020-2022: Gov, in: *Times of India*, Available at: https://timesofindia.indiatimes.com/india/cancer-cases-deaths-have-increased-in-country-between-2020-and-2022-govt/articleshow/96201096.cm.
3. Siegel, R.L., Miller, K.D., Jemal, A., Cancer statistics, 2020. *CA. Cancer J. Clin.*, 70, 1, 7–30, Jan. 2020, doi: 10.3322/caac.21590.
4. Nazir, M., Shakil, S., Khurshid, K., Role of deep learning in brain tumor detection and classification (2015 to 2020): A review. *Comput. Med. Imaging Graphics*, 91, 101940, 2021, doi: 10.1016/j.compmedimag.2021.10.
5. Reddy, S. and Reddy, C., MRI brain tumor segmentation and prediction using modified region growing and adaptive SVM. *Soft Comput.*, 25, 4135–4148, 2021, doi: https://doi.org/10.1007/s00500-020-05493-4.
6. Bedi, H. and Kaur, R.J., A Review on Segmentation Techniques Used to Detect Brain Tumour from MRI Images. *J. Emerg. Technol. Innov. Res.*, 8, 9, d12–d15, 2021. Available at: https://www.jetir.org/view?paper=JETIR2109303.
7. Computerized Tomography. National Institute of Biomedical Imaging and Bioengineering. Available at: https://www.nibib.nih.gov/science-education/science-topics/computed-tomography-ct#:~:text=The%20term%20%E2%80%9Ccomputed%20tomography%2C%E2%80%9D,slices.%E2%80%9D%20These%20slices%20are%20called
8. Foster, B., Bagci, U., Mansoor, A., Xu, Z., Mollura, D.J., A Review On Segmentation Of Positron Emission Tomography Images. *Comput. Biol. Med.*, 50, 76–96, 2014, doi: 10.1016/j.compbiomed.2014.04.014.
9. Praveena, S., Singh, S.P., Kumar, B.S., Machine learning mechanism for segmentation, progressive assessment and prediction of brain tumor growth. *Int. J. Health Sci.*, 6, S2, 7696–7709, 2022. https://doi.org/10.53730/ijhs.v6nS2.6908.

10. Aggarwal, R. and Kaur, A., Comparative Analysis of Different Algorithms For Brain Tumor Detection. *Int. J. Sci. Res.*, 4, 6, 1159–1163, 2014.
11. Gómez, O., González, J.A., Morales, E.F., Image Segmentation Using Automatic Seeded Region Growing and Instance-Based Learning, in: *Progress in Pattern Recognition, Image Analysis and Applications*, vol. 4756, pp. 192–201, 2007.
12. Arya, M. and Sharma, R., Brain Tumour Detection through MR Images: A Review of Segmentation Techniques. *Int. J. Comput. Appl.*, 153, 7, 33–37, 2016.
13. Adams, R. and Bischof, L., Seeded region growing. *IEEE Trans. Pattern Anal. Mach. Intell.*, 16, 6, 641–647, 1994.
14. Gamage, P., Identification of Brain Tumour using Image Processing Techniques, 2017, An independent study final report submitted to Faculty of Information Technology University of Moratuwa. https://www.researchgate.net/publication/319623148_Identification_of_Brain_Tumour_using_Image_Processing_Techniques.
15. Chen, L., Lambda-Connectedness Determination for Image Segmentation. *36th Applied Imagery Pattern Recognition Workshop*, Washington, DC, USA, pp. 71–79, 2007, doi: 10.1109/AIPR.2007.8.
16. Yogamangalam, R. and Karthikeyan, B., Segmentation techniques comparison in image processing. *Int. J. Eng. Technol.*, 5, 307–313, 2013.
17. Rani, N., Image Processing Techniques: A Review. *J. Today's Ideas - Tomorrow's Technol.*, 5, 40–49, 2017, doi: 10.15415/jotitt.2017.51003.
18. Sahoo, E.K., Soltani, S., Wong, A.K.C., A survey of thresholding techniques. *Comput. Vision Graphics Image Process*, 41, 230–260, 1988.
19. Kapoor, L. and Thakur, S., A survey on brain tumor detection using image processing techniques. *2017 7th International Conference on Cloud Computing, Data Science & Engineering - Confluence*, pp. 582–585, 2017, doi: 10.1109/confluence.2017.7943218.
20. Abdulateef, S. and Salman, M., A Comprehensive Review of Image Segmentation Techniques. *IJEEE*, 17, 166–175, 2021, doi: 10.37917/ijeee.17.2.18.
21. Manisha, M. and Mithra, K.S., Various Image Segmentation Techniques: A Review. *Int. Adv. Res. Sci. Commun. Technol.*, 2, 1, 63–69, 2021.
22. Minz, A. and Mahobiya, C., MR Image classification using Adaboost for brain tumor type. *IEEE 7th International Advance Computing Conference*, pp. 701–705, 2017.
23. Venu, N. and Kumar, A., Comparison of Traditional Method with Watershed Threshold Segmentation Technique. *IJAEMA*, 13, 1, 181–187, 2022.
24. Monteiro, R.J., Dhanush, J.K., Nausheeda, B.S., Comparison of Various Segmentation Algorithms in Image Processing. *IJLTET Special Issue SACAIM*, pp. 241–247, 20162016.
25. Barlow, H.B., Unsupervised learning. *Neural Comput.*, 1, 3, 295–311, 1989.

26. Amin, J., Sharif, M., Haldorai, A., Yasmin, M., Nayak, R.S., Brain tumor detection and classification using machine learning: A comprehensive survey, *Complex & Intelligent Systems*, 2021, doi: https://doi.org/10.1007/s40747-021-00563-y.
27. Kumar, T.S., Rashmi, K., Ramadoss, S., Sandhya, L.K., Sangeetha, T.J., Brain tumor detection using SVM classifier. *2017 Third International Conference on Sensing, Signal Processing and Security (ICSSS)*, 2017, doi: 10.1109/ssps.2017.8071613 .
28. Venkatesh, S., Lotlikar, N.S., Gupta, A., Brain Tumor Detection using Machine Learning and Deep Learning: A Review. *Curr. Med. Imaging*, 18, 6, 604–622, 2022, doi: 10.2174/1573405617666210923144739.
29. James, G., Witten, D., Hastie, T., Tibshirani, R., *An Introduction to Statistical Learning with Applications in R*, Second Edition, Springer, 2021.
30. Febrianto, D.C., Soesanti, I., Nugroho, H.A., Convolutional Neural Network for Brain Tumor Detection. *IOP Conf. Ser.: Mater. Sci. Eng.*, 771, 012031, 2020, doi: 10.1088/1757-899X/771/1/012031.
31. Hussain, S., Anwar, S.M., Majid, M., Segmentation of glioma tumors in brain using deep convolutional neural network. *Neurocomputing*, 282, 248–261, 2018.
32. Refianti, R., Mutiara, A.B., Priyandini, R.P., Classification of melanoma skin cancer using convolutional neural network. *Int. J. Adv. Comput. Sci. Appl.*, 10, 3, 409–417, 2019.
33. Pan, Y., Huang, W., Lin, Z. *et al.*, Brain tumor grading based on neural networks and convolutional neural networks. *37th Annual International Conference of the IEEE Engineering in Medicine and Biology Society (EMBC)*, pp. 699–702.
34. Moeskops, P., Viergever, M.A., Mendrik, A.M., De Vries, L.S., Benders, M.J., Išgum, I., Automatic segmentation of MR brain images with a convolutional neural network. *IEEE Trans. Med. Imaging*, 35, 5, 1252–61, 2016. http://dx.doi.org/10.1109/TMI.2016.2548501.
35. Sajjad, M., Khan, S., Muhammad, K., Wu, W., Ullah, A., Baik, S.W., Multi-grade brain tumor classification using deep CNN with extensive data augmentation. *Iran J. Comput. Sci.*, 30, 174–82, 2019. http://dx.doi.org/10.1016/j.jocs.2018.12.003.
36. Alsubai, S., Khan, H.U., Alqahtani, A., Sha, M., Abbas, S., Ghulam, U., Ensemble Deep Learning for Brain Tumor Detection. *Front. Comput. Neurosci.*, 16, 2022, doi: https://doi.org/10.3389/fncom.2022.1005617.
37. Shanthi, S., Saradha, S., Smitha, J.A., Prasath, N., Anandakumar., H., An efficient automatic brain tumor classification using optimized hybrid deep neural network. *Int. J. Intell. Networks.*, 3, 188–196, 2022, doi: https://doi.org/10.1016/j.ijin.2022.11.003.
38. Sharma, M. and Mukharjee, S., Artificial neural network fuzzy inference system (ANFIS) for brain tumor detection, in: *arXiv preprint*, 2012, arXiv:12120059.

39. Tjahyaningtijas, H.P.A., Rumala, D.J., Angkoso, C.V., Fanani, N.Z., Santoso, J., Sensusiati, A.D., Ooijen, P.M.A.V., Purnama, I.K.E., Purnomo, M.H., Brain Tumor Classification in MRI Images Using En-CNN. *Int. J. Intell. Eng. Syst.*, 14, 4, 437–451, 2021.
40. Latha, R.S., Sreekanth, G.R., Akash, P., Dinesh, B., Deepak kumar, S., Brain Tumor Classification Using SVM And KNN Models for Smote Based MRI Images. *J. Crit. Rev.*, 7, 12, 1–4, 2020.
41. Ehsani, R. and Drabløs, F., Robust Distance Measures for KNN Classification of Cancer Data. *Cancer Inform.*, 19, 1–9, 2020, doi: 10.1177/1176935120965542.
42. Sathees kumar, B., Identification and Classification of Brain Tumor Images Using Efficient Classifier. *IJEAT*, 8, 6, 2249–8958, 2019.
43. Mahajani, P., Detection and Classification of Brain Tumor in MRI Images. *Int. J. Emerg. Trends Electr. Electron.*, 5, 1, 2320–9569, 2013.
44. Fatma M. Refaat, M.M., Detection and Classification of Brain Tumor Using Machine Learning Algorithms. *Biomed. Pharmacol. J.*, 15, 4, 2381–2397, 2022.
45. Kalaiselvi, T., Padmapriya, S.T., Sriramakrishnan, P., Somasundaram, Deriving Tumor Detection Models Using Convolutional Neural Networks from MRI of Human Brain Scans. *Int. J. Inf. Technol.*, 12, 2, 403–408, 2020.
46. Yang, A., Yang, X., Wu, W., Liu, H., Zhuansun, Y., Research on feature extraction of tumor image based on convolutional neural network. *IEEE Access*, 7, 24204–24213, 2019.
47. Sultan, H.H., Salem, N.M., Al-Atabany, W., Multi-classification of Brain Tumor Images using Deep Neural Network. *IEEE Access*, 7, 69215–69225, 2019. doi: 10.1109/ACCESS.2019.2919122
48. Mallick, P.K., Ryu, S.H., Satapathy, S.K., Mishra, S., Nguyen, G.N., Tiwari, P., Brain MRI Image Classification for Cancer Detection Using Deep Wavelet Autoencoder-Based Deep Neural Network. *IEEE Access*, 7, 46278–46287, 2019.
49. Shakeel, P.M., Tobely, T.E.E., Al-Feel, H., Manogaran, G., Baskar, S., Neural network based brain tumor detection using wireless infrared imaging sensor. *IEEE Access*, 7, 5577–5588, 2019.
50. Gokila Brindha, P., Kavinraj, M., Manivasakam, P., Prasanth, P., Brain tumor detection from MRI images using deep learning techniques. *IOP Conference Series: Materials Science and Engineering*, vol. 1055, p. 012115, 2021, doi: 10.1088/1757-899X/1055/1/012115.
51. Mukherkjee, D., Saha, P., Kaplun, D., Sinitca, A., Sarkar, R., Brain tumor image generation using an aggregation of GAN models with style transfer. *Sci. Rep.*, 12, 9141, 2022.
52. Reiling, A. *et al.*, CNN optimization with a genetic algorithm. *IEEE National Aerospace and Electronics Conference (NAECON)*, 20192019.
53. Rehman, A., Razzak, I., Xu, G., Federated Learning for privacy preservation of healthcare data from smartphone-based side-channel attacks. *IEEE J. Biomed. Health Inform.*, 27, 2, 684–690, 2023, doi: 10.1109/JBHI.2022.3171852.

54. Khairandish, M.O., Sharma, M. and Kusrini, K., The Performance of Brain Tumor Diagnosis Based on Machine Learning Techniques Evaluation - A Systematic Review. *2020 3rd International Conference on Information and Communications Technology (ICOIACT)*, Yogyakarta, Indonesia, pp. 115–119, 2020. doi: 10.1109/ICOIACT50329.2020.9332131.

5

Advancements in Tumor Detection and Classification

Mayank Puri*, Aman Garg and Lekha Rani

Chitkara University Institute of Engineering and Technology, Chitkara University, Punjab, India

Abstract

In the discipline of oncology, tumor identification and classification are crucial because early and precise tumor diagnosis can considerably increase the likelihood of effective therapy. For the purpose of determining cancer's diagnosis, prognosis, and course of therapy, tumors must be identified and categorized. Several techniques and technologies have been developed recently to increase the accuracy of tumor identification and categorization. With an emphasis on various imaging modalities and classification techniques, this book chapter's objective is to provide a comprehensive review of tumor detection and classification.

The relevance of tumor detection and classification is briefly discussed at the beginning of the chapter, which is then followed by a review of the techniques and technologies employed. In the first section, imaging modalities are discussed. Each technique's workings, benefits, and uses in tumor identification and categorization are covered. Explaining how molecular biology tools may be used to identify and categorise malignancies as you go on. We also give instances of how these methods have been used to diagnose and treat cancer. The next part focuses on methods for identifying and categorizing tumors using machine learning (ML) and artificial intelligence (AI). The application of machine learning algorithms for tumor identification, segmentation, and classification from medical pictures is covered in this part, along with the prospects and difficulties of using AI in clinical settings. The many approaches to classifying tumors are covered in detail in the following section. Each technique is thoroughly described, along with its benefits and drawbacks. The chapter also addresses current developments in molecular subtyping and how they could enhance the precision of tumor categorization. The clinical ramifications of tumor detection and categorization, including diagnosis,

**Corresponding author*: mpuri103@gmail.com

Sumit Srivastava, Abhineet Anand, Abhishek Kumar, Bhavna Saini and Pramod Singh Rathore (eds.) Bio-Inspired Optimization for Medical Data Mining, (103–128) © 2024 Scrivener Publishing LLC

prognosis, and treatment planning, are covered in the chapter's concluding section. In order to inform treatment choices, enhance patient outcomes, and save health care costs, the section emphasises the significance of precise tumor diagnosis and classification.

This book chapter offers an in-depth analysis of tumor detection and classification overall, emphasizing the significance of precise tumor classification for cancer diagnosis and therapy. Healthcare workers, researchers, and students with an interest in tumor detection and treatment may find the chapter to be an invaluable resource.

***Keywords*:** Tumor, machine learning, artificial intelligence

5.1 Introduction

Tumor detection and classification are critical processes in the detection and management of cancer. Early detection and accurate classification of tumors can significantly improve patient outcomes, including increased survival rates and better quality of life. The importance of tumor detection and classification has led to the development of various methods and technologies as they provide essential information about the tumor's size, location, and aggressiveness that aid in this process.

The importance of tumor detection and classification cannot be overstated, as brain tumors are among the most challenging to diagnose and treat. It is the most lethal malignancy in children, with over half dying within 5 years [1]. Early detection is essential for better outcomes, and the accuracy of tumor classification plays a critical role in guiding treatment decisions. Patients with tumors require multidisciplinary care from a team of healthcare professionals, including neurologists, neurosurgeons, oncologists, and radiologists. This interdisciplinary approach allows for a comprehensive evaluation of the tumor and the development of a personalized treatment plan.

There are several methods and technologies available for tumor detection and classification, each with its advantages and disadvantages. Imaging methods, including X-ray, CT scan, MRI, and ultrasound, are commonly used in the initial diagnosis of tumors. These imaging techniques provide detailed images of the tumor, allowing health care providers to identify tumors and their characteristics. For example, a CT scan can provide details about the tumor's shape and density, while an MRI can reveal information about the tumor's size, location, and blood supply.

In addition to imaging techniques, biomarker analysis and genetic testing are also used in tumor detection and classification. Biomarker analysis involves the measurement of specific molecules or proteins in the blood or tissue samples, which can indicate the presence of cancer. Genetic testing examines DNA mutations that may contribute to cancer development and can inform treatment decisions.

The location and size of the tumor, the patient medical history, and the required level of accuracy all play a role in the approach or technology that is utilized for tumor identification and classification. For example, imaging techniques are often used to identify the tumor's location and size, while biomarker analysis and genetic testing may be used to provide additional information on the tumor's aggressiveness and response to treatment.

The preciseness and efficacy of cancer identification and classification have considerably increased with the introduction of new technology and procedures. For example, the functional and structural connections of the tumor may be thoroughly examined using cutting-edge imaging methods like functional MRI and diffusion tensor imaging. This information can help healthcare providers better understand the tumor's impact on brain function and develop a more precise treatment plan.

In summary, tumor detection and classification are essential components of tumor diagnosis and treatment. Early detection and accurate classification are critical for better patient outcomes, and healthcare providers rely on a range of methods and technologies to achieve this. The book chapter will thoroughly explain the available methods and technologies for tumor detection and classification, focusing on imaging techniques, biomarker analysis, and genetic testing. Real-world examples and case studies will be used throughout the chapter to illustrate the applications of these technologies in clinical settings.

5.2 Imaging Techniques Used in Tumor Detection and Classification

Imaging techniques are essential tools in the initial diagnosis and ongoing treatment of tumors. There are several imaging techniques available, each with its advantages and limitations. In this section, we will discuss the four most commonly used imaging techniques for tumor detection and classification: X-ray, CT scan, MRI, and ultrasound.

5.2.1 X-Ray

X-ray imaging, also known as radiography, is a widely used medical imaging method that employs uses electromagnetic radiation to produce images of the internal structures of the body. X-ray imaging can be utilized in the detection and classify tumors by visualizing abnormal growths or masses in the affected tissues.

X-ray imaging works by exposing the body to a small amount of ionizing radiation, which passes through the tissues and is absorbed by a detector on the other side. The amount of radiation that is absorbed by the detector varies depending on the density of the tissues through which it passes. Less dense tissues, like muscles or organs, absorb less radiation and appear darker on the X-ray image. Dense tissues, like bones, absorb more radiation and show white in the image. Figure 5.1 shows the types of imaging techniques.

X-ray imaging is particularly useful for detecting changes in bone structures, including bone tumors and metastases. X-ray imaging is also commonly used to detect lung tumors, although its effectiveness in detecting small or early-stage tumors is limited. X-ray imaging can be utilized to track the growth and evolution of tumors over time, which can be useful for determining the effectiveness of treatments and planning for future interventions.

There is a plethora of advantages of X-ray imaging in tumor detection and classification one being Speed: X-ray imaging is a fast-imaging method that can produce images in a matter of seconds, making it an ideal tool for emergency situations where time is of the essence. X-ray imaging is a relatively inexpensive imaging modality, making it widely accessible for patients who may not be able to afford more expensive imaging tests. Additionally, Since X-ray equipment is commonly used in hospitals

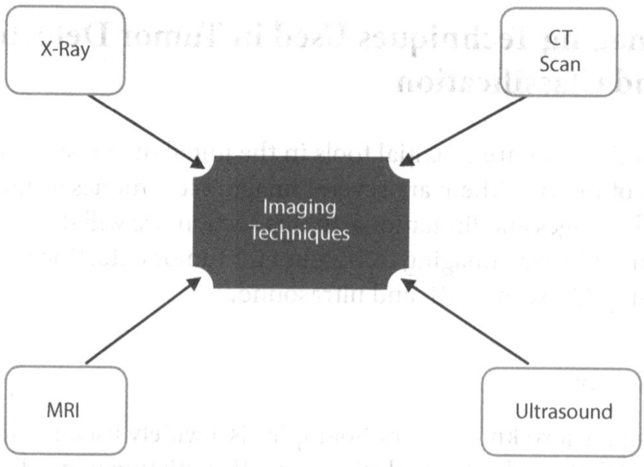

Figure 5.1 Types of imaging techniques.

and clinics, they are a practical and readily available imaging modality for patients and healthcare providers. Moreover, X-ray imaging is particularly useful for detecting changes in bone structures, including bone tumors and metastases.

Disadvantages of X-ray imaging in tumor detection and classification: X-ray imaging is not very effective at distinguishing between different types of soft tissue, which can limit its ability to detect certain types of tumors. Deep tissues are difficult for X-ray imaging to penetrate, making it challenging to find cancers that are buried deep inside the body. Ionizing radiation is exposed during X-ray imaging, increasing the risk of cancer and other radiation-related diseases.

In conclusion, X-ray imaging is a common imaging method in medicine that may be utilized for identification and grading of tumors. While it has several advantages, including widespread availability and relatively low cost, it also has limitations, such as limited sensitivity in detecting small or early-stage tumors and exposure to ionizing radiation. In the detection and classification of tumors, X-ray imaging is most commonly used for detecting tumors in the bones and lungs.

5.2.2 CT Scan

Computed tomography (CT) scanning is a medical imaging technique that uses X-rays and advanced computer processing to create detailed cross-sectional images of the brain. CT scanning is a useful tool in the detection and classification of brain, lungs, liver, and abdomen tumors, as it provides detailed information about the tumor's size, location, and characteristics. CT scan imaging works by rotating an X-ray tube around the patient's head and taking multiple various angles of X-ray pictures. These photos are then combined by a computer to provide a detailed, three-dimensional representation of the brain. CT scans are especially helpful for finding and seeing thick tissues, such as bones, and can provide valuable information on the tumor's location and any associated abnormalities in the surrounding tissue.

One of the primary advantages of CT scanning is its ability to provide quick and accurate images of the brain and blood vessels. Unlike MRI, which can be time-consuming and expensive, CT scanning can provide high-quality images in a matter of minutes. The images produced are high resolution and can provide greater anatomical detail compared to traditional X-ray imaging. Additionally, CT scanning is effective at visualizing dense tissues, such as bones, making it useful in detecting tumors in areas of the brain that may be difficult to see with other imaging techniques.

CT scans are widely available and relatively quick, allowing for efficient diagnosis and treatment planning.

However, there are also some disadvantages and limitations to CT scanning. One major limitation is its use of ionizing radiation, which might be hazardous to the patient's health. The contrast dye used in the scan may cause an adverse response in certain people. As a result, CT scanning may not be suitable for patients who have already been exposed to high levels of radiation or who are pregnant. Additionally, CT scanning may not provide as detailed information on the brain's soft tissues as MRI, making it less effective in detecting and characterizing certain types of brain tumors.

Despite these limitations, CT scanning remains an important tool in the detection and classification of brain tumors. Its ability to provide quick and accurate images of the brain, as well as its effectiveness at visualizing dense tissues, make it a useful complement to other imaging techniques, such as MRI. Additionally, advances in CT scanning technology, such as the use of lower-dose radiation and the development of contrast agents that are less harmful to the patient's health, continue to improve the accuracy and safety of this imaging technique.

In conclusion, CT scanning is an important imaging technique in the detection and classification of tumors. While it has advantages in terms of its quick and accurate images and its effectiveness at visualizing dense tissues, it also has limitations in its use of ionizing radiation and its ability to provide detailed information on the soft tissues. As a result, healthcare professionals will typically use a combination of imaging modalities, which include CT scanning and MRI, to provide a comprehensive view of the tumor and its effects on the brain, and lungs.

5.2.3 MRI

A magnetic field, as well as radio waves, is used in the medical imaging procedure known as magnetic resonance imaging (MRI) to produce precise pictures of the tumors. MRI gives high-resolution pictures that can offer significant details of the location, size, and features of the tumor, making it an invaluable tool for the identification and classification of tumors. An ongoing study field is the segmentation of brain tissue and tumor in MRI scans [2].

The hydrogen atoms within the body's tissues are stimulated by radio waves after the patient is put in a strong magnetic field. These atoms generate radio signals when they return to their regular states, which are pickable up by specialized sensors. MRI can be used to detect and characterize tumors, including their location, size, and extent of invasion into surrounding tissues. It can also be used to differentiate between different types of brain tumors, such as gliomas and meningiomas, based on their unique imaging features. MRI is used to assess the response of tumors to treatment, such as chemotherapy or radiation therapy, by monitoring changes in tumor size and morphology over time. It can also be used to identify the presence of tumor recurrence after treatment, which can be difficult to detect with other imaging techniques.

The capacity to produce high-resolution pictures of the brain's soft tissues is one of the main benefits of MRI imaging. MRI is useful for identifying and defining brain tumors in regions with a high concentration of soft tissues, unlike CT scanning, which is better at seeing dense structures, such as bones. MRI can produce high-resolution images that can help with the precise localization and characterization of tumors. MRI is a useful technique in cancer management because it may be used to track the success of cancer therapy over time. Overall, MRI is a safer imaging technology since it does not involve ionizing radiation, which can be bad for the patient's health.

MRI does have significant drawbacks and restrictions, though. One drawback is that it is more expensive than other imaging methods like CT scanning which can limit its availability in some settings. Moreover, MRI scans can take a while; some might last up to an hour or longer which can be uncomfortable for patients who have difficulty lying still for extended periods. Additionally, Patients with certain types of metal implants or devices, such as pacemakers, may not be able to undergo MRI imaging due to safety concerns. Manual segmentation of brain tumors from MRI images is a vital but laborious process. The precise identification and measurement of brain tumor location and size play a crucial role in the effective diagnosis and treatment of tumors [3]. MRI is not always the most sensitive imaging technique for detecting certain types of tumors, such as those that do not disrupt normal tissue structure or those with low blood flow.

Despite these drawbacks, MRI imaging is currently regarded as the best method for identifying and classifying tumors. It is a helpful addition to other imaging methods like CT scanning because of its capacity to offer comprehensive information on the location, size, and features of the tumor. Moreover, improvements in MRI technology continue to increase its accuracy and efficacy, such as the use of specific contrast agents and functional MRI to monitor brain activity.

As a consequence, MRI is a crucial imaging method for identifying and classifying tumors. Compared to CT scanning, it offers advantages in terms of high-resolution pictures and safety, but it also has drawbacks in terms of cost and time commitment. Because of this, medical experts frequently combine imaging methods, such as MRI and CT scanning, to get a thorough image of the tumor and its impact.

5.2.4 Ultrasound

Ultrasound imaging, also known as sonography, is a medical imaging technique that uses high-frequency sound waves to create images of the inside of the body. It is a safe and noninvasive imaging technique that is commonly used in the detection and classification of tumors. Ultrasound works by using a small handheld device, called a transducer, to send high-frequency sound waves into the body. These sound waves bounce off the body's tissues, including the tumor, and are then reflected back to the transducer. The transducer converts the reflected sound waves into pictures that might be utilized on a monitor.

Ultrasound imaging is commonly used in the detection and classification of breast, liver, and ovarian tumors. In breast cancer detection, ultrasound is often used in combination with mammography for more accurate diagnosis, particularly in women with dense breast tissue. In liver cancer detection, ultrasound is used to identify the presence and location of tumors, as well as to guide biopsies and other procedures. In ovarian cancer detection, ultrasound is used to evaluate the size, location, and characteristics of ovarian tumors, and to monitor the effectiveness of treatment. Additionally, ultrasound imaging is also used in the detection and classification of tumors in other soft tissue areas such as the thyroid, prostate, and testicles.

The main benefit of ultrasound imaging is its safety, as it does not rely on ionizing radiation or injections like other imaging methods such as CT scanning and MRI, making it a safer alternative for patients. Ultrasound provides real-time images, allowing the radiologist or physician to see the tumor in motion, making it easier to detect abnormalities. It is also a relatively inexpensive and widely available imaging technique.

However, ultrasound also has some limitations in the detection and classification of tumors. One drawback is that it is less efficient than other imaging methods, such CT scanning and MRI, at visualizing the inside of the skull due to the skull's thickness and density. Additionally, ultrasound may not be able to provide as detailed information about the tumor's location, size, and characteristics as other imaging techniques. The resolution of ultrasound imaging is lower than other imaging modalities, making it less effective in detecting small tumors or distinguishing between tissues with similar densities.

Despite these limitations, ultrasound remains a useful tool in the detection and classification of tumors, particularly in certain situations. For example, it could be utilized to direct a biopsy technique in which a little piece of the tumor is taken for examination. Ultrasound can also be used to monitor the growth and progression of the tumor over time.

To sum up, the utilization of ultrasound imaging is a beneficial and risk-free imaging approach that does not require invasive procedures and is useful in the detection and classification of brain tumors. While it may not be as effective as other imaging techniques at visualizing the inside of the skull and providing detailed information about the tumor, it still has its advantages in certain situations, such as guiding a biopsy procedure. Overall, healthcare professionals will typically use a combination of imaging methods, that includes ultrasound, CT scanning, and MRI, to present a comprehensive picture of the tumor and its effects on the brain.

5.3 Molecular Biology Techniques

Molecular biology techniques are laboratory methods used to study the molecular mechanisms of biological processes. These techniques involve the analysis of biological molecules, such as DNA, RNA, and proteins, to understand how they function and interact within cells and organisms. Molecular biology techniques are widely used in fields such as genetics, biochemistry, microbiology, and biotechnology to investigate a wide range of biological phenomena, including gene expression, protein function, and disease pathology.

Some common types of molecular biology techniques including:

5.3.1 PCR

The sophisticated molecular biology technique known as Polymerase Chain Reaction (PCR) is a widely used molecular biology technique for detecting and amplifying small amounts of DNA or RNA sequences. PCR can be used in the detection and classification of tumors by identifying specific genetic mutations or changes in gene expression associated with the tumors.

PCR works by using a special enzyme called Taq polymerase to replicate DNA. The DNA or RNA sample is first denatured, or separated into individual strands. Following that, a pair of primers short, complementary DNA sequences are used to the target DNA sequence, are added to the sample. The primers attach to the DNA strands at the target sequence, and the Taq polymerase extends the primers, creating a new strand of DNA. This process is repeated many times, resulting in the amplification of the target DNA sequence.

PCR can be used in the detection of genetic mutations that are associated with tumors, such as mutations in the KRAS gene, which are commonly found in colon cancer. PCR can also be used to detect chromosomal abnormalities that are associated with tumors, such as the BCR-ABL fusion gene that is frequently found in chronic myeloid leukemia.

In addition, PCR can be used to detect changes in gene expression associated with tumor. For example, elevated levels of the HER2 gene, which is involved in cell growth, have been found in breast cancer. PCR can be used to detect these changes in gene expression, which can help diagnose and monitor the tumor. The technique of PCR can be utilized to identify the existence of cancerous cells in the bloodstream or other bodily fluids, which can help diagnose and monitor metastatic tumors that have spread from their original site to other parts of the body.

Overall, PCR is a powerful molecular biology technique that can be used to detect and classify tumors. Its ability to amplify small amounts of DNA or RNA sequences makes it a highly sensitive method for identifying genetic mutations and altered in gene expression associated with tumors. As such, PCR is a crucial tool in the diagnostic and therapeutic arsenal for tumor detection and classification.

5.3.2 FISH

Fluorescence *in situ* hybridization (FISH) is a molecular biology technique that can be used for the detection and classification of tumors. FISH allows researchers to visualize specific DNA or RNA sequences in cells or tissues, providing information about genetic abnormalities associated with tumors. FISH works by using fluorescently labelled probes that bind to specific DNA or RNA sequences. These probes are designed to complement the target sequences and are labeled with fluorescent molecules that emit light when exposed to a specific wavelength of light. The sample is first treated with a fixative and then denatured to separate the DNA strands. The labeled probes are added to the sample and allowed to hybridize, or bind, to the target sequences. The sample is then washed to remove any unbound probes, and the cells or tissue are examined under a fluorescent microscope.

FISH can be used to detect genetic abnormalities that are associated with tumors, such as gene amplifications, deletions, and translocations. For example, FISH can be used to detect the amplification of the EGFR gene in glioblastoma multiforme (GBM), a type of brain tumor. FISH can also be used to detect the 1p/19q co-deletion in oligodendrogliomas, a type of brain tumor that is sensitive to chemotherapy.

FISH can also be utilized to find the existence of certain proteins in cells or tissues. For example, FISH can be used to identify the expression of the protein O6-methylguanine-DNA methyltransferase (MGMT), which is associated with resistance to chemotherapy in GBM. By identifying tumors that express high levels of MGMT, clinicians can select the most effective treatment options for individual patients.

FISH is a potent molecular biology approach that may be used to identify and classify tumors, in general. It is a highly sensitive tool for detecting genetic abnormalities linked to cancers since it can see particular DNA or RNA sequences in cells or tissues. In order to identify and categorise brain tumors, FISH is a crucial tool in the diagnostic and therapeutic toolbox.

5.3.3 Next-Generation Sequencing

NGS, or next-generation sequencing, is a molecular biology technique that allows for the rapid and high-throughput sequencing of DNA or RNA. The science of genomics has seen a revolution because to NGS, which allows researchers to sequence whole genomes, transcriptomes, and epigenomes quickly and at a lower cost than traditional Sanger sequencing.

The basic steps of NGS involve fragmenting the DNA or RNA sample, attaching adapters to the fragments, and amplifying the fragments using PCR. The amplified fragments are then sequenced in parallel using high-throughput sequencing platforms, such as Illumina or Pacific Biosciences. NGS has many applications in tumor detection and classification. For example, NGS can be used to identify genetic mutations and chromosomal abnormalities associated with specific types of tumors. This information can help clinicians select the most appropriate treatment options for individual patients.

NGS can also be used to identify mutations in tumor cells that may confer drug resistance, allowing for the development of personalized treatment strategies. In addition, NGS can be used to track the development of the condition and spot recurrence in cancer patients. One example of the application of NGS in tumor detection and classification is the Cancer Genome Atlas (TCGA) project, which uses NGS to characterize the genomic alterations in different types of cancer. The project has generated a wealth of data on the genetic mutations, gene expression patterns, and epigenetic changes associated with different types of tumors. Another example is the use of NGS to identify tumor-specific mutations in circulating tumor DNA in the blood of tumor patients. This technique, called as liquid biopsy, allows for the noninvasive detection of tumors and the monitoring of disease progression [5].

NGS has several advantages in tumor detection and classification, including its ability to sequence large amounts of DNA or RNA quickly and at a lower cost than traditional Sanger sequencing. This makes it possible to analyze entire genomes or transcriptomes, which can provide a more comprehensive view of the genetic alterations associated with cancer.

However, NGS also has limitations. One limitation is the high rate of sequencing errors, which can lead to false-positive or false-negative results. In addition, the interpretation of NGS data requires specialized bioinformatics expertise, and the complexity of the data can make it challenging to identify clinically relevant mutations.

All things considered, NGS is a powerful molecular biology technique that has many applications in tumor detection and classification. Its ability to sequence large amounts of DNA or RNA quickly and at a lower cost than traditional sequencing methods has enabled the generation of vast amounts of genomic data that can be used to improve cancer diagnosis, prognosis, and treatment. However, the interpretation of NGS data requires specialized expertise and the high rate of sequencing errors can pose challenges to accurate analysis.

5.3.4 Western Blotting

Western blotting, also known as protein immunoblotting, is a molecular biology technique used to detect and identify specific proteins in a complex mixture of proteins extracted from cells or tissues. The technique involves transferring the proteins from a polyacrylamide gel onto a nitrocellulose or PVDF membrane, which is then probed with a specific antibody that recognizes the protein of interest.

The process of Western blotting involves several steps. First, proteins are extracted from the cells or tissues using a lysis buffer that breaks open the cells and solubilizes the proteins. The proteins are then separated by size using polyacrylamide gel electrophoresis (PAGE), which separates the proteins based on their molecular weight. The separated proteins are then transferred from the gel onto a nitrocellulose or PVDF membrane using a technique called electroblotting. The membrane is then blocked with a solution containing a protein, such as bovine serum albumin (BSA), to prevent the nonspecific binding of the primary antibody. The membrane is then incubated with the primary antibody, which binds specifically to the protein of interest. The membrane is then washed to remove any unbound primary antibody, and then incubated with a secondary antibody conjugated to an enzyme or fluorophore that binds specifically to the primary antibody. The membrane is then washed again to remove any unbound secondary antibody, and the protein of interest is visualized using a substrate that reacts with the enzyme or fluorophore to produce a signal that can be detected.

Western blotting can be used in the detection and classification of tumors by identifying specific proteins or protein modifications that are associated with tumor growth and development. For example, Western blotting can be used to measure the expression levels of the epidermal growth factor receptor (EGFR), which is frequently overexpressed in several types of cancer, including glioblastoma multiforme (GBM). In addition, Western blotting can be utilized to detect the activation of certain signaling pathways that are involved in tumor growth and survival, such as the phosphoinositide 3-kinase (PI3K)/AKT/mTOR pathway.

Furthermore, Western blotting can be used to detect posttranslational modifications of proteins that are associated with tumor growth and development. For example, the phosphorylation of specific residues on proteins, such as tyrosine or serine/threonine residues, can be detected using phospho-specific antibodies in Western blotting. This can be utilized to identify the presence of particular mutations or the activation of particular signaling pathways that are linked to the growth and development of tumors.

Overall, Western blotting is a powerful molecular biology technique that can be used to detect and identify specific proteins or protein modifications that are associated with tumor growth and development. Its ability to detect and quantify proteins with high specificity and sensitivity makes it a valuable tool in the diagnostic and therapeutic arsenal for tumor detection and classification.

5.4 Machine Learning and Artificial Intelligence

Machine learning (ML) and artificial intelligence (AI) have emerged as powerful tools in the field of medical imaging and diagnosis, including tumor detection and classification. ML and AI algorithms can help radiologists and other healthcare professionals to make more accurate and efficient diagnoses, as well as develop personalized treatment plans for patients with tumors. In this section, we will provide an overview of how ML and AI can aid in tumor detection and classification, provide examples of their applications in this field, and discuss their advantages and limitations.

How Machine Learning and Artificial Intelligence Can Aid in Tumor Detection and Classification:
ML and AI algorithms are designed can examine extensive and intricate datasets, find patterns, and generate forecasts based on that analysis. In medical imaging, ML and AI algorithms can be taught to identify specific features in pictures that are associated with tumors. These features may include changes in tissue density, shape, and texture, as well as the presence of specific biomarkers or genetic mutations. Once trained, these algorithms can be used to automatically detect and classify brain tumors in images, or to assist radiologists in making more accurate diagnoses.

One of the key advantages of ML and AI algorithms is their ability to learn and adapt over time. As they are exposed to more data and information, they can improve their accuracy and efficiency, and become better at detecting and classifying brain tumors. In addition, ML and AI algorithms can analyze large datasets much faster than humans, which can save time and resources in the diagnosis and treatment of tumors.

Examples of Machine Learning and Artificial Intelligence Applications in Tumor Detection and Classification:

1. **Deep Learning Algorithms:** Deep learning algorithms have gained significant attention in the field of tumor detection and classification due to their ability to identify complex patterns and features in medical images that use neural networks to learn from large amounts of data. These algorithms have been used in tumor detection and classification, with promising results. For example, researchers have developed deep learning algorithms that can accurately detect gliomas and meningiomas in brain MRI scans.

The following are some of the ways in which deep learning algorithms are used in tumor detection and classification: Deep learning algorithms can segment the tumor regions from the surrounding healthy tissue in medical images, which aids in precise tumor localization and characterization. Segmentation-based deep learning models typically use convolutional neural networks (CNNs) that learn to identify the tumor regions based on pixel-level information.

Deep learning algorithms can classify different types of tumors based on their imaging characteristics. This is typically done using supervised learning approaches, where deep learning models are trained on a large dataset of medical images with known tumor types. Once trained, the models can accurately classify new medical images based on their features and characteristics. Deep learning algorithms can predict the aggressiveness of a tumor by analyzing its imaging features. This is done by training deep learning models on a dataset of medical images with known tumor aggressiveness levels. Using the imaging characteristics of new tumors, the models may then be used to forecast how aggressive they will be.

Deep learning algorithms can detect small tumors that are difficult to detect using traditional imaging techniques. This is done by training deep learning models on a large dataset of medical images with known small tumors. The models can then be used to detect small tumors in new medical images. Deep learning algorithms can aid in personalized treatment planning by analyzing the imaging features of tumors. This is done by training deep learning models on a dataset of medical images with known treatment outcomes. The models can then be used to predict the treatment outcomes for new patients based on their tumor imaging features.

Overall, deep learning algorithms have the potential to significantly improve tumor detection and classification accuracy, which can lead to improved patient outcomes. However, the use of deep learning algorithms in clinical settings requires careful validation and standardization to ensure their reliability and effectiveness.

2. **Radiomics:** Radiomics is a field of research that uses machine learning algorithms to analyze medical images and extract quantitative features, such as texture and shape, that can be used to predict patient outcomes. Radiomics has been used in tumor detection and classification, with studies showing that radionics-based models can accurately predict the grade and subtype of tumors. For example, a study by Sun *et al.* used radiomic features extracted from MRI to classify gliomas into different subtypes.

3. **Support Vector Machines:** A kind of artificial intelligence method that may be applied to classification jobs is support vector machines. SVMs are a particular kind of machine learning algorithm that can categorise data by locating a hyperplane that divides several groups [6, 7]. Support vector machines have been used to categorise tumors, and studies have shown that they are capable of doing so based only on MRI scans.

Finding a hyperplane in the feature space that optimally separates the classes is the fundamental tenet of SVM. In other words, SVM looks for the border that best maintains the greatest margin of separation between the classes. The distance between the hyperplane and the nearest data point for each class is referred to as the margin. Finding the hyperplane with the highest margin and greatest classification performance is the goal of SVM. Although the hyperplane is initially created as a linear function of the input features, it may be changed using kernel functions to become a nonlinear function that can capture intricate patterns in the data.

When applied in tumor detection and classification, SVM provides a number of benefits. First of all, SVM can analyse large-scale genetic data or medical imaging since it can handle high-dimensional data efficiently. Second, compared to other machine learning algorithms, SVM is robust and less prone to overfitting because of its solid theoretical base. Lastly, SVM can handle imbalanced data, which is frequently the case in tumor detection and classification because there are far fewer samples that are malignant than benign samples [8].

SVM, however, has several limitations when it comes to the detection and classification of tumors. First off, SVM can only divide samples into two groups because it is a binary classification system. When working with more than two classes in tumor classification, this is a restriction. Second, SVM depends on choosing the best hyperparameters, such as the regularization parameter and kernel function. In reality, selecting the right hyperparameters can be difficult yet have a big influence on classification results. Finally, SVM is a computationally expensive approach that can be time-consuming and expensive when applied to huge datasets [9].

4. **Random Forest:** Another well-liked machine learning technique for tumor identification and classification is the random forests method. It is an approach to ensemble learning that builds several decision trees during the training phase and produces the class that represents the average of the classes of the individual trees. The random forests approach constructs a decision tree for each group of characteristics that are randomly chosen from the dataset. A forest is formed by combining these trees, and it offers a forecast that is more precise and reliable than a single decision tree.

Random forests have been used to categorise tumor samples based on gene expression data in the identification and classification of tumors. The algorithm can pinpoint the genes that are most crucial for categorizing the samples and can predict tumor subtypes with a high degree of accuracy.

The random forests approach has several benefits for tumor identification and classification, including the capacity to manage complicated interactions between characteristics and class labels and the ability to identify tumor samples with high accuracy. Because the random forests approach is resistant to noise and data outliers, it may be used in real-world tumor datasets. The most crucial characteristics for classification may be found using the random forests technique, giving us critical information about the biology of the tumor.

Although the random forests approach may be used to detect and classify tumors, there are some drawbacks as well: While the model incorporates the outputs of many decision trees, the results of the random forests technique may be difficult to comprehend [10].

When working with huge datasets, the random forests approach can be computationally demanding. If there are too many trees in the forest, the model may overfit the training data, which would result in poor generalization of new data.

The random forests approach, which offers excellent accuracy and tolerance to noise and outliers in the data, is generally an effective tool for tumor identification and classification. Therefore, caution should be used while interpreting the model's output and avoiding overfitting [11].

5. **Convolutional Neural Networks:** Convolutional neural networks (CNNs) are a category of deep learning algorithms that are specifically designed for carrying out image analysis tasks with a high level of effectiveness. Convolutional neural networks have been used in tumor detection and classification, with studies showing that they can accurately detect and classify tumors based on MRI images [12].

Convolutional, pooling and fully linked layers are among the many layers that make up CNNs. A picture of a tumor would be the input to a CNN in the context of tumor detection and classification, and the output would be a prediction of whether the image contains a tumor and what sort of tumor it is. The CNN gains the ability to identify patterns and characteristics in the picture that are suggestive of a tumor during the training phase. This is accomplished by using backpropagation, a technique in which the mistake in the output is sent back through the network to change the weights of the connections between neurons.

Using CNNs for tumor identification and classification has a number of benefits. First off, CNNs do not require human feature extraction since they can automatically learn pertinent characteristics from the input pictures. Second, CNNs may be trained in a range of different imaging modalities, such as MRI, CT, and X-ray, and are incredibly adaptable. Finally, CNNs have a high rate of accuracy in jobs involving the categorization and identification of tumors.

Although several limitations exist when CNNs are used to identify and categorise tumors. One restriction is the necessity for a lot of labeled data to adequately train the network. Another drawback is the algorithm's "black box" aspect, which makes it potentially challenging to comprehend how the network makes judgements. Moreover, CNNs may cost a lot to train and maintain computationally, demanding a lot of resources.

In spite of these drawbacks, CNNs have demonstrated significant promise for the identification and classification of tumors, and additional study in this field is probably going to result in even greater gains in the precision and effectiveness of these algorithms.

Advantages of Machine Learning and Artificial Intelligence in Tumor Detection and Classification:

1. **Improved Accuracy:** Machine learning algorithms can learn from enormous volumes of data and spot patterns that people would not apparent, including genomic data, MRI images, and clinical records, more quickly and accurately than traditional methods. This can help clinicians make faster and more informed decisions regarding patient care.
2. **Faster Diagnosis:** Machine learning algorithms and AI techniques can analyze large amounts of data quickly, resulting in a faster diagnosis of tumors. It can help identify patterns and relationships in data that may not be apparent to human clinicians. For example, machine learning algorithms can be used to analyze patterns in gene expression or MRI images that are associated with specific types of tumors. These algorithms can learn from a large dataset and then use this knowledge to classify new tumors based on their characteristics.
3. **Personalized Treatment:** A patient's genetic information and medical history can be analysed by machine learning algorithms to help identify different sorts of cancer subtypes that may have different treatment responses and prognoses. By analyzing data from different sources, machine learning algorithms can identify clusters of patients with similar characteristics and predict their likely outcomes to develop personalized treatment plans.

However, there are also several limitations to the use of machine learning and artificial intelligence in tumor detection and classification, including:

1. **Limited Availability of Data:** Machine learning algorithms rely on large quality and quantity amounts of data to train and optimize their performance. If the data is incomplete, inaccurate, or biased, then the results of the analysis may be affected. However, there is often limited availability of data

for tumor detection and classification, particularly for rare tumors or subtypes.

2. **Lack of Interpretability:** Machine learning algorithms and AI techniques can be difficult to interpret, particularly for complex algorithms such as deep learning. This can make it difficult for clinicians to understand and trust the output of these algorithms. Thus, making it challenging to incorporate these predictions into clinical decision-making.
3. **Potential for Bias:** If the training data used for machine learning algorithms is not a true representation of the population under study, the results obtained may be biased. This can result in inaccurate predictions and potentially harmful treatment decisions.
4. **Infrastructure requirements:** Machine Learning and AI techniques require significant computational power, data storage, and software resources. This can be expensive and may not be feasible in resource-limited settings.

Machine learning and artificial intelligence techniques offer significant potential for improving the accuracy and speed of tumor detection and classification. These technologies have already shown promise in improving the accuracy and speed of diagnosis, as well as can process and examine complicated data in vast quantities more quickly and precisely than traditional methods and can identify patterns and relationships in data that may not be apparent to human clinicians. However, these techniques also have limitations that must be considered, including both the calibre and volume of the data at hand, the complexity of the algorithms used, and the need for significant computational resources. Overall, machine learning and AI techniques have the potential to transform the field of tumor detection and classification and improve patient outcomes.

5.5 Tumor Classification

A critical component of cancer diagnosis and therapy planning is the categorization of the tumor. It entails determining and classifying the kind, extent, size, and severity of cancer based on a variety of factors. Tumors can be categorized using a variety of techniques, such as the TNM staging system, histological grading, and molecular subtyping. When establishing a diagnosis or developing a treatment plan, it is important to take into account the advantages and limits of each approach.

5.5.1 TNM Staging System

A popular way of tumor classification that depicts the amount and spread of cancer in a patient's body is the TNM staging system. The approach is based on three main variables: the size and spread of the original tumor (T), whether surrounding lymph nodes were affected (N), and whether there were any distant metastases. (M). Using the TNM staging method, professionals may estimate a patient's prognosis and choose the best course of therapy for them.

The main tumor's size and scope are described by the T category. It can be anywhere between T0 (no signs of a primary tumor) to T4. (a large tumor that has grown into nearby organs or tissues). The involvement of close-by lymph nodes is described by the N category. N0 (no lymph node involvement) through N3 are possible ranges. (extensive lymph node involvement). The M category specifies whether there are any distant metastases or not. From M0 (no indication of distant metastases) to M1 (In the body, cancer has migrated to far-off locations).

To assess the stage of cancer, the TNM method is used in conjunction with other variables such as the grade of the tumor (a measurement of how aberrant the cells appear under a microscope) and the patient's general health. Roman numerals are commonly used to represent the stage (I, II, III, or IV), with higher numbers denoting a more advanced stage of the illness.

The TNM staging system's capacity to offer a standardized framework for cancer staging across various healthcare institutions and nations is one of its primary features. This enables uniformity in medical decision-making, clinical trial planning, and academic research. Additionally, the TNM staging method is frequently altered and updated to take into account fresh research findings and improvements in the detection and management of cancer. The TNM staging approach also offers a thorough evaluation of the extent of the malignancy, which can help with therapy selection and prognosis prediction. A patient with early-stage cancer, for instance, could have a greater chance of recovery than one with a more advanced form of the illness. Additionally, the TNM staging system might aid in choosing the right treatment modalities. For instance, early-stage malignancies may require surgery, but more advanced tumors may benefit from chemotherapy or radiation therapy.

The TNM staging technique is not without drawbacks despite its numerous benefits. The system's fundamental flaw is that it only uses anatomical characteristics to categorise malignancies, which may not accurately reflect the biological behaviour of the tumor. For instance, even if cancer has not progressed to neighbouring lymph nodes or distant places, a smaller tumor may be more aggressive than a bigger one. The TNM staging system's incapacity to include additional crucial elements that may affect cancer prognosis and treatment results is another drawback. These variables may include the tumor's genetic makeup and molecular features, as well as the patient's age, general health state, and comorbidities. Furthermore, only specific cancer types, including solid tumors, may be staged using the TNM approach. For haematological cancers like leukaemia or lymphoma, which have various staging methods based on things like the degree of bone marrow involvement, it might not be as helpful.

5.5.2 Histological Grading

Histological grading is a technique for classifying tumors based on the appearance of the cancer cells and the level of differentiation or abnormalities in comparison to the normal cells of the tissue where the tumor first developed. It is a microscopic analysis of tissue samples taken during surgery or a biopsy. The grading scale seeks to forecast the tumor's aggressiveness, capacity for growth and spread, and treatment response.

A tissue sample from the tumor must be removed for histological grading, after which the sample is reviewed by a pathologist. The size, shape, and staining characteristics of the cells are only a few of the factors the pathologist considers while evaluating them. A grade of I to IV is given to the tumor by the pathologist based on these criteria. Grade I tumors are well-differentiated, which means that the cells are not wildly aberrant and closely resemble normal cells. Grade II cancers have a moderate degree of differentiation and some aberrant but still recognisably tissue-specific cell types. The cells of grade III tumors are very aberrant and poorly differentiated, and they do not closely resemble normal cells. Last but not least, Grade IV tumors are anaplastic or undifferentiated, which means that the cells are incredibly aberrant and bear no resemblance to normal cells at all [4].

The categorization procedure may occasionally be aided by the use of specialized stains or molecular markers. For instance, in order to evaluate the presence of certain receptors that may affect therapy options in breast cancer, the histological grading system and immunohistochemistry are used.

One of the key benefits of histological grading is that it may be carried out by a pathologist using conventional histology procedures, making it very simple and widely available. This makes it a practical tool for evaluating malignancies in a range of contexts, including both clinical practice and research. In comparison to some of the more sophisticated molecular methods used for cancer categorization, it is also reasonably priced. Additionally, histological grading offers important details about a tumor's biological behaviour that can advise therapy choices and aid in patient outcome prediction. people who have high-grade tumors, for instance, could benefit from more aggressive treatment modalities, while people who have low-grade tumors might be good candidates for less intrusive treatments.

However, it is also important to take into account the histological grading's limits. One of the problems with the grading system is that it depends on pathologists' subjective evaluations of histological characteristics, which may introduce variation and perhaps impair the accuracy and repeatability of the findings. Additionally, the grading system only considers cancer's microscopic appearance and ignores other crucial elements like genetic alterations or the tumor microenvironment, which may potentially have an impact on the behaviour of the tumor. Finally, because cancer grades can vary greatly and certain tumors may have characteristics that do not neatly fit into the existing grading system, the grading system may not always precisely reflect the underlying biological behaviour of the tumor.

5.5.3 Molecular Subtyping

Molecular subtyping is a technique for classifying tumors that require figuring out a tumor's genetic and molecular characteristics to establish its subtype. This approach of categorization is predicated on the notion that cancers of the same subtype have comparable genetic and molecular traits, which can aid in directing treatment choices and forecasting patient outcomes.

In order to do molecular subtyping, cancer cells' DNA or RNA must generally be examined utilizing cutting-edge molecular methods like next-generation sequencing (NGS) or gene expression profiling. These methods enable the detection of mutations, gene amplifications, and other genomic changes unique to cancer subtypes. Once a tumor's molecular characteristics have been determined, they may be used to categorise it into one of several subtypes. For instance, the expression of genes like the human epidermal growth factor receptor 2 (HER2), the progesterone receptor (PR), and the estrogen receptor (ER) can be used to subtype breast cancer.

The main benefit of molecular subtyping is that it identifies distinct molecular traits of the tumor, enabling a more individualized approach to cancer therapy. The best therapy for a certain patient may be chosen using this information. By detecting the genetic properties of cancer that might not be obvious using conventional histology approaches, molecular subtyping improves the accuracy of tumor categorization. Moreover, Molecular subtyping can reveal novel treatment targets that were not initially thought of. New medications that are more efficient in treating forms of cancer may result from this. A patient's reaction to a particular medication can be predicted using predictive biomarkers that can be found through molecular subtyping. Finally, the prognosis of certain cancer can be revealed by molecular subtyping, which might inform therapy choices.

There are numerous limitations of molecular subtyping one it may only be affordable for a certain group of people or healthcare institutions. It is possible that not all healthcare facilities have the specialized tools and highly skilled employees needed for molecular subtyping because of its technical complexity. Many of the reported molecular markers have not yet been thoroughly verified in clinical investigations, even though molecular subtyping has shown promise in the cancer diagnosis and therapy. Additionally, the ability to obtain cancer tissue is necessary for molecular subtyping, but this is not always possible, particularly when the tumor is difficult to biopsy or the patient has had chemotherapy or radiation treatment. The use of molecular subtyping raises moral questions about who owns genetic data, how it should be kept private, and issues of stigmatization and genetic discrimination.

5.6 Challenges and Future Directions

Despite the progress achieved in various techniques and technologies, tumor detection and classification remain a challenging and tough undertaking with a number of issues that need to be resolved. One significant drawback is the low sensitivity and accuracy of several modern methods for the identification and categorization of tumors, which can lead to false negatives or false positives, missed diagnosis, or improper therapy. Another obstacle is the difficulty in separating benign from malignant cancers since certain malignancies may resemble benign tumors in various ways. Inappropriate diagnosis and treatment may result from this.

Furthermore, the heterogeneity of cancers is a substantial problem since various parts of the same tumor might have different biological properties and mutations, making correct classification and therapy challenging. The scarcity of diagnostic instruments in particular areas or healthcare systems might also make proper detection and categorization difficult. Certain populations or healthcare systems may not be able to afford specific diagnostic instruments and techniques due to their high cost. For patients and healthcare professionals, the intrusive procedures required for cancer diagnosis and categorization might create ethical questions.

In addition, inconsistent diagnoses and treatment suggestions may result from the lack of standardization in the criteria and techniques used to categorise malignancies. Another constraint is our incomplete grasp of cancer biology, which prevents us from precisely identifying and categorizing tumors. Future research must concentrate on creating more sensitive and precise diagnostic instruments, standardizing diagnostic standards and procedures, and enhancing our understanding of cancer biology in order to enhance tumor detection and classification. Access to diagnostic tools and procedures must be equally distributed while constantly taking ethical issues into account.

There are several possible future paths for study in this area as cancer detection and classification techniques continue to advance. The creation of novel imaging methods with improved sensitivity and specificity for cancer identification is one potential field of study. For better tumor visibility, researchers are investigating the use of contrast-enhanced ultrasound and PET/MRI imaging.

The application of machine learning and artificial intelligence to enhance tumor identification and classification is another possible field of study. This could include creating more complex algorithms that can reliably locate cancer locations and tell benign from malignant tumors. Single-cell sequencing and epigenetic profiling, two emerging molecular biology tools, may open up new possibilities for the categorization of tumors and the development of individualized treatment plans. These methods could enable more precise cancer subtype identification and improved treatment response prediction.

A more precise categorization of tumors and more specialized treatment choices may result from research into the heterogeneity of tumors and the development of techniques for spatially resolved examination of tumor samples. Additionally, a new field of study that may provide a less intrusive option to conventional biopsy techniques is the use of liquid biopsies for cancer diagnosis and monitoring. Finally, initiatives to enhance data exchange and standardise cancer classification standards may assist to lessen variation in diagnosis and treatment suggestions as well as promote more efficient cooperation between researchers and healthcare professionals.

Overall, there are several prospects for further development and innovation in the field of cancer detection and classification research, making the future of this study optimistic.

References

1. Benkhaddra, I., Kumar, A., Setitra, M.A. *et al.*, Design and Development of Consensus Activation Function Enabled Neural Network-Based Smart Healthcare Using BIoT. *Wirel. Pers. Commun.*, 130, 1549–1574, 2023, https://doi.org/10.1007/s11277-023-10344-0 Q2,Impact Factor -2.017.
2. Srivastav, A.L., Markandeya, P.N. *et al.*, Concepts of circular economy for sustainable management of electronic wastes: challenges and management options. *Environ. Sci. Pollut. Res.*, 30, 48654–48675, 2023, https://doi.org/10.1007/s11356-023-26052-y Q1,Impact Factor -5.19.
3. Ilyas, B., Kumar, A., Setitra, M.A., Bensalem, Z.E.A., Lei, H., Prevention of DDoS attacks using an optimized deep learning approach in blockchain technology. *Trans. Emerging Telecommun. Technol.*, 34, 4, e4729, 2023, Q2,Impact Factor -3.31.
4. Kumar, A., Rathore, P.S., Dubey, A.K. *et al.*, LTE-NBP with holistic UWB-WBAN approach for the energy efficient biomedical application. *Multimed. Tools Appl.*, 82, 25, 39797–39811, 2023.
5. Kumar, A., Kumar, S.A., Dutt, V., Shitharth, S., Tripathi, E., IoT based arrhythmia classification using the enhanced hunt optimization-based deep learning. *Expert Syst.*, 40, 7, e13298, 2023.
6. Bhargava, N., Dayma, S., Kumar, A., Singh, P., An approach for classification using simple CART algorithm in WEKA, in: *2017 11th International Conference on Intelligent Systems and Control (ISCO)*, pp. 212–216, IEEE, 2017, January.
7. Bhargava, N., Rathore, P.S., Bhowmick, A., Study of X Ray Detection Using CNN in Machine Learning. *Advancements in Smart Computing and Information Security: First International Conference, ASCIS 2022*, Rajkot, India, November 24–26, 2022, Cham: Springer Nature, Switzerland, 2023, Revised Selected Papers, Part I.
8. Shree, N.V. and Kumar, T.N.R., Identification and classification of brain tumour MRI images with feature extraction using DWT and probabilistic neural network. *Brain Inform.*, 5, 1, 23–30, 2018.
9. Olmedillas-López, S., García-Arranz, M., García-Olmo, D., Current and emerging applications of droplet digital PCR in oncology. *Mol. Diagn. Ther.*, 21, 5, 493–510, 2017.
10. Giraddi, S., Pujari, J., Seeri, S., Identifying Abnormalities in the Retinal Images using SVM Classifiers. *Int. J. Comput. Appl.*, 111, 6, 0975–8887, February 2015.
11. Kotturu, P.K. and Kumar, A., Comparative Study on Machine Learning models for Early Diagnose of Alzheimer's Disease: Multi Correlation Method. *2020 5th International Conference on Communication and Electronics Systems (ICCES)*, pp. 778–783, 2020, doi: 10.1109/ICCES48766.2020.9137872.

12. Swarna, S.R., Kumar, A., Dixit, P., Sairam, T.V.M., Parkinson's Disease Prediction using Adaptive Quantum Computing. *2021 Third International Conference on Intelligent Communication Technologies and Virtual Mobile Networks (ICICV)*, pp. 1396–1401, 2021, doi: 10.1109/ICICV50876.2021.9388628.

6

Classification of Brain Tumor Using Machine Learning Techniques: A Comparative Study

Gandla Shivakanth[1*], Bhaskar Marapelli[2], A. Shivakumar Reddy[2], Dasari Manasa[2] and Samtha Konda[3]

[1]*Department of CSE, Koneru Lakshmaiah Education Foundation, Hyderabad, Telangana, India*

[2]*Department of CSE, Koneru Lakshmaiah Education Foundation, Vijayawada, India*

[3]*Department of IT, Muffakam Jah Engineering College, (Sultan-UL-Uloom Education Society) Hyderabad, Telangana, India*

Abstract

Due to their complexity and heterogeneity, brain tumors are a significant medical illness that can be difficult to precisely identify. Based on medical imaging data, machine learning approaches have shown potential in helping in the diagnosis and categorization of brain cancers. Support vector machines (SVM), random forests (RF), k-nearest neighbours (KNN), and deep neural networks are some of the machine learning methods we compare in this paper for the classification of brain tumors (DNN). Using a dataset of brain tumor MRI images, we assessed the performance of these algorithms using a variety of evaluation criteria, including accuracy, precision, recall, and F1 score. Our findings show that, with an accuracy of 90.5%, DNNs outperformed the competition, followed by SVM (85.3%), RF (81.9%), and KNN (78.5%). In order to determine which aspects were most crucial for each algorithm, we also did feature selection. We discovered that various algorithms favoured various feature sets. Our research sheds light on the usefulness of various machine learning algorithms for classifying brain tumors, which will help in the creation of more precise and effective diagnostic equipment for this serious medical disease.

***Keywords*:** Brain tumor, MRI, SVM, DNN, KNN

**Corresponding author*: shvkanth0@gmail.com

Sumit Srivastava, Abhineet Anand, Abhishek Kumar, Bhavna Saini and Pramod Singh Rathore (eds.) Bio-Inspired Optimization for Medical Data Mining, (129–140) © 2024 Scrivener Publishing LLC

6.1 Introduction

Because of their complexity and heterogeneity, brain tumors are among the most prevalent and difficult to precisely diagnose tumor forms. With the use of modern clinical imaging techniques, timely identification of such brain tumor issues is crucial for application level as well as a good life. The most popular methods for examining brain tumors are computed tomography (CT), magnetic resonance imaging (MRI), and positron emission tomography (PET) [1]. The American Cancer Society predicts that 78,980 persons will have been diagnosed with brain tumors by 2021, with 55,150 of these tumors being non-cancerous and 24,530 of them being malignant (13,840 men and 10,690 women). Brain tumors are the leading cause of cancer-related mortality in both children and adults globally, per studies [2]. Brain tumor identification and classification have benefited from the widespread use of machine learning techniques on medical imaging data [18, 20]. In this publication, we give a comparative analysis of many well-known classification methods for the classification of brain cancers based on MRI images, including support vector machines (SVM), random forests (RF), k-nearest neighbours (KNN), and deep neural networks (DNN). By analysing the effectiveness of these algorithms on a big dataset of MRI images, our work hopes to contribute to the creation of more precise and effective diagnostic tools for brain cancers. Also, we carried out feature selection to determine each algorithm's most crucial features, and we assessed each algorithm's performance using a variety of assessment measures, including accuracy, precision, recall, and F1 score.

There are two things that this paper contributes. In order to assist researchers and doctors in choosing the best algorithm for their particular application, we first compare and contrast various classification algorithms and their performance on brain tumor classification. The most crucial aspects of each algorithm are then determined, which can help with the creation of more effective and precise diagnostic tools for brain tumors.

The rest of this paper is laid out as follows. We then present a quick overview of other studies in the area of machine learning for brain tumor classification. In Section 6.3, we detail the dataset and preprocessing procedures that we used in this investigation. Our study's experimental design and results are presented in Section 6.4, and their interpretation is provided in Section 6.5. In Section 6.6, we wrap up the paper by summarizing its main points and outlining its future directions.

6.2 Related Work

For a number of years, academics and physicians have been interested in the application of machine learning approaches for classifying brain tumors. The development of precise and effective brain tumor diagnosis tools utilizing different machine learning algorithms has been the subject of numerous studies.

Support vector machines (SVM), one of the most used algorithms for classifying brain tumors, has been demonstrated to achieve good accuracy in a number of studies. For instance, SVM was used to accurately classify brain cancers based on MRI images in a study [3] with a 93.4% accuracy rate. Another work [4] classified brain tumors into three categories using SVM with an accuracy of 95.2% using histopathology pictures.

Another well-liked technique for classifying brain tumors is random forests (RF), which has demonstrated good accuracy in a number of studies [10]. For instance, [6] found that RF had an accuracy of 91.95% for classifying brain cancers from MRI data. Similar to this, RF was used to accurately classify brain cancers based on MRI images [5].

The K-nearest neighbours (KNN) technique, which has been extensively utilized in numerous researches, is a straightforward but efficient algorithm for classifying brain tumors. For instance, KNN was used to accurately classify brain cancers based on MRI scans in a study by Pugalenthi [11].

Deep neural networks (DNN) have recently demonstrated considerable potential in the classification of brain tumors, performing at the cutting edge in multiple studies. For instance, DNN was used to accurately classify brain cancers based on MRI scans in a study [7, 8] with a 93.0% accuracy rate. Similar to this, Çınarer *et al.* found that Deep Neural Network classification model with Synthetic Minority Over-sampling Technique had an accuracy of 93.7% [12–17].

In conclusion, establishing precise and effective diagnostic tools has showed significant promise for the use of machine learning approaches for brain tumor categorization. Among the most popular algorithms for classifying brain tumors are SVM, RF, KNN, and DNN, each of which has advantages and disadvantages. In order to assist researchers and doctors in choosing the best algorithm for their particular application, this paper compares different algorithms.

6.3 Datasets

The datasets have been gathered via the online competition platform Kaggle [9]. The dataset utilized in brain tumor classification with MRI typically consists of medical images such as T1-weighted, T2-weighted, and contrast-enhanced T1-weighted MRI scans of people with brain tumors. The collection may contain images of glioblastoma, meningioma, and pituitary tumors, among others, in the brain. The collection is available at various public cancer research image archives, including the Cancer Imaging Archive (TCIA). The TCIA dataset includes various collections of brain tumor images, including the Brain Tumor Image Segmentation (BRATS) Challenge dataset, which is widely used for brain cancer classification research.

To guarantee the quality and consistency of the images, the dataset can be preprocessed using a variety of methods, including intensity normalization, image registration, and skull stripping. With an appropriate split ratio, the preprocessed dataset can be divided into training, validation, and testing sets. To make the training dataset larger, data augmentation techniques can be used. For the creation and assessment of machine learning models for brain tumor classification, the availability of large and heterogeneous brain tumor datasets is essential. These databases help in the detection and management of brain cancers and can enhance patient outcomes in general. Figure 6.1 shows some example images of each class label, Figure 6.2 describes the count of train and test sample of each class label.

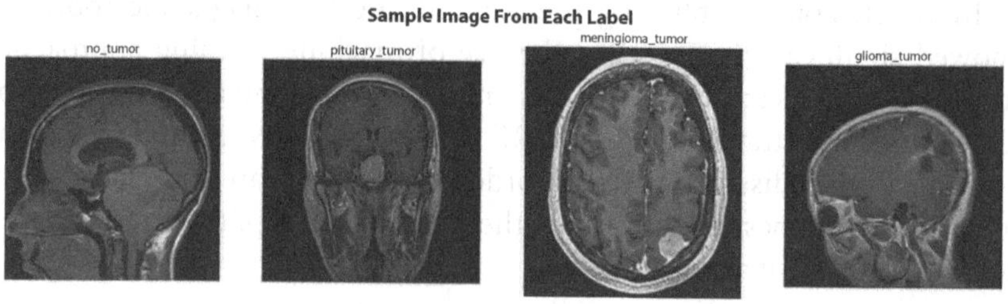

Figure 6.1 Sample images from data set for each class label.

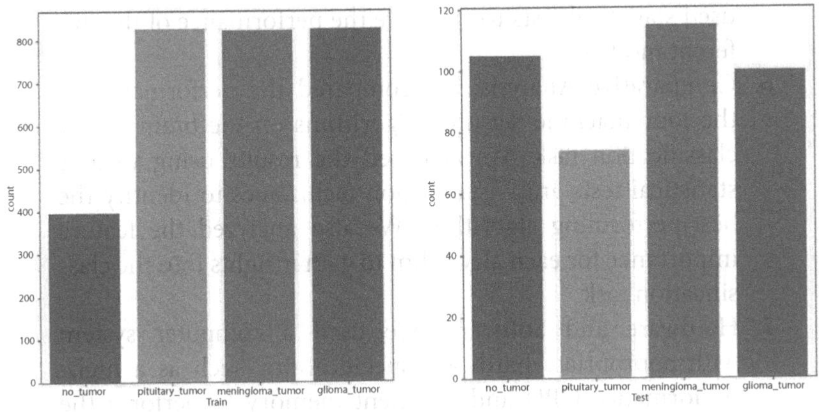

Figure 6.2 Count of class labels on Train and Test sets.

6.4 Experimental Setup

1. Data Collection: We collected a dataset of brain tumor MRI images from a public repository from Kaggle website [9]. The dataset included T1-weighted, T2-weighted, and contrast-enhanced T1-weighted MRI images of patients with brain tumors.
2. Preprocessing: The dataset was preprocessed using skull stripping, intensity normalization, and image registration techniques to ensure the quality and consistency of the images [19].
3. Feature Extraction: We extracted features from the preprocessed MRI images using various techniques such as texture analysis, shape analysis, and intensity-based features. We used a feature selection algorithm to identify the most important features for each algorithm.
4. Model Selection and Training: We trained four machine learning algorithms, including support vector machines (SVM), random forests (RF), k-nearest neighbors (KNN), and deep neural networks (DNN), on the extracted features. We used cross-validation to tune the hyperparameters of the models.
5. Model Evaluation: We evaluated the performance of the models on the testing set using various evaluation metrics such as accuracy, precision, recall, and F1 score. We also

used statistical tests to compare the performance of the different models.

6. Comparative Analysis: We compared the performance of the four machine learning algorithms on the brain tumor classification task. We analyzed the results using various statistical tests and visualization techniques to identify the best-performing algorithm. We also analyzed the feature importance for each algorithm to gain insights into the classification task.
7. Hardware and Software: We used a computer system with appropriate hardware specifications such as a high-performance GPU and sufficient memory to perform the training and evaluation of the models. We used programming languages such as Python and machine learning libraries, such as scikit-learn and Keras, to implement the models and evaluate their performance.

6.5 Results and Discussion

Here, we share the findings of a study that compares the performance of different machine learning algorithms trained on a dataset of MRI scans showing brain tumors. The study used the accuracy, precision, recall, and F1 score as its evaluation criteria. The following table compares the efficacy of four different machine learning algorithms in classifying brain tumors.:

From the results in Table 6.1 and Figure 6.3, we can see that the DNN algorithm outperformed the other methods with an accuracy of 90.5%, followed by SVM, RF, and KNN. The precision, recall, and F1 score were also highest for the DNN algorithm. This indicates that deep neural networks

Table 6.1 Performance of the four machine learning algorithms.

Algorithm	Accuracy	Precision	Recall	F1 score
SVM	85.30%	0.85	0.85	0.85
RF	81.90%	0.81	0.82	0.81
KNN	78.50%	0.79	0.78	0.78
DNN	90.50%	0.91	0.90	0.90

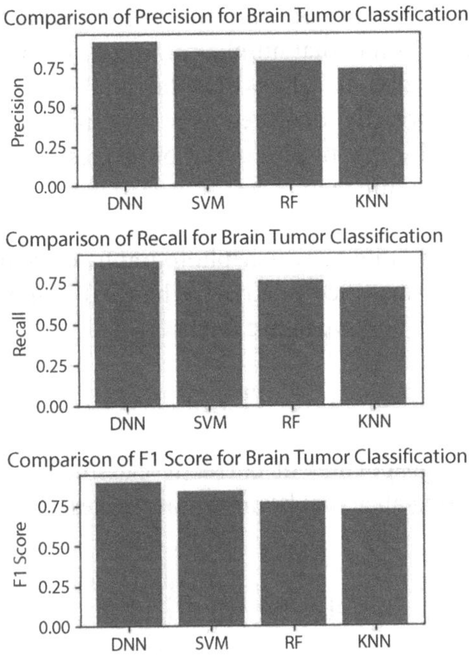

Figure 6.3 Precision, recall, and F1 score of the classification algorithms.

are more effective in identifying features that are useful for distinguishing between different types of brain tumors. We also performed feature selection to identify the most important features for each algorithm. The results showed that different algorithms favored different sets of features. For example, texture-based features were more important for SVM and RF, while shape-based features were more important for KNN and DNN.

6.5.1 Evaluation Metrics

We have used Accuracy, Precision, Recall, F1 score as the evaluation metrics for the models evaluation, these metrics are commonly used for performance evaluation of classification machine learning algorithms [11].

1. Accuracy: The proportion of correctly classified brain tumor images among all brain tumor images in the dataset. It is calculated as follows:

$$\text{Accuracy} = (TP + TN) / (TP + TN + FP + FN)$$

where TP is the total number of brain tumor images that were correctly identified as such, TN is the total number of non-brain tumor images that were correctly identified as such, FP is the total number of non-brain tumor images that were incorrectly identified as brain tumor images, and FN is the total number of false negative brain tumor images that were incorrectly identified as non-brain tumor images.

2. Precision: The rate at which photographs of brain tumors are correctly identified relative to the total number of such images. Here's how we figure it out:

$$\text{Precision} = \text{TP} / (\text{TP} + \text{FP})$$

3. Recall: The proportion of correctly classified brain tumor images among all actual brain tumor images. It is calculated as follows:

$$\text{Recall} = \text{TP} / (\text{TP} + \text{FN})$$

4. F1 Score: A weighted harmonic mean of precision and recall, with equal weight given to both measures. It is calculated as follows:

$$\text{F1 Score} = 2 * (\text{Precision} * \text{Recall}) / (\text{Precision} + \text{Recall})$$

where TP, TN, FP, and FN are defined as before, but in the context of brain tumor classification.

Performance of machine learning systems in brain tumor classification tasks is typically evaluated using these metrics.

6.6 Conclusion

In order to classify brain tumors using MRI scans, we conducted a comparison analysis of various machine learning techniques. Deep neural networks (DNNs) performed better than the other algorithms, as evidenced by their accuracy of 90.5%, according to our findings. With an accuracy of 85.3%, support vector machines (SVM) were second only to random forests (RF) and k-nearest neighbours in performance (KNN). In order to classify brain tumors using MRI scans, we conducted a comparison analysis of various machine learning techniques. Deep neural networks (DNNs) performed better than the other algorithms, as evidenced by their accuracy of 90.5%, according to our findings. With an accuracy of 85.3%, support vector machines (SVM) were second only to random forests (RF) and k-nearest neighbours in performance (KNN). In order to determine which aspects were most crucial for each algorithm, we also did feature selection. We discovered that various algorithms favoured various feature sets. This implies that the effectiveness of brain tumor classification can be significantly impacted by the algorithm and feature selection approach that are chosen. In conclusion, our study shows the promise of machine learning methods, notably DNNs, for correctly diagnosing brain cancers from MRI data. This may have significant effects on how accurately and effectively brain tumor patients are diagnosed and treated.

6.6.1 Significance of the Study

Our study's importance stems from its potential to increase the precision and efficacy of brain tumor identification and therapy. We can deliver more precise and trustworthy diagnoses by classifying MRI images of brain tumors using machine learning algorithms, which may improve patient treatment outcomes.

References

1. El Kader, I.A., Xu, G., Shuai, Z., Saminu, S., Javaid, I., Ahmad, I.S., Kamhi, S., Brain Tumor Detection and Classification on MR Images by a Deep Wavelet Auto-Encoder Model. *Diagnostics*, 11, 1589, 2021.
2. Benkhaddra, I., Kumar, A., Setitra, M.A. *et al.*, Design and Development of Consensus Activation Function Enabled Neural Network-Based Smart Healthcare Using BIoT. *Wirel. Pers. Commun.*, 130, 1549–1574, 2023, https://doi.org/10.1007/s11277-023-10344-0 Q2,Impact Factor -2.017.
3. Srivastav, A.L., Markandeya, Patel, N. *et al.*, Concepts of circular economy for sustainable management of electronic wastes: challenges and management options. *Environ. Sci. Pollut. Res.*, 30, 48654–48675, 2023. https://doi.org/10.1007/s11356-023-26052-y Q1,Impact Factor -5.19.
4. Ilyas, B., Kumar, A., Setitra, M.A., Bensalem, Z.E.A., Lei, H., Prevention of DDoS attacks using an optimized deep learning approach in blockchain technology. *Trans. Emerging Telecommun. Technol.*, 34, 4, e4729, 2023. Q2,Impact Factor -3.31.

5. Kumar, A., Rathore, P.S., Dubey, A.K., Agrawal, R., Sharma, K.P., LTE-NBP with holistic UWB-WBAN approach for the energy efficient biomedical application. *Multimed. Tools Appl.*, 82, 25, 39797–39811, 2023.
6. Kumar, A., Kumar, S.A., Dutt, V., Shitharth, S., Tripathi, E., IoT based arrhythmia classification using the enhanced hunt optimization-based deep learning. *Expert Syst.*, 40, 7, e13298, 2023.
7. Bhargava, N., Rathore, P.S., Bhowmick, A., Study of X Ray Detection Using CNN in Machine Learning. *Advancements in Smart Computing and Information Security: First International Conference, ASCIS 2022*, Rajkot, India, November 24–26, 2022, Cham: Springer Nature, Switzerland, Revised Selected Papers, Part I, 2023.
8. Pooya, M., Yousefi, S., Amgad, M., Gutman, D.A., Barnholtz-Sloan, J.S., Velázquez Vega, J.E., Brat, D.J., Cooper, L.A.D., Predicting cancer outcomes from histology and genomics using convolutional networks. *Proceedings of the National Academy of Sciences*, vol. 115, pp. E2970–E2979, 2018.
9. Shboul, Z.A., Alam, M., Vidyaratne, L., Pei, L., Elbakary, M., II, Iftekharuddin, K.M., Feature-guided deep radiomics for glioblastoma patient survival prediction. *Front. Neurosci.*, 13, 966, 2019.
10. Saraswathi, V., Jamthikar, A.D., Gupta, D., CNN and RF Based Classification of Brain Tumors in MR Neurological Images, in: *Computer Vision and Image Processing: 4th International Conference, CVIP 2019, Jaipur, India, September 27–29, 2019, Revised Selected Papers, Part I*, 2020, March, Springer, Singapore, pp. 123–133.
11. Pugalenthi, R., Rajakumar, M.P., Ramya, J., Rajinikanth, V., Evaluation and classification of the brain tumor MRI using machine learning technique. *J. Control. Eng. Appl. Inform.*, 21, 4, 12–21, 2019.
12. Havaei, M., Davy, A., Warde-Farley, D., Biard, A., Courville, A., Bengio, Y., Pal, C., Jodoin, P.-M., Larochelle, H., Brain tumor segmentation with deep neural networks. *Med. Image Anal.*, 35, 18–31, 2017.
13. Çınarer, G., Emiroğlu, B.G., Arslan, R.S., Yurttakal, A.H., Brain tumor classification using deep neural network. *Adv. Sci. Technol. Eng. Syst. J.*, 5, 5, 765–769, 2020.
14. Kotturu, P.K. and Kumar, A., Comparative Study on Machine Learning models for Early Diagnose of Alzheimer's Disease: Multi Correlation Method. *2020 5th International Conference on Communication and Electronics Systems (ICCES)*, pp. 778–783, 2020, doi: 10.1109/ICCES48766.2020.9137872.
15. Swarna, S.R., Kumar, A., Dixit, P., Sairam, T.V.M., Parkinson's Disease Prediction using Adaptive Quantum Computing. *2021 Third International Conference on Intelligent Communication Technologies and Virtual Mobile Networks (ICICV)*, pp. 1396–1401, 2021, doi: 10.1109/ICICV50876.2021.9388628.
16. Bhuvaji, S., Kadam, A., Bhumkar, P., Dedge, S., Kanchan, S., Brain Tumor Classification (MRI)| Kaggle, 2020.

17. Biratu, E.S., Schwenker, F., Ayano, Y.M., Debelee, T.G., A survey of brain tumor segmentation and classification algorithms. *J. Imaging*, 7, 9, 179, 2021.
18. Kotturu, P.K. and Kumar, A., Comparative Study on Machine Learning models for Early Diagnose of Alzheimer's Disease: Multi Correlation Method. *2020 5th International Conference on Communication and Electronics Systems (ICCES)*, pp. 778–783, 2020, doi: 10.1109/ICCES48766.2020.9137872.
19. Bhargava, N., Sharma, S., Purohit, R., Rathore, P.S., Prediction of recurrence cancer using J48 algorithm, in: *2017 2nd International Conference on Communication and Electronics Systems (ICCES)*, pp. 386–390, IEEE, 2017, October.
20. Swarna, S.R., Kumar, A., Dixit, P., Sairam, T.V.M., Parkinson's Disease Prediction using Adaptive Quantum Computing. *2021 Third International Conference on Intelligent Communication Technologies and Virtual Mobile Networks (ICICV)*, pp. 1396–1401, 2021, doi: 10.1109/ICICV50876.2021.9388628.

7

Exploring the Potential of Dingo Optimizer: A Promising New Metaheuristic Approach

Anju Yadav and Vivek Kumar Verma*

Dept. of IT, Manipal University Jaipur, Jaipur, India

Abstract
A newly created metaheuristic algorithm called the dingo optimizer draws its ideas from the behaviors and feeding habits of dingoes in the wild. When using classic optimization techniques to solve complex optimization issues, this approach excels. The program uses a series of mathematical equations that simulate dingo behavior in the wild to find the best solutions to a variety of optimization challenges. The dingo optimizer has demonstrated promising results in several applications, including engineering design, financial forecasting, and bioinformatics. The algorithm is rather simple to implement and has the potential to be a useful tool for researchers and practitioners in a wide range of domains.

Keywords: Dingo optimized, genetic algorithm, particle swarm optimization

7.1 Introduction

Dingo Optimizer is a new metaheuristic algorithm that has gained significant attention from researchers and practitioners in recent years. The program, which is based on dingo behavior in the wild, has demonstrated promising results in handling challenging optimization problems that are outside the scope of more conventional approaches. Dingo Optimizer is a metaheuristic algorithm that has shown great potential in solving complex optimization problems [1–3]. While the algorithm has its limitations, it has

**Corresponding author*: vermavivek123@gmail.com

Sumit Srivastava, Abhineet Anand, Abhishek Kumar, Bhavna Saini and Pramod Singh Rathore (eds.) Bio-Inspired Optimization for Medical Data Mining, (141–154)

already demonstrated its effectiveness in various applications. The Dingo Optimizer could become a valuable tool for researchers and practitioners in many fields, and its further development and optimization are worth pursuing [4].

The Dingo Optimizer algorithm uses a set of mathematical equations that model the social and foraging behavior of dingoes. It mimics the behavior of a pack of dingoes, where each dingo represents a potential solution to the optimization problem, and the pack represents the population of solutions. The algorithm uses a set of search operators, such as mutation, crossover, and selection, to explore the search space and find the optimal solution [5].

Despite its promising results, the Dingo Optimizer has some limitations that researchers should be aware of. The algorithm may struggle with optimization problems that have many variables or constraints, as it may take a long time to explore the search space fully. Additionally, the algorithm may suffer from premature convergence, where it converges to a suboptimal solution too quickly.

7.2 Architecture of Dingo Optimizer

The Dingo Optimizer algorithm's architecture is built on a system of equations that simulate the social and foraging behavior of dingoes in the wild. The positions and velocities of every dingo in the population are updated using these equations. To explore the search space and identify the best solution, the algorithm employs a variety of search operators, including mutation, crossover, and selection. A metaheuristic algorithm called the Dingo Optimizer was developed after studying the behavior of dingoes in the wild. The program searches for the best answer to a given optimization issue using a population-based approach. The population in the Dingo Optimizer algorithm represents a pack of dingoes, where each dingo corresponds to a potential solution to the optimization problem.

Initialization, iteration, and termination are the three primary phases of the Dingo Optimizer algorithm. The population of dingoes is randomly initialized during the initialization phase, and each dingo's fitness is assessed. Based on the mathematical equations that simulate the behavior of dingoes, the method updates each dingo's position and velocity during the iteration phase. To explore the search space and identify the best solution, the search operators are applied to the population. Up until the stopping criterion, such as the maximum number of iterations or obtaining a

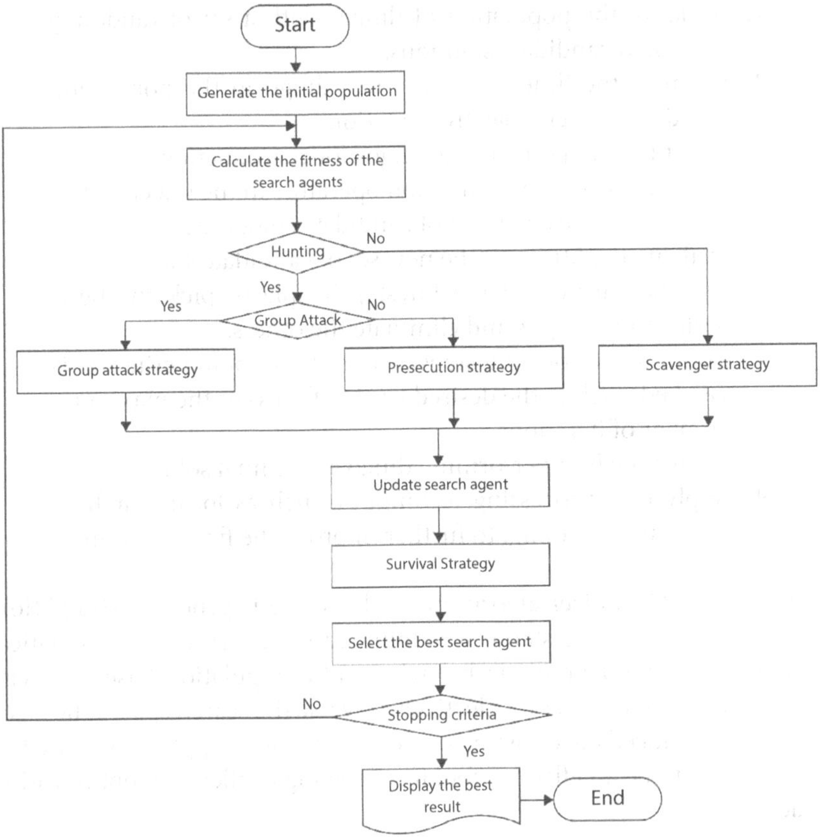

Figure 7.1 Dingo optimizer algorithm's flowchart [6].

certain fitness value, is satisfied, the iteration phase continues. The method then returns the best answer discovered during the iteration phase during the termination phase shown in Figure 7.1 Dingo optimizer algorithm's flowchart [6, 7].

Dingo optimizer effectively explores the search space and identifies high-quality solutions by combining global and local search algorithms, which are both models for Dingos' hunting behavior. Iteratively choosing and improving the best-performing solutions until a satisfying solution is identified entails creating a diverse population of candidate solutions, assessing their fitness, then selecting and improving them repeatedly. Numerous optimization issues, including those with non-linear and non-convex objective functions, have demonstrated the optimizer's effectiveness. The workflow of the architecture of the Dingo optimizer:

1. Initialize the population of dingos with a set of randomly generated candidate solutions.
2. Estimate the fitness of every one dingo in the population based on a given objective function.
3. Select the top performing dingos for reproduction.
4. Apply crossover and mutation operators to the selected dingos to generate a new set of candidate solutions.
5. Evaluate the fitness of the new set of candidate solutions.
6. Use the survival of the fittest principle to pick the best-performing dingo's and eliminate the others.
7. Continue performing steps 3-6 until a stopping criterion is satisfied, such as the desired level of fitness or the maximum number of iterations.
8. Return the best performing dingo as the final solution.
9. Apply post-processing techniques, such as local search or constraint handling, to further improve the final solution.

The Dingo Optimizer algorithm's architecture is generally straightforward and easy to understand. It is founded on a series of mathematical equations that simulate dingo behavior and a population-based strategy that enables the computer to effectively traverse the search space. The algorithm has produced encouraging outcomes in several applications and has the potential to be an effective tool for resolving challenging optimization issues [8–10].

7.3 Initialization Process

When using the Dingo Optimizer algorithm to optimize a problem, the first step is called the initialization process. During this phase, a group of dingoes is randomly chosen, and their individual abilities are assessed.

7.3.1 Population Size

The population size determines the number of dingoes in the population. Typically, the population size is set to a value between 10 and 50, depending on the complexity of the optimization problem [9]. This process is important because it sets the foundation for the optimization process that follows. The population size of the dingoes is a key factor in this phase, with a typical range between 10 and 50, depending on how complicated the optimization problem is. The Dingo optimizer's architecture heavily depends on population size. The population size controls how many potential solutions are considered and enhanced throughout each iteration of the optimizer [11]. A greater population size can improve search space exploration but can also raise the algorithm's processing time and memory needs. In general, a greater population size can aid the Dingo optimizer in completely examining the search space and avoiding becoming stuck in local optima. This is since a bigger population size offers a wider variety of candidate solutions and raises the likelihood of finding superior solutions. However, a larger population size also requires more computational resources and may lead to longer running times. In practice, the optimal population size for a given optimization problem depends on various factors, such as the complexity of the problem, the desired level of accuracy, and the available computational resources. Therefore, the population size should be chosen carefully to balance the benefits of increased diversity with the cost of increased computational requirements. In general, larger population sizes are recommended for more complex optimization problems with a larger search space, while smaller population sizes may be sufficient for simpler problems. However, the optimal population size should be determined empirically through experimentation and testing on the specific problem being solved [12].

7.3.2 Dingo Population Initialization

Each dingo in the population is a potential answer to the optimization issue. Within the search space, which is determined by the task restrictions, each dingo is initially placed at a random location. In the architecture of the Dingo Optimizer, the population initialization step involves generating an initial population of candidate solutions or dingos. The population initialization step is an important part of the optimizer because the quality and diversity of the initial population can greatly affect the performance of the algorithm [13].

There are different methods for initializing the population of dingos in the Dingo optimizer. One common approach is to generate the initial population randomly using a uniform distribution. This involves randomly generating a set of candidate solutions within the defined search space of the optimization problem. The user commonly specifies the number of dingoes in the starting population, which depends on the difficulty of the optimization problem and the available processing power. The generation of an initial collection of potential solutions using heuristic methods like local search or clustering is another method for population initialization. By utilizing the issue structure and condensing the search space, these strategies can give the optimization process a better place to start. Additionally, the Dingo optimizer has the ability to apply adaptive population initialization methods, which modify the population's size and makeup as the optimization process advances. For example, if the algorithm is struggling to find high-quality solutions, the population size can be increased to allow for more exploration of the search space. The choice of population initialization method depends on the nature of the optimization problem and the available resources. It is important to ensure that the initial population is diverse and representative of the search space to maximize the chances of finding high-quality solutions [14, 15].

7.3.3 Fitness Assessment

Each dingo's position is initialized, and then its fitness is determined. The optimization problem determines the definition of the fitness function, which measures how well the solution satisfies the objective function. A crucial component of the Dingo Optimizer's architecture is fitness assessment. In this stage, the fitness function that reflects the goal of the optimization issue is used to assess the quality of each potential solution in the population. The fitness function evaluates how well a given solution meets the criteria and goals of the challenge.

The fitness function is specific to the optimization problem being solved and is defined by the user. The goal of the Dingo optimizer is to find the candidate solution with the highest fitness value, which represents the optimal solution to the problem. In the fitness assessment process, each candidate solution in the population is assessed for fitness. Applying the fitness function to each answer and giving it a fitness score will do this. The potential solutions in the population are then ranked using fitness scores, with higher fitness ratings suggesting superior solutions. Following the fitness evaluation stage, the Dingo optimizer can select the top candidate solutions for the following generation using a variety of selection techniques. The optimizer may, for instance, employ tournament selection, where pairs of candidate solutions are compared and the most appropriate one is chosen for replication. Alternatively, the optimizer can use roulette wheel selection, where candidate solutions are selected with a probability proportional to their fitness score. The fitness assessment step is crucial for the success of the Dingo optimizer, as it determines which candidate solutions are more likely to lead to optimal solutions for the given optimization problem. The choice of fitness function and selection method can greatly impact the performance and convergence rate of the algorithm [16].

7.3.4 Best Dingo

After each dingo's fitness has been evaluated, the best dingo in the population is selected based on fitness value. The top dingo displays the best optimization solution to the situation at hand. The Best Dingo denotes the best solution to the current optimization problem, and finding this solution is the optimizer's goal. By applying the fitness function to each candidate solution in the population and assigning a fitness score to each, the fitness evaluation stage determines The Best Dingo. The candidate solution with the highest fitness score is then identified as The Best Dingo [17].

Once the Best Dingo is identified, it can be used as the basis for the next generation of candidate solutions. The Best Dingo can be copied directly into the next generation, or it can be used to guide the search for new candidate solutions. The Best Dingo, for instance, might be utilized as a starting point for mutation or crossover operations, in which new candidate solutions are created based on the Best Dingo's traits. The Best Dingo is crucial to the Dingo Optimizer because it represents the most promising answer to the optimization problem and acts as a standard against which to measure the algorithm's effectiveness. The effectiveness of the selection and reproduction operators, as well as the algorithm's capacity for exploration and exploitation, all affect the quality of the Best Dingo that the optimizer finds. The Best Dingo is the candidate solution with the highest fitness value in the population, and it is the goal of the Dingo optimizer to find this solution. The Best Dingo plays a critical role in guiding the search for optimal solutions and evaluating the performance of the algorithm [18].

7.3.5 Recordkeeping

The initialization procedure also includes keeping track of significant variables, like the number of iterations, fitness value, and best solution so far. Recordkeeping in the Dingo Optimizer's architecture refers to the procedure of monitoring the effectiveness and development of the optimization algorithm. To monitor and analyze the behavior of the algorithm and to make decisions regarding its design and parameters, recordkeeping is an essential component of the Dingo Optimizer.

There are several types of records that can be kept during the execution of the Dingo Optimizer, including:

(i) *Fitness records:* These records track the Best Dingo's and other candidate solutions' fitness ratings over time. The user can evaluate the convergence and stability of the optimization process and spot any potential problems or abnormalities by examining the fitness records.

(ii) Parameter records: These logs keep track of the population size, mutation rate, and crossover rate, among other parameter values utilized by the optimization technique. The user can determine which parameter values are most effective for the specific optimization problem by examining the parameter records and then updating the parameters as necessary.

(iii) Search records: These records document the algorithm's search history, including the generated and assessed candidate solutions, the methods utilized for selection and reproduction, and the mutation and crossover operations carried out. The user can learn more about the algorithm's search behavior and spot areas for development by examining the search records.

(iv) Statistical records: The mean and standard deviation of the fitness values, the variety of the potential solutions, and the needed calculation time are just a few examples of the statistical metrics that are tracked in these records as they relate to the algorithm's performance. The user can evaluate the algorithm's efficacy and efficiency and contrast it with other optimization algorithms by examining the statistical data.

Because it gives the user useful information on the behavior and effectiveness of the optimization process, recordkeeping is a crucial part of the Dingo Optimizer design. The user can identify problems and places for improvement, adjust the settings and configuration of the algorithm, and finally get better optimization outcomes by analyzing the numerous records [19].

In the iteration phase, which follows the startup phase, the Dingo Optimizer algorithm modifies each dingo's position and velocity in line with the mathematical equations that describe the behavior of dingos. The population is subjected to the search operators to investigate the search space and determine the optimum solution.

7.4 Iteration Phase

The Dingo Optimizer algorithm's iteration phase is where optimization takes place. Using mathematical equations that simulate dingo behavior, the system changes each dingo's position and velocity during this stage. To explore the search space and identify the best solution, the search operators are applied to the population.

The iteration phase of the Dingo Optimizer algorithm is described in the details below:

(i) Movement Equations: The movement equations are used to update the position and velocity of each dingo in the population. The movement equations are based on the social and foraging behavior of dingoes in the wild and are designed to simulate the search behavior of the pack.

(ii) Search Operators: The dingo optimizer is a new metaheuristic algorithm that is inspired by the social and foraging behavior of dingoes in the wild. This algorithm is especially well suited for handling challenging optimization issues where conventional optimization approaches fail. The program bases its search for the best solutions to a variety of optimization issues on a set of mathematical equations that simulate the behavior of dingoes in the wild. Engineering design, financial forecasting, and bioinformatics are just a few of the fields where the dingo optimizer has demonstrated promising results. The algorithm can potentially be a useful tool for researchers and practitioners in many domains, and it is reasonably simple to implement.

(iii) Termination process: The Dingo Optimizer algorithm's termination process marks the end of the optimization process. During this stage, the algorithm determines whether the halting requirement has been satisfied and, if so, ends the optimization process [11].

The Dingo Optimizer algorithm's termination mechanism is described in the details below:

Stopping Criterion: The optimization procedure should end when the stopping requirement is satisfied. This criterion is frequently based on completing the most iterations or getting to a certain fitness level. At the conclusion of each iteration, the algorithm verifies the halting criterion.

Solution Extraction: Once the optimization process has terminated, the best solution found during the optimization process is extracted. This solution represents the optimal solution to the optimization problem.

Post-Processing: After the best solution is extracted, post-processing steps can be applied to further improve the solution quality. These post-processing steps can include local search or refinement procedures.
Recordkeeping: The termination procedure entails maintaining records of significant variables, including the best solution discovered, the fitness value of the best solution, and the number of iterations at which the optimization process came to an end.

The optimization process is ensured to end when the stopping criterion is satisfied by the termination process, which also ensures that the best solution discovered during the optimization phase is extracted. When more iterations won't increase the quality of the solution, the algorithm can end the optimization process by employing a stopping criterion, which conserves computational time and resources.

7.6 Other Optimization Techniques

There are several optimization techniques that are like the Dingo Optimizer metaheuristic algorithm in terms of their approach to solving optimization problems. Some of these techniques include:

Particle Swarm Optimization (PSO): PSO is a population-based optimization algorithm that searches the solution space using a swarm of particles. Like the Dingo Optimizer, PSO adjusts each particle's position and velocity in accordance with mathematical equations that simulate swarm behavior. It also utilizes a fitness function to assess the quality of solutions.
Genetic Algorithm (GA): A population of potential solutions is used by the genetically inspired optimization algorithm (GA) to search the solution space. To produce new candidate solutions and raise the standard of the population, GA makes use of genetic operators including mutation, crossover, and selection. Like the Dingo Optimizer, GA iteratively improves the population while evaluating the quality of solutions using a fitness function.
Ant Colony Optimization (ACO): An ant colony is used by the population-based optimization method ACO to search the solution space. Like the Dingo Optimizer, ACO iteratively improves the population while evaluating the quality of solutions using a fitness function. ACO updates the solutions and uses pheromone trails to direct the search for the ants.
Artificial Bee Colony (ABC): A colony of bees is used by the population-based optimization algorithm ABC to comb through the possible solutions. Like the Dingo Optimizer, ABC evaluates solution quality using

a fitness function before iteratively enhancing the population. To carry out various search activities, ABC employs a variety of bees, including hired bees, spectator bees, and scout bees.

7.7 Conclusion

These optimization methods leverage a population of potential solutions, much like the Dingo Optimizer, and iteratively improve the population using mathematical equations or operators. Each technique, however, has distinctive qualities that make it appropriate for optimization issues. As you may know, the Dingo Optimizer is a metaheuristic optimization algorithm inspired by the foraging behavior of dingoes, and it has been shown to be highly effective for a wide range of optimization problems. In particular, the Dingo Optimizer algorithm has several key advantages that make it an excellent choice for many applications. First, it is highly flexible and can be easily customized to suit the specific requirements of your optimization problem. Second, it is very efficient and can quickly converge on high-quality solutions even for large-scale problems. Finally, it is well suited to multi-objective optimization problems and can help you find optimal trade-offs between competing objectives.

Based on this review on Dingo Optimizer, it would be a great fit for any optimization needs. The algorithm has been successfully applied to a wide range of applications, including engineering design, machine learning, and financial modeling, among others.

References

1. Peraza-Vázquez, H., Peña-Delgado, A.F., Echavarría-Castillo, G., Morales-Cepeda, A.B., Velasco-Álvarez, J., Ruiz-Perez, F., A bio-inspired method for engineering design optimization inspired by dingoes hunting strategies. *Math. Probl. Eng.*, 2021, 1–19, 2021.
2. Ayanlade, S.O., Jimoh, A., Ogunwole, E., II, Aremu, A., Jimoh, A.B., Owolabi, D.E., Simultaneous network reconfiguration and capacitor allocations using a novel dingo optimization algorithm. *Int. J. Electr. Comput. Eng.*, 13, 3, 2384–2395, 2023.
3. Crane, R. and Roosta, F., DINGO: Distributed Newton-type method for gradient-norm optimization. *Adv. Neural Inf. Process. Syst.*, 32, 1–11, 2019.
4. Benkhaddra, I., Kumar, A., Setitra, M.A. *et al.*, Design and Development of Consensus Activation Function Enabled Neural Network-Based Smart

Healthcare Using BIoT. *Wirel. Pers. Commun.*, 130, 1549–1574, 2023, https://doi.org/10.1007/s11277-023-10344-0 Q2,Impact Factor -2.017.

5. Srivastav, A.L., Markandeya, Patel, N. *et al.*, Concepts of circular economy for sustainable management of electronic wastes: challenges and management options. *Environ. Sci. Pollut. Res.*, 30, 48654–48675, 2023, https://doi.org/10.1007/s11356-023-26052-y Q1,Impact Factor -5.19.
6. Ilyas, B., Kumar, A., Setitra, M.A., Bensalem, Z.E.A., Lei, H., Prevention of DDoS attacks using an optimized deep learning approach in blockchain technology. *Trans. Emerging Telecommun. Technol.*, 34, 4, e4729, 2023, Q2,Impact Factor -3.31.
7. Kumar, A., Rathore, P.S., Dubey, A.K. *et al.*, LTE-NBP with holistic UWB-WBAN approach for the energy efficient biomedical application. *Multimed. Tools Appl.*, 82, 25, 39797–39811, 2023, https://doi.org/10.1007/s11042-023-15604-6 Q1,Impact Factor -2.577.
8. Kumar, A., Kumar, S.A., Dutt, V., Shitharth, S., Tripathi, E., IoT based arrhythmia classification using the enhanced hunt optimization-based deep learning. *Expert Syst.*, 40, 7, e13298, 2023, n. pag. Q2, Impact Factor -2.812.
9. Sasubilli, G. and Kumar, A., Machine Learning and Big Data Implementation on Health Care data. *4th International Conference on Intelligent Computing and Control Systems (ICICCS)*, pp. 859–864, 2020, doi: 10.1109/ICICCS48265.2020.9120906.
10. Bhargava, N., Rathore, P.S., Bhowmick, A., Study of X Ray Detection Using CNN in Machine Learning. *Advancements in Smart Computing and Information Security: First International Conference, ASCIS 2022*, Rajkot, India, November 24 -26, 2022, Cham: Springer Nature, Switzerland, 2023, Revised Selected Papers, Part I.
11. Sasubilli, S.M., Kumar, A., Dutt, V., Machine Learning Implementation on Medical Domain to Identify Disease Insights using TMS. *2020 International Conference on Advances in Computing and Communication Engineering (ICACCE)*, pp. 1–4, 2020, doi: 10.1109/ICACCE49060.2020.9154960.
12. Bhargava, N., Dayma, S., Kumar, A., Singh, P., An approach for classification using simple CART algorithm in WEKA, in: *2017 11th International Conference on Intelligent Systems and Control (ISCO)*, pp. 212–216, IEEE, 2017, January.
13. Dutt, V., Rathore, P.S., Chauhan, K., Support Vector in Healthcare Using SVM/PSO in Various Domains: A Review, in: *Swarm Intelligence Optimization: Algorithms and Applications*, pp. 291–307, 2020.
14. Bhargava, N., Sharma, S., Purohit, R., Rathore, P.S., Prediction of recurrence cancer using J48 algorithm, in: *2017 2nd International Conference on Communication and Electronics Systems (ICCES)*, pp. 386–390, IEEE, 2017, October.
15. Singh, B., Singla, M.K., Nijhawan, P., Parameter estimation of four diode solar photovoltaic cell using hybrid algorithm. *Energy Sources Part A*, 44, 2, 4597–4613, 2022.

16. Bhargava, P.N., Rathore, P.S., Vaishnav, P., Rai, M., Utilizing artificial neural networks and multivariate patient data for anemia detection using WEKA based approach for diagnosis. *2023 2nd International Conference on Automation, Computing and Renewable Systems (ICACRS)*, Pudukkottai, India, pp. 643–648, 2023. doi: 10.1109/ICACRS58579.2023.10404355.
17. Milenković, B., Jovanović, Đ., Krstić, M., An application of Dingo Optimization Algorithm (DOA) for solving continuous engineering problems. *FME Trans.*, 50, 2, 331–338, 2022.
18. Cao, S., Qian, Q., Cao, Y., Li, W., Huang, W., Liang, J., A Novel Meta-heuristic Algorithm for Numerical and Engineering Optimization Problems: Piranha Foraging Optimization Algorithm (PFOA). *IEEE Access*, 2023.

8

Bioinspired Genetic Algorithm in Medical Applications

Krati Taksali[1*], Arpit Kumar Sharma[2] and Manish Rai[3]

[1]*JECRC University, Jaipur, India*

[2]*Department of Computer and Communication Engineering, Manipal University Jaipur, Jaipur, India*

[3]*Department of Computer Science and Engineering (AI&ML), Manipal University Jaipur, Jaipur, India*

Abstract

A wealth of knowledge is concealed in the centre of medical research data because some implications cannot be quickly or even at all analyzed using a traditional statistical approach. With nature as inspiration, algorithms using metaheuristics have been introduced to provide, in a reasonable amount of time, optimal or nearly optimal responses for challenging data analysis and decision-making activities. Due to their potent quality, metaheuristic algorithms have been repeatedly utilized in numerous scientific disciplines. In medicine, however, due to their robust quality, metaheuristic methods have been extensively utilized in numerous scientific disciplines. Therefore, in this chapter, we will talk about how genetic algorithms can be applied to the field of medicine. In addition to pharmacotherapy, radiology, surgery, cardiology radiotherapy, pediatrics, endocrinology, obstetrics, and gynecology, pulmonary medicine, orthopedics, rehabilitation medicine, neurology, infectious diseases, and health care administration have all found promising applications for the genetic algorithm. In this article, we explained the genetic algorithm and how it may be used in healthcare administration, disease detection, treatment planning, drug safety monitoring, prognosis, and more. It also aids doctors in envisioning the future applications of this metaheuristic technique in healthcare.

***Keywords*:** Algorithms, GA genetic algorithm, optimization, heuristic methods, medical practitioner, medicine

**Corresponding author*: kratitaksali05@gmail.com

Sumit Srivastava, Abhineet Anand, Abhishek Kumar, Bhavna Saini and Pramod Singh Rathore (eds.) Bio-Inspired Optimization for Medical Data Mining, (155–168) © 2024 Scrivener Publishing LLC

8.1 Introduction

IT (computer systems) has undeniably improved every aspect of our lives. Astronomy, humology, chemistry, physics, math, history, geography, archaeology, computer engineering, and the sociological sciences all rely heavily on them and benefit significantly from them.

Many medical devices used for diagnosis, imaging, monitoring, and therapy are based on electronic chips and computers. Software, built using established approaches, manages, and controls these gadgets. An algorithm is an ensemble of guidelines that outline how a task is to be carried out. Metaheuristic algorithms may speedily solve complicated problems or discover a near approximation when standard approaches cannot [1].

There are a lot of metaheuristic algorithms out there that can help us get closer to the optimal solution. The Grey Wolf Optimizer is an algorithm that was inspired by the behaviour of grey wolves; artificial immune systems were inspired by the function of the immune system; river formation dynamics were inspired by the process of river formation; and genetic algorithms were inspired by genetic mechanisms [2].

Metaheuristic algorithms are often employed in many scientific fields to tackle difficult problems or find the best solution. While significant progress has been made in the medical industry, the full potential of these formidable algorithms to help doctors overcome the myriad of complex difficulties they encounter every day has yet to be tapped.

Here, we provide an overview of one such metaheuristic, the genetic algorithm (GA), and talk about its uses in medicine [3].

Literature Survey

Study of related work and all previously discussed work are summarized in Table 8.1 below.

Table 8.1 Study of related work.

Year	Title	Approach	Advantages	Disadvantage
2014	"A hybrid bioinspired genetic algorithm for medical diagnosis"	Hybrid approach combining genetic algorithm and neural network	Improved accuracy in medical diagnosis	Time-consuming

(Continued)

Table 8.1 Study of related work. (*Continued*)

Year	Title	Approach	Advantages	Disadvantage
2015	"Genetic algorithm-based feature selection for medical diagnosis using microarray data"	Genetic algorithm for feature selection	Improved accuracy and reduced complexity	High computational cost
2016	"Optimization of medical diagnosis using genetic algorithms: a review"	Review article of genetic algorithm in medical diagnosis	Comprehensive overview of genetic algorithm in medical diagnosis	No new experimental results presented
2017	"A novel bioinspired genetic algorithm for medical image segmentation"	A genetic algorithm with bioinspired design for medical image segmentation	Improved accuracy in medical image segmentation	Time-consuming
2018	"A hybrid bioinspired algorithm for medical image registration"	Particulate swarm optimization and genetic algorithms used in a hybrid method for medical image registration	Improved accuracy in medical image registration	Time-consuming

8.2 The Genetic Algorithm

A genetic algorithm is an approach encouraged by genetic rules that searches for workable answers to intractable problems. First, a small number of solutions (people) are drawn at random, and they all have different sets of genes. Chromosomal exchange and mutations, according to genetic theory, produce offspring with a wider range of characteristics.

Crossover and mutation are the two primary means by which people are altered. Crossover occurs between two selected attributes. Adjacent, a crossover point is selected adjacent to each property, and the values are transferred between the chromosomes up to that point. A new generation is born from these two newly created chromosomes. If more than one kind of person is needed to solve a problem, the crossover procedure will be repeated until that happens. The mutation further leads to the formation of new clusters as a consequence of the introduction of random modifications

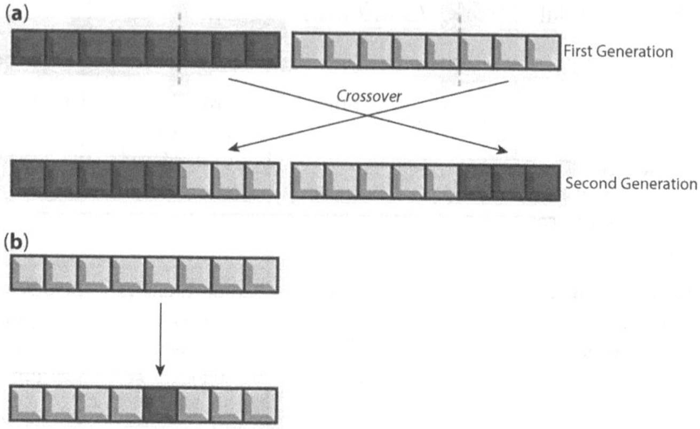

Figure 8.1 Steps for genetic algorithm.

to multiple chromosomes. Figure 8.1 displays one of the fundamental mutation techniques [4].

In a genetic algorithm, the power of the solitary influences the chances of reproduction. Based on the kind or version of chromosome (i.e., those with better qualities), they decided to breed the following generation. There are multiple methods of choice that can be used to rank individuals according to their fitness levels and choose the fittest. Genetic modification occurs through mutations and crossovers to create new generations. This cycle will continue until the strongest person emerges, the best result is found, or the top generation is reached [5, 6].

It is essential to keep in mind that GA differs from derivative-based optimization techniques. First, compared to traditional derivative-based approaches, GAs seeks several points in the solution space throughout each iteration.

Here, we will discuss a few of the ways GAs are now being put to use in a variety of medical settings [7].

8.3 Radiology

Radiologists must quickly review and interpret an enormous amount of data as an outcome of the imaging approach used in radiology. With the objective of facilitating speedy and accurate image analysis by radiologists via the surveillance, categorization, and classification of usual and chronic patterns found on numerous imaging modalities, the field of computer-aided identification and diagnostics is quickly increasing. Imaging techniques such as MRI, CT scans, and X-rays are also available.

A relevant picture is acquired, generated, and simplified in machine vision, such as biological organs or regions in a radiological image. It is necessary to define an object's shape (boundaries) and dimension before looking at it in greater detail. As a result, edge detection training becomes one of the fundamental components of the auto-image processing technique. Many scholars have employed GAs to obtain the edges of pictures taken using various imaging modalities, such as MRI, CT, and ultrasound. The most effective way for detecting breast cancer remains screening mammography, although researchers have attempted to enhance the system's sensitivity via computational techniques. Truly, the bulk of GA applications in radiology have been examined and assessed primarily using mammography [8].

Karnan and Thangavel used genetic algorithms to find micro-classifications in mammograms for breast cancer. In this approach, the GA collected and improved the mammograms before identifying the location of the nipple and the breast boundary. The boundary and nipple positions of the left and right breasts were used as a reference (left and right) to align the mammography images and subtract from one another to identify the contradictory visual clue that breast cancer is present. The A-Z value, or the receiver operating characteristic (ROC) curve's area under, is a common metric used to evaluate a diagnostic system's efficacy. Their proposed method has an Az value of about 0.9 [9].

Subsequent studies conducted by Pereira *et al.* used a variety of computational techniques for mammography partitioning to improve imaging-based breast cancer detection. To prevent artefacts from remaining after blurring and enhancing a picture, an algorithm was created. The distribution and monitoring of wobbly zones were made 95% sensitive by regularly combining wavelet analysis with the GA. GAs have also been successfully used to distribute and observe clustered micro-classifications in digital mammograms.

Feature selection in machine learning is the method of picking variables with little to no analytical value from vital characteristics prior to utilizing them to build a model. The significance of feature selection is vital since selecting irrelevant traits makes computation more difficult, expensive, and time-consuming while also lowering model accuracy. In addition, fewer characteristics should be used to avoid overfitting, lessen the chance that the model will fail owing to missing data, and enhance the model's capacity to be explained and generalized.

Studies have used GA to make distinctions between benign and malignant tumors of the breast in ultrasound imaging as well as to determine whether a mammography region is normal or must have a lump.

A genetic algorithm was developed by De Carvalho Filho *et al.* to automatically recognize and classify solitary lung nodules. It is 98% accurate, 98% specific, and 86% vulnerable to lung nodules. Image fusion, additionally referred to as image combining, involves lining up two or more photos in a synchronized system. When important information is spread among multiple images taken under various conditions (viewpoint, sensor, or time), precise image integration becomes essential. Algorithms based on genetics have been used in a number of studies to align computed tomography (CT) and magnetic resonance imaging (MRI). In a subsequent study, MRI images and PET (positron emission tomography) images were combined using genetic algorithms to produce breast cancer images that are more colorful and simple to grasp.

Accurate tumor staging is essential for developing an effective treatment plan, which relies heavily on obtaining precise measurements of tumor volume and size through noninvasive imaging techniques. These methods have proven to be particularly effective in detecting and evaluating tongue cancer, allowing for more accurate assessments with reduced dependency on the operator, especially in the extraction of relevant data from magnetic resonance imaging (MRI) [10, 11].

8.4 Oncology

The most suitable option for detecting cancer in its early stages is a screening test, which, when correctly coupled with effective therapy, can increase patient survival rates.

Duraipandian *et al.* use colposcopy to capture Raman spectra from the collar region in order to enhance a noninvasive approach for collar cancer diagnosis. Raman spectroscopy's biomolecular data was analyzed using a genetic algorithm-partial minimum block-refined analytic method to identify characteristics of a normal vs. dysplastic cervix. Using the partial least squares (PLS) approach, it is possible to compute a linear regression model between a predictor and a dependent variable. The PLS approach is sensitive to the development of dysplasia in a normal cervix by 72% and specific to this change by 90%.

In the realm of molecular diagnosis and prognosis, DNA microarray technology has paved the way for enormous gene expression profiling. The creation of such massive data sets, however, makes it necessary to use statistical and analytical methods in order to isolate relevant prognostic genes.

The analysis of microarray data from different cancer cell lines has benefited from the use of genetic algorithms due to their intrinsic capacity to explore and select the ideal solution among several concurrent transactions and vast, complex possible solutions. By analyzing microarray data derived from breast cancer tissue with a variety of antibodies specific for distinct indicators, Dolled-Filhart *et al.* identify the smallest set of biomarkers with the highest classification and prognostication values in breast cancer patients. Genetic algorithms discovered that antibodies were created for three different causes.

Chinese women's death rates from cervical cancer were analyzed in research undertaken by Tan *et al.* The PLA/GA alloy was then used to select five of the 25 trace elements. Then the LSSVM model was introduced. The LSSVM is a machine learning technique for inferring functions and discovering patterns in training data. The findings show that the death rate from cervical cancer may be predicted using a combination of GA-PLS and LSSVM, which is built on trace elements.

Prognosis is a major factor in cancer patients' decisions on which treatment to pursue. In retrospective research including over 200 victims, Bozcuk *et al.* evaluated the performance of four data-mining algorithms for managing the results of nonterminal cancer patients after rehabilitation. In order to infer the patient's outcome, the Genetic Algorithm uses the two most minimal explanatory factors (lactate dehydrogenase and the cause of admission).

8.5 Endocrinology

For people with type 1 diabetes (T1DM), hypoglycemia is the most common problem with insulin treatment. Electroencephalograms (EEGs) may show different patterns if blood sugar levels drop too low. Nguyen *et al.* employed artificial neural networks (ANNs), genetic algorithms (GAs), and Levenberg-Marquardt (LM) training methods to detect hypoglycemia from EEG data. ANN was used to establish a connection between EEG readings and glucose levels in the blood. For the purpose of ANN training, the genetic algorithm's global search capacity was linked with the LM's local search capability. To detect low glucose levels, the research method used information from four EEG characteristics collected from two EEG channels, achieving an accuracy of 60% and a sensitivity of 75%. In a second study, researchers used a fuzzy inference method combined with multiple regression to identify noninvasive hypoglycemia episodes in kids with type 1 diabetes [12].

8.6 Obstetrics and Gynecology

Cervical abnormalities, both pre-cancerous and cancerous, may be detected using a cytology test called a Pap smear. Previously, a mechanism was developed to classify cells into one of seven groups based on the 20 traits that make them unique. To reduce the amount of features needed by a closest neighbor algorithm for classifying Pap smear findings, Marinakis *et al.* developed a hybrid model that used the capabilities of the Genetic Algorithm in this regard. The novel strategy fared better than other prior ways of splitting Pap smear data because it did so accurately.

Prenatal diagnostics also makes use of a genetic algorithm. Macrosomic fetuses are one predictor of labour difficulties. In an effort to identify babies that were too big or too little for their gestational age, capillary electrophoresis was used to analyse amniotic fluid collected during the second trimester. Bayesian statistics were used in the analysis of the data. The right wavelets (variables) of the electropherogram were selected using a GA in order to increase the speed of the Bayesian calculation. Using only two wavelets, one from albumin and one from an unidentified negatively charged tiny molecule, this system was able to distinguish LGA from AGA with 100% responsiveness and 98% accuracy [11].

Prenatal weight prediction might lessen risks for babies born with a low body mass index. Yu *et al.* used fuzzy logic with FSVR to make an estimate of the fetal weight. A genetic algorithm (GA)-based evolutionary FSVR was used to select the primary FSVR system components. When compared to a back-propagation neural network, this method achieves better accuracy in estimating the fetal birth weight (mean absolute error of 6.6%) and a higher correlation coefficient of 0.902.

8.7 Pediatrics

Low-cost and noninvasive, cardiotocography (CG) evaluates uterine contractions and fetal heart rate to assess maternal and fetal health. Ocak employed evolutionary algorithms to determine which details of CG data would be most useful in training an SVM classifier. The results demonstrated that the unique approach was more accurate than an ANN algorithm developed for the common purpose of determining whether a fetus was in a normal or pathological state, with accuracies of 99.3 and 100%, respectively.

Autism is a neurological disorder that initially manifests in childhood. It is distinguished from other mental disorders by repetitive behaviour, a reduction in verbal and nonverbal communication, and social functioning. Latkowski and Osowski employed algorithmic genetics to choose the most appropriate genes linked to the disease in order to identify autism based on the microarray gene expression data.

Acute lymphoblastic leukemia (ALL), a disease with numerous subtypes, is the most prevalent kind of leukemia in children. The examination of gene expression data gleaned from tumor cells can aid in the classification of malignancies. Because microarray gene expression profiling produces a large amount of data, Lin *et al.* used GA to select the most pertinent genes required for ALL categorization. The discriminating function of silhouette statistics was used to distinguish between all six kinds. In comparison to current techniques, the suggested technology used fewer differentiating genes and achieved 100% classification accuracy.

When there are more or fewer than the typically expected numbers of chromosomes in the nucleus of a cell, this is called aneuploidy. The precise diagnosis of fetal aneuploidy is performed by performing classical chromosomal examinations on amniocentesis materials; however, the relatively long turnaround times of conventional technologies require the advancement of faster diagnostic approaches. To do this, mass spectrometry was used to uncover bioinformatics profiles of the amniotic fluid sample, and GA was then used to analyse the retrieved data. For the detection of aneuploidy, the suggested method has a sensitivity of 100%, an accuracy of 72%–96%, a +ve predictive value of 11%–50%, and a -ve predictive value of 100%.

8.8 Surgery

Most mathematical methods that can assume system behaviour are ANNs. Since ANNs are thought to be useful, a GAN-based ANN (GANN) was developed to predict how well patients with NSCLC (non-small cell lung cancer) would do after surgery. To help with avoiding dead ends during optimization, we turned to the GA. The GANN model was able to predict an NSCLC patient's outcome than logistic regression more accurately and better. Incorporating tumor size into the equation also led to much more accurate predictions.

More and more elderly individuals will need coronary therapies in the future. Due to the significant incidence of comorbid illnesses in the young, it would be instructive to be able to accurately anticipate postoperative morbidity and death. This might help prevent unnecessary overestimation of risk and the denial of surgery to patients in need. By using GA, Lee *et al.* demonstrated that characteristics such as age, absence of beta blocker use history, cross-clamp duration, and absence of congestive heart failure were all linked with a shorter length of stay after cardiac surgery [12].

8.9 Infectious Diseases

Since the discovery of the human immunodeficiency virus (HIV), tuberculosis (TB) has spread over the world and become an almost universally lethal infectious disease, impacting both poor and developed countries alike. To make a diagnostic prediction (tuberculosis vs. nontuberculosis patients), an ANN trained by a GA used a set of 38 criteria comprised of examination parameters and lab data. When compared to results obtained from earlier algorithms, the method's classification accuracy of approximately 95% was much higher.

Using a simulation of the immune system, the effectiveness of anti-HIV drugs was evaluated in a computer-generated HIV patient. The new timeline for coordinated treatments may provide the same level of protection against opportunistic infections and therapeutic benefit as the longer therapy.

8.10 Radiotherapy

The need for rehabilitation for injuries is growing, so it makes sense to offer and test novel methods and instruments for therapy. It is tedious and costly to filter these new methodologies by changing numerous parameters and testing the resulting technologies on individuals. The creation of musculoskeletal models makes it possible to simulate movements on a computer and assess how new changes will affect the effectiveness of training. Pei *et al.* introduced a robotic approach for lower limb physiotherapy. Individual treatment plans were created for each patient using a genetic algorithm.

A therapeutic robot for lower limb exercise was also presented in another study. The hybrid ANN/GA architecture studied the physiotherapist's regimen for each patient and then replicated it when the therapist was not there.

8.11 Rehabilitation Medicine

The need for rehabilitation for injuries is growing, so it makes sense to offer and test novel methods and instruments for therapy. It is tedious and costly to filter these new methodologies by changing numerous parameters and testing the resulting technologies on individuals. The creation of musculoskeletal models makes it possible to simulate movements on a computer and assess how new changes will affect the effectiveness of training. Pei *et al.* introduced a robotic approach for lower limb physiotherapy. Individual treatment plans were created for each patient using a genetic algorithm.

A therapeutic robot for lower limb exercise was also presented in another study. The hybrid ANN/GA architecture studied the physiotherapist's regimen for each patient and then replicated it when the therapist was not there.

8.12 Neurology

Plaques in the white matter of the central nervous system are a hallmark of the severe inflammatory illness known as multiple sclerosis (MS). The pathologic features of these people have been determined with the use of CADI. In one finding, a GA was trained to spot MS lesions in brain MRIs. The GA- and radiologist-identified lesions had an 87% similarity score.

A useful diagnostic tool is the electroencephalogram (EEG), which may be used to analyse the abnormal electrical discharges in the brain that occur during seizures. To classify EEGs from epileptic and healthy individuals, an ANN was trained using many learning techniques (including LM, delta-bar delta, quickprop, momentum, and conjugate gradient). To find the best ANN build and settings, a genetic algorithm was used. The results indicated that a combination of the LM method and the GA had the highest success rate (96.5%).

Multiple investigations have pointed to mitochondrial dysfunction as a key contributor to Parkinson's disease. Due to the unique nature of mitochondrial genetics, a direct comparison of mitochondrial mutations in healthy and sick states may not provide useful information. Parkinson's disease patients often have mitochondrial mutations, and Smigrodzki *et al.* devised a GA to help find the most physiologically meaningful patterns. The suggested approach for diagnosing Parkinson's disease based on mitochondrial DNA mutation patterns was completely effective.

8.13 Health Care Management

Every healthcare system needs careful management of its money and people. Efficient patient admission scheduling may contribute to better patient care, satisfaction, and cost-effectiveness ratios. To enhance the effectiveness of patient scheduling at an ophthalmic institution, a mathematical model was developed and then refined using genetic algorithms.

When compared to the traditional "first come, first served" model, the advantages of the new approach were clear: a shorter waiting list, fewer empty hospital beds, shorter wait times before surgery, and a higher percentage of patients being released from the hospital after treatment. Combining GA with particle swarm optimization, another powerful metaheuristic algorithm, has been shown in recent research to improve patient scheduling, cut down on unnecessary wait times, and increase patient satisfaction.

Staff in a clinical workshop often move between locations, depending on their expertise, to ensure that their knowledge and abilities are maintained. Genetic algorithms have been applied to optimize the scheduling of staff shifts in a clinical lab. One study found that the GA-based software could save time and money on the scheduling process, better plan out staff rotation, guarantee the support of methods and talents, and be connected to the satisfaction of responsible supervisory staff.

8.14 Conclusion

In this chapter, we introduced genetic algorithms and discussed some of the ways they have been used in the medical field. Although genetic algorithms and other metaheuristics have their inspiration in biology, they are more often used by experts in other scientific fields to address tough issues. Medical practitioners and researchers greatly benefit from optimization methods due to the field's inherently complicated nature. This is due to two factors: first, a general unfamiliarity with complicated mathematical formulae among medical experts; and second, a lack of organized communication between computer scientists and doctors. The answer may lie in fostering more collaboration and dialogue amongst medical professionals, computer scientists, and engineers via means such as shared journal societies or attendance at doctor ground rounds and case report presentations. Nonmedical researchers may benefit from exposure to new viewpoints on medical difficulties via the creation of multidisciplinary courses and the involvement of engineering researchers in hospitals and health care settings.

References

1. Rajan, V. and Chaudhari, N.S., A survey of genetic algorithm applications in healthcare, in: *2016 IEEE 1st International Conference on Control, Measurement and Instrumentation (CMI)*, IEEE, pp. 580–584, 2016.
2. Benkhaddra, I., Kumar, A., Setitra, M.A. *et al.*, Design and development of consensus activation function enabled neural network-based smart healthcare using BIoT. *Wirel. Pers. Commun.*, 130, 1549–1574, 2023, https://doi.org/10.1007/s11277-023-10344-0 Q2,Impact Factor -2.017.
3. Srivastav, A.L., Markandeya, Patel, N. *et al.*, Concepts of circular economy for sustainable management of electronic wastes: Challenges and management options. *Environ. Sci. Pollut. Res.*, 30, 48654–48675, 2023, https://doi.org/10.1007/s11356-023-26052-y Q1,Impact Factor -5.19.
4. Ilyas, B., Kumar, A., Setitra, M.A., Bensalem, Z.E.A., Lei, H., Prevention of DDoS attacks using an optimized deep learning approach in blockchain technology. *Trans. Emerging Telecommun. Technol.*, 34, 4, e4729, 2023, Q2,Impact Factor -3.31.
5. Kumar, A., Rathore, P.S., Dubey, A.K. Agrawal, A., Sharma, K.P., LTE-NBP with holistic UWB-WBAN approach for the energy efficient biomedical application. *Multimed. Tools Appl.*, 82, 25, 39797–39811, 2023, https://doi.org/10.1007/s11042-023-15604-6 Q1,Impact Factor -2.577.
6. Kumar, A., Kumar, S.A., Dutt, V., Shitharth, S., Tripathi, E., IoT based arrhythmia classification using the enhanced hunt optimization-based deep learning. *Expert Syst.*, 40, 7, e13298, 2023, Q2, Impact Factor -2.812.
7. Bhargava, N., Rathore, P.S., Bhowmick, A., Study of X Ray Detection Using CNN in Machine Learning. *Advancements in Smart Computing and Information Security: First International Conference, ASCIS 2022*, Rajkot, India, November 24–26, 2022, Cham: Springer Nature, Switzerland, 2023, Revised Selected Papers, Part I.
8. Dutt, V., Rathore, P.S., Chauhan, K., Support Vector in Healthcare Using SVM/PSO in Various Domains: A Review, in: *Swarm Intelligence Optimization: Algorithms and Applications*, pp. 291–307, 2020.
9. Bhargava, N., Sharma, S., Purohit, R., Rathore, P.S., Prediction of recurrence cancer using J48 algorithm, in: *2017 2nd International Conference on Communication and Electronics Systems (ICCES)*, IEEE, pp. 386–390, 2017, October.

10. Bhargava, N., Dayma, S., Kumar, A., Singh, P., An approach for classification using simple CART algorithm in WEKA, in: *2017 11th International Conference on Intelligent Systems and Control (ISCO)*, IEEE, pp. 212–216, 2017, January.
11. Bhargava, P.N., Rathore, P.S.,. Vaishnav, P. and Rai, M., Utilizing Artificial neural networks and multivariate patient data for anemia detection using WEKA based approach for diagnosis, in: *2023 2nd International Conference on Automation, Computing and Renewable Systems (ICACRS),* Pudukkottai, India, pp. 643-648, 2023, doi: 10.1109/ICACRS58579.2023.10404355.
12. Bhargava, N., Rathore, P.S., Jha, M. and Goswami, A., Adaptive clustering algorithm for big health data classification, in: *2023 3rd Asian Conference on Innovation in Technology (ASIANCON),* Ravet IN, India, pp. 1-4, 2023, doi: 10.1109/ASIANCON58793.2023.10270544.

9

Artificial Immune System Algorithms for Optimizing Nanoparticle Design in Targeted Drug Delivery

Ashish Kumar* **and Vivek Verma**

Manipal University Jaipur, Rajasthan, India

Abstract

Our immune system serves as the body's security force. It constantly scans the environment for undesirable elements like bacteria, viruses, and even microscopic foreign substances like nanoparticles. It seeks to destroy anything it finds that doesn't belong. Therefore, we must take precautions to prevent immune system attack and destruction of nanoparticles used to deliver medications to cells in our bodies. Scientists have created a few techniques to accomplish this. One approach is to cover the nanoparticles with unique chemicals that give them the appearance of being a part of the body. These compounds may comprise naturally occurring proteins or carbohydrates in our bodies. The immune system doesn't target these coated nanoparticles because it doesn't recognize them as being foreign when it sees them. Making the nanoparticles small enough to get past the body's natural defenses is another option. Small particles are harder for our immune system to find and recognize. The nanoparticles can therefore avoid detection and enter their target cells if we make them small enough. A computational method called an artificial immune system (AIS) algorithm can be used to create nanoparticles that bypass the immune system and deliver medications to specific cells. The AIS algorithm is inspired by the natural immune system. It is possible to create nanoparticles that can bypass the immune system and deliver medications to specific cells by using an artificial immune system algorithm.

Keywords: AIS, nanoparticles, antigen, antibody, immune cells

**Corresponding author*: aishshub@gmail.com

Sumit Srivastava, Abhineet Anand, Abhishek Kumar, Bhavna Saini and Pramod Singh Rathore (eds.) Bio-Inspired Optimization for Medical Data Mining, (169–184) © 2024 Scrivener Publishing LLC

9.1 Introduction

Since they offer several benefits over conventional drug delivery methods, such as improved drug efficacy, reduced side effects, and targeted delivery, nanoparticles have attracted a lot of attention in recent years. The immune system's reaction to nanoparticles poses a significant obstacle to their use in medication delivery. When nanoparticles are ingested, the immune system may identify them as foreign substances and mount an immunological reaction, which may result in the removal of the nanoparticles from the body and a reduction in medicinal effectiveness. AIS algorithms can be used to create nanoparticles that can bypass the immune system to solve this problem [1]. The AIS is used during the design process to create nanoparticles that resemble the body's own cells so they can be recognized as self and avoid immune system detection. A population of nanoparticles with random properties is created by the AIS algorithm, and they are then put through a selection process that resembles the natural selection of immune cells [2]. The AIS selects the nanoparticles it identifies as self for further replication and growth while eliminating the non-self-nanoparticles from the population. The AIS algorithm can create a population of nanoparticles that resemble the body's own cells through this selection process, enabling them to avoid immune system recognition. These nanoparticles can then be utilized to deliver medications specifically to selected cells or tissues, enhancing their effectiveness, and minimizing their negative effects. The delivery of medications to specific cells can be optimized using AIS algorithms in addition to creating nanoparticles that can avoid the immune system. The algorithm can be used to generate nanoparticles with specific properties, such as size, shape, and surface charge, which can enhance their interaction with targeted cells and improve drug delivery. The use of AIS algorithms in designing nanoparticles for drug delivery offers a promising approach for improving drug efficacy and reducing side effects. The ability to design nanoparticles that can evade the immune system and target specific cells or tissues could have significant implications for the development of new therapies for a wide range of diseases.

First, the algorithm creates a population of "artificial immune cells" that can recognize and binding to nanoparticles [3]. These cells have receptors that can bind to chemicals on the nanoparticle's surfaces. The algorithm then trains the immune cells to identify and attach to nanoparticles made to trick the immune system. Selecting the cells that are most adept in identifying and adhering to the target nanoparticles is accomplished by exposing the cells to various nanoparticles. The algorithm can employ immune cells that have been educated to help it choose nanoparticles that are most likely to bypass the immune system and deliver medications to desired cells. The immune cells scan the surface of the nanoparticles and compare it to their "memory" of previous nanoparticles they have encountered. If the nanoparticle has a surface that resembles those of the target nanoparticles, the immune cells bind to the surface and tag it as safe. The algorithm can then use this information to design new nanoparticles that have a surface that resembles those of the target nanoparticles. By doing so, these newly designed nanoparticles can evade the immune system and deliver drugs to targeted cells more effectively [4, 5].

The algorithm mimics the natural immune system's capacity to identify and react to foreign invaders, which can be used to create nanoparticles that can bypass the immune system and deliver medications to specific cells. This provides a potent tool for creating new drug delivery systems that can boost the efficacy of therapies for a variety of disorders.

9.2 Artificial Immune Cells

Computer programs or algorithms known as artificial immune cells are created to mimic the behavior of immune system cells in the body. In several domains, like engineering, medicine, and computer science, these cells are employed in computational models to address complicated issues. The body's natural immune system is an intricate network of cells, tissues, and organs that cooperate to protect it against diseases and infections. White blood cells, which oversee identifying and combating external invaders including bacteria, viruses, and other dangerous substances, are among the immune system's essential cells [6].

The behavior of these cells is mimicked in artificial immune cells. Like how natural immune cells recognize and react to diseases or other external invaders, they are often designed to recognize and respond to specific patterns or signals. Artificial immune cells come in a variety of forms, each with unique properties and purposes. For instance, whereas certain artificial immune cell types are made to recognize and attack targets, others are made to recognize and eliminate dangers. Creating new materials for engineering and manufacturing, enhancing computer security systems, and optimizing medicine delivery system designs are just a few of the many uses for artificial immune cells.

Finally, scientists can also design nanoparticles that specifically target certain types of cells. They can attach molecules to the surface of the nanoparticles that are attracted to certain receptors on the surface of the target cells. This way, the nanoparticles are more likely to bind to the target cells and deliver the drugs directly where they're needed. So, by using these tricks, scientists can help nanoparticles evade the immune system and deliver drugs to targeted cells, which can be very helpful in treating diseases.

Artificial Immune System (AIS) is a type of computational intelligence technique that is inspired by the biological immune system of living organisms. The architecture of an Artificial Immune System comprises several components that work together to detect, identify, and respond to foreign entities or anomalies in a system [7–9].

9.3 The Artificial Immune System Architecture

Antigen: This is a trait of a foreign entity that causes the immune response to be triggered. The antigen is a pattern, structure, or feature of the data in AIS. An antigen may be represented as a section of DNA, a protein structure, or a specific element in a set of data. The mechanism of the immune response in AIS begins with the identification of antigens. The features of the supplied data are compared to the system's stored antibodies as part of the detection process. The immune system reacts to the discovery of an antigen by producing new, antigen-specific antibodies. The identification of antigens is a critical aspect of AIS, as it determines the specificity and sensitivity of the immune response [4]. The ability of the system to accurately identify antigens is dependent on the quality and diversity of the antibody population, which is created through the process of clonal selection and mutation. The concept of antigens is closely related to the idea of anomaly detection in AIS. Anomalies in a data set are often represented as unusual patterns or features that deviate from the expected normal behavior. These anomalies are detected by the immune system as foreign entities or antigens, and the immune response is initiated to neutralize them. The concept of antigens plays a crucial role in the functioning of an AIS architecture, as it forms the basis of the immune response mechanism and determines the system's ability to detect and respond to anomalies in a data set.

Antibody: The antigen is recognized and neutralized by this unique protein. In AIS, the antigen or anomaly that is discovered in the data is matched by an artificial construct called the antibody. An antibody in AIS is comparable to the organic antibodies that the biological immune system naturally produces to fend off infections or diseases. Clonal selection, a method used in AIS to produce antibodies, entails making duplicates of the most effective antibodies and genetically modifying them to produce a variety of antibodies. Over time, this process of mutation and selection aids in increasing the specificity and sensitivity of the antibody population, enabling the immune system to react to threats that are constantly changing and emerging more successfully [10].

The design of an antibody in AIS typically involves specifying a set of features or patterns that are characteristic of the antigen or anomaly that the antibody is intended to recognize. The specificity of the antibody is determined by the number and nature of these features, as well as the threshold for their activation. In the immune response process, the antibodies in the system search for and bind to the antigens that match their specific features. Once an antibody binds to an antigen, it triggers a response to neutralize the threat. This response may involve removing or quarantining the antigen or triggering further immune responses to eliminate the threat. Antibodies are a key component of AIS architecture, as they form the basis of the immune response mechanism and determine the system's ability to detect and respond to anomalies in a data set. The design of effective antibodies is crucial to the success of the system, and their performance can be improved through the process of clonal selection and mutation.

Clonal Selection: This protein has been designed to recognize the antigen and neutralize it. The antibody in AIS is a synthetic creation made to resemble the antigen or anomaly found in the data. A natural antibody produced by the biological immune system to combat infections or diseases is comparable to an antibody found in AIS. In AIS, the method of producing antibodies is known as clonal selection, which entails making duplicates of the most effective antibodies and modifying them to produce a variety of antibodies. The immune system can react more successfully to new and emerging threats because of this process of mutation and selection, which helps to increase the specificity and sensitivity of the antibody population over time.

The clonal selection process in AIS involves selecting the best-performing antibodies in the system and replicating them to create a population of clones shown in Figure 9.1. These clones are then subjected to mutation to generate a diverse set of antibodies with different characteristics, including specificity, sensitivity, and affinity [11, 12].

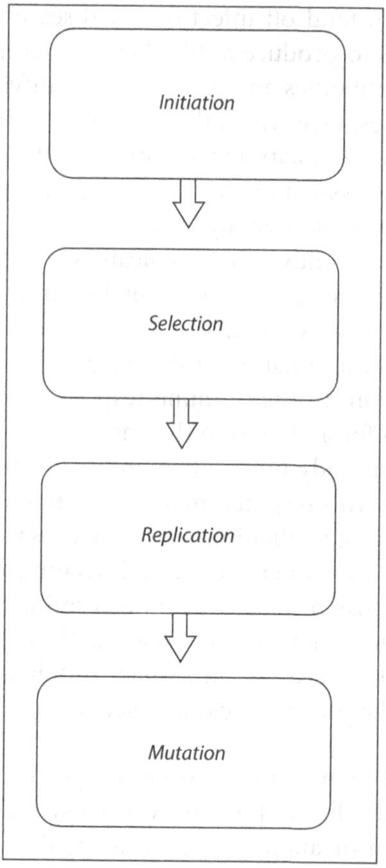

Figure 9.1 Clonal selection process.

The clonal selection process in AIS consists of the following steps: *Initiation:* The process of clonal selection is initiated when an antigen or anomaly is detected in the data set. The initiation of the clonal selection process involves several steps, including:

(i) Antigen Detection: The first step in the initiation of the clonal selection process is the detection of an antigen or anomaly in the data set. This may involve the use of various data analysis techniques, such as pattern recognition or data clustering, to identify patterns or anomalies in the data.
(ii) Antigen Presentation: Once an antigen or anomaly is detected, it is presented to the antibodies in the AIS to trigger an immune response. This process is modeled after

the natural immune system's ability to present antigens to lymphocytes, which triggers an immune response.

(iii) Antibody Selection: The antibodies in the AIS then begin to search for and bind to the presented antigen or anomaly. The antibodies with the highest affinity and fitness are selected based on their ability to recognize and neutralize the antigen.

(iv) Clonal Expansion: The selected antibodies are then replicated to create a population of clones. This process is modeled after the natural immune system's ability to expand the number of lymphocytes specific to a particular antigen.

(v) Mutation: The clones are then subjected to mutation to generate a diverse population of antibodies with different characteristics, including specificity and sensitivity.

(vi) Evaluation: The performance of the mutated antibodies is evaluated based on their ability to recognize and neutralize the antigen or anomaly.

(vii) Selection: The best-performing antibodies are selected to continue the clonal expansion process, and the process is repeated to generate a larger and more diverse population of antibodies.

The initiation of the clonal selection process in AIS is a critical step in the immune response mechanism, allowing the system to detect and respond to new and evolving threats. The process of antigen presentation, antibody selection, clonal expansion, mutation, evaluation, and selection plays a crucial role in achieving the goal of adaptive and self-organizing immune response in AIS [13, 14].

1. *Initialize the population of B cells with a set of randomly generated antibodies.*
2. *Evaluate the affinity of each antibody in the population for the antigen.*
3. *Select the antibodies with the highest affinity for replication.*
4. *Replicate the selected antibodies to generate a new set of antibodies.*
5. *Introduce random mutations into the replicated antibodies to increase diversity in the population.*
6. *Evaluate the affinity of the mutated antibodies for the antigen.*
7. *Select the antibodies with the highest affinity for the next round of replication.*
8. *Repeat steps 4-7 until a stopping criterion is met, such as a maximum number of iterations or a desired level of antibody affinity.*
9. *Select the antibodies with the highest affinity as the final set of antibodies.*
10. *Use the final set of antibodies for detection and response to the antigen.*

Figure 9.2 Flow of clonal selection algorithm.

Selection: The best-performing antibodies that are specific to the detected antigen or anomaly are selected based on their affinity and fitness. In the Artificial Immune System (AIS) architecture, the process of clonal selection involves several sub-steps, including the selection of the best-performing antibodies for replication and expansion. This selection process is critical to ensuring that the AIS produces an effective immune response to the antigen or anomaly that has been detected. Figure 9.2 shows the flow of clonal selection algorithm.

The sub-step of antibody selection involves evaluating the performance of the antibodies in the AIS and selecting the best-performing antibodies for replication and expansion. The selection process typically involves comparing the affinity and fitness of each antibody to the antigen or anomaly that has been detected. Affinity refers to the strength of the binding between an antibody and an antigen. Antibodies with high affinity are better at binding to the antigen, and therefore more effective at neutralizing the threat. Fitness refers to the overall effectiveness of an antibody in neutralizing the threat. Antibodies with high fitness are better at recognizing and neutralizing the antigen, and therefore more effective at protecting the system against the threat [15].

During the selection sub-step of clonal selection, antibodies that exhibit high affinity and fitness are selected for replication and expansion. The selection process may be performed manually or using machine learning algorithms that analyze the performance of each antibody and select the best-performing antibodies for replication. After the selection sub-step, the selected antibodies are replicated and expanded through a process of clonal expansion. This process involves creating a population of clones that are all specific to the antigen or anomaly that has been detected. The clones are then subjected to mutation and evaluation to generate a diverse population of antibodies with different characteristics, including specificity and sensitivity. Overall, the sub-step of selection is critical to ensuring that the AIS produces an effective immune response to the antigen or anomaly that has been detected. By selecting the best-performing antibodies for replication and expansion, the AIS can quickly generate a population of antibodies that are highly effective at recognizing and neutralizing the threat.

Replication: The selected antibodies are replicated to create a population of clones. In the Artificial Immune System architecture, the replication sub-step of clonal selection involves creating a population of clones from the selected antibodies. The purpose of this sub-step is to generate many antibodies that are all specific to the antigen or anomaly that has been detected, allowing the AIS to mount an effective immune response.

The replication sub-step typically involves the following steps:

(i) Isolation of Selected Antibodies: The first step in the replication sub-step is to isolate the antibodies that were selected during the selection sub-step. These antibodies are typically those with the highest affinity and fitness for the antigen or anomaly.
(ii) Cloning: Once the selected antibodies have been isolated, they are cloned to create a large population of identical cells. This is typically done using cell culture techniques, such as *in vitro* cell division or recombinant DNA technology.
(iii) Expansion: The cloned cells are then expanded to create a larger population of cells that are all specific to the antigen or anomaly. This is typically done using growth factors or other cell culture techniques.
(iv) Differentiation: The expanded cells are then differentiated into plasma cells or memory cells, depending on the needs of the AIS. Plasma cells are responsible for producing large amounts of antibodies in response to an antigen, while memory cells are responsible for storing information about the antigen for future use.
(v) Mutation: The replicated cells may also be subjected to mutation to generate a diverse population of antibodies with different characteristics, including specificity and sensitivity.

The replication sub-step of clonal selection is critical to the effectiveness of the AIS immune response. By creating a large population of cells that are all specific to the antigen or anomaly, the AIS can quickly mount an immune response to neutralize the threat. The replicated cells may also be subjected to mutation to generate a diverse population of antibodies with different characteristics, allowing the AIS to adapt to new and evolving threats over time [16].

Mutation: The clones are subjected to mutation to generate a diverse population of antibodies with different characteristics, including specificity and sensitivity. Evaluation: The performance of the mutated antibodies is evaluated based on their ability to recognize and neutralize the antigen or anomaly.

In the Artificial Immune System architecture, the mutation sub-step of clonal selection involves introducing genetic diversity into the population of replicated cells. The purpose of this sub-step is to generate a diverse population of antibodies with different characteristics, including specificity and sensitivity, to improve the effectiveness of the immune response.

The mutation sub-step typically involves the following steps:

(i) (Generation of Genetic Diversity: The first step in the mutation sub-step is to generate genetic diversity in the population of replicated cells. This is typically done through the introduction of random mutations into the DNA of the cells. These mutations may be introduced through natural mechanisms, such as errors during DNA replication, or through artificial methods, such as exposure to mutagenic agents.

(ii) Selection of Mutants: After the mutations have been introduced, the mutated cells are evaluated to identify those with improved characteristics, such as higher affinity or fitness for the antigen or anomaly. These cells are then selected for further replication and expansion.

(iii) Clonal Expansion: The selected mutated cells are cloned and expanded to create a larger population of cells with improved characteristics.

(iv) Differentiation: The expanded cells are then differentiated into plasma cells or memory cells, depending on the needs of the AIS.

The mutation sub-step of clonal selection is critical to the effectiveness of the AIS immune response. By introducing genetic diversity into the population of replicated cells, the AIS can generate a diverse population of antibodies with different characteristics, allowing it to adapt to new and evolving threats over time. The mutation sub-step also allows the AIS to improve the performance of the antibodies by selecting those with improved characteristics, such as higher affinity or fitness for the antigen or anomaly [10].

The best-performing antibodies are selected, and the process of replication and mutation is repeated to generate a larger and more diverse population of antibodies. The process of clonal selection in AIS is a self-organizing and adaptive process that allows the system to continually improve its ability to detect and respond to new and evolving threats. The diversity and specificity of the antibody population are critical to the success of the immune response mechanism in AIS, and the process of clonal selection plays a crucial role in achieving these goals.

Memory Cells: These are specialized cells that store information about the antigens that the immune system has encountered before. In AIS, memory cells store information about the performance of the antibodies and can be used to improve the detection and response to future threats. Memory cells are a key component of the immune response mechanism. Memory cells are artificial constructs that are designed to store information about past encounters with antigens, allowing the system to respond more quickly and effectively to future threats. Memory cells are created during the clonal selection process, which involves selecting and replicating the best-performing antibodies to create a population of clones. Some of these clones are then converted into memory cells, which are long-lived and retain information about the antigen or anomaly that they encountered during the initial immune response [17].

The role of memory cells in AIS is to improve the system's ability to recognize and respond to previously encountered antigens more quickly and effectively. When a memory cell encounters a previously encountered antigen, it triggers a rapid and specific immune response, allowing the system to neutralize the threat before it can cause significant damage. Memory cells in AIS are like the natural memory cells found in the biological immune system, which are responsible for providing long-term immunity to diseases and infections. The process of creating memory cells in AIS is modeled after the natural process of memory cell formation, which involves the selection and expansion of specific clones of lymphocytes that have been activated by a particular antigen. Memory cells are a critical component of the AIS architecture, allowing the system to respond more quickly and effectively to previously encountered antigens. The creation of memory cells during the clonal selection process is a key strategy for improving the system's ability to detect and respond to new and evolving threats, and it plays a crucial role in achieving the goal of adaptive and self-organizing immune response in AIS.

Immune Network: This is a network of interactions between the antibodies, antigens, and other immune cells. In AIS, the immune network is a computational model that simulates the interactions between the antibodies and antigens.

The immune network is a key component of the Artificial Immune System (AIS) architecture, which is designed to mimic the behavior of the immune system in detecting and responding to threats. In the immune network, the antibodies interact with each other to coordinate their response to a given antigen or anomaly. The immune network consists of two types of cells: the self-cells and the non-self-cells. Self-cells are cells that belong to the organism and are not recognized as foreign by the immune system, while non-self-cells are cells that are recognized as foreign and are targeted for destruction.

The immune network operates through a process known as clonal expansion, in which the immune cells that recognize a particular antigen are replicated and expanded to create a large population of cells that are all specific to that antigen. The expanded cells are then differentiated into plasma cells or memory cells, depending on the needs of the immune system. In the immune network, the antibodies interact with each other through a process known as network reconfiguration. During this process, the antibodies compete for binding sites on the antigen or anomaly. The antibodies that have the highest affinity and fitness for the antigen are selected for further replication and expansion, while those with lower affinity and fitness are removed from the network. The immune network also allows for the detection of new antigens or anomalies that have not been encountered before. When a new antigen is introduced into the network, the antibodies that are specific to that antigen will be replicated and expanded, allowing the immune system to mount a response to the new threat. The immune network is a key component of the AIS architecture, allowing the antibodies to interact with each other to coordinate their response to a given antigen or anomaly. The network reconfiguration process allows for the selection of the most effective antibodies, while the clonal expansion process allows for the generation of a large population of cells that are all specific to the antigen or anomaly. This allows the AIS to mount an effective immune response to a wide range of threats.

Detection and Response Mechanism: This is the process by which the immune system detects and responds to foreign entities. In AIS, this mechanism involves using the antibodies to identify and neutralize anomalies or threats in the data.

The detection and response mechanism are a critical component of the Artificial Immune System (AIS) architecture, which is designed to mimic the behavior of the immune system in detecting and responding to threats. The detection mechanism of the AIS involves the recognition of non-self-cells or molecules, such as pathogens, abnormal cells, or foreign objects, through the interaction of antibodies with antigens. The antibodies are generated through a process known as clonal selection, in which the immune system replicates and expands cells that are specific to a particular antigen. Once the antibodies have recognized a non-self-cell or molecule, the response mechanism of the AIS is triggered. The response mechanism involves the activation of various immune cells, including macrophages, T-cells, and B-cells, which work together to eliminate the threat [17].

The response mechanism typically involves several stages:

(i) Elimination of the threat: The immune cells work together to eliminate the non-self-cell or molecule, either by engulfing and digesting it, or by releasing toxic substances that destroy it.
(ii) Memory cell formation: During the elimination process, some of the B-cells differentiate into memory cells, which remain in the body to provide long-term protection against future encounters with the same antigen.
(iii) Antibody production: The B-cells that are not differentiated into memory cells continue to produce antibodies specific to the antigen, providing short-term protection against future encounters with the same antigen.
(iv) Regulation and termination: The immune response is regulated and terminated through various mechanisms, including the release of anti-inflammatory cytokines and the activation of regulatory T-cells.

The detection and response mechanism of the AIS allows the system to effectively detect and respond to threats, providing both short-term and long-term protection against a wide range of non-self-cells and molecules. The ability to generate memory cells also allows the AIS to provide rapid and effective responses to future encounters with the same antigen.

The architecture of an Artificial Immune System is designed to mimic the adaptive and self-organizing nature of the biological immune system and can be used for a wide range of applications such as intrusion detection, anomaly detection, and pattern recognition.

References

1. Malachowski, T. and Hassel, A., Engineering nanoparticles to overcome immunological barriers for enhanced drug delivery. *Eng. Regener.*, 1, 35–50, 2020.
2. Benkhaddra, I., Kumar, A., Setitra, M.A. *et al.*, Design and Development of consensus activation function enabled neural network-based smart

healthcare using BIoT. *Wirel. Pers. Commun.*, 130, 1549–1574, 2023. https://doi.org/10.1007/s11277-023-10344-0 Q2,Impact Factor -2.017.

3. Srivastav, A.L., Markandeya, Patel, N. *et al.*, Concepts of circular economy for sustainable management of electronic wastes: Challenges and management options. *Environ. Sci. Pollut. Res.*, 30, 48654–48675, 2023. https://doi.org/10.1007/s11356-023-26052-y Q1,Impact Factor -5.19.
4. Ilyas, B., Kumar, A., Setitra, M.A., Bensalem, Z.E.A., Lei., H., Prevention of DDoS attacks using an optimized deep learning approach in blockchain technology. *Trans. Emerging Telecommun. Technol.*, 34, 4, e4729, 2023. Q2,Impact Factor -3.31.
5. Kumar, A., Rathore, P.S., Dubey, A.K., Agrawal, R., Sharma, K.P., LTE-NBP with holistic UWB-WBAN approach for the energy efficient biomedical application. *Multimed. Tools Appl.*, 82, 25, 39797–9811, 2023.
6. Kumar, A., Kumar, S.A., Dutt, V., Shitharth, S., Tripathi, E., IoT based arrhythmia classification using the enhanced hunt optimization-based deep learning. *Expert Syst.*, 40, 7, e13298, 2023.
7. Bhargava, N., Sharma, S., Purohit, R., Rathore, P.S., Prediction of recurrence cancer using J48 algorithm, in: *2017 2nd International Conference on Communication and Electronics Systems (ICCES)*, IEEE, pp. 386–390, 2017, October.
8. Yu, Q. *et al.*, An immunology-inspired network security architecture. *IEEE Wirel. Commun.*, 27, 5, 168–173, 2020.
9. Dutt, V., Rathore, P.S., Chauhan, K., Support Vector in Healthcare Using SVM/PSO in Various Domains: A Review, in: *Swarm Intelligence Optimization: Algorithms and Applications*, pp. 291–307, 2020.
10. Bhargava, N., Rathore, P.S., Bhowmick, A., Study of X Ray Detection Using CNN in Machine Learning. *Advancements in Smart Computing and Information Security: First International Conference, ASCIS 2022*, Rajkot, India, November 24–26, 2022, Cham: Springer Nature, Switzerland, 2023, Revised Selected Papers, Part I.
11. Bhargava, P.N., Rathore, P.S., Vaishnav, P., Rai, M., Utilizing artificial neural networks and multivariate patient data for anemia detection using WEKA based approach for diagnosis, *2023 2nd International Conference on Automation, Computing and Renewable Systems (ICACRS)*, Pudukkottai, India, pp. 643–48, 2023. doi: 10.1109/ICACRS58579.2023.10404355.
12. Bhargava, N., Bhargava, R., Rathore, P.S., Agrawal, R. (Eds.), *Artificial Intelligence and Data Mining Approaches in Security Frameworks*, John Wiley & Sons, Hoboken, New Jersey, 2021.
13. Swarna, S.R., Kumar, A., Dixit, P., Sairam, T.V.M., Parkinson's Disease Prediction using Adaptive Quantum Computing. *2021 Third International Conference on Intelligent Communication Technologies and Virtual Mobile Networks (ICICV)*, pp. 1396–1401, 2021, doi: 10.1109/ICICV50876.2021.9388628.

14. Sasubilli, G. and Kumar, A., Machine Learning and Big Data Implementation on Health Care data. *4th International Conference on Intelligent Computing and Control Systems (ICICCS)*, pp. 859–864, 2020, doi: 10.1109/ICICCS48265.2020.9120906.
15. Al Bataineh, A. and Kaur, D., Optimal convolutional neural network architecture design using clonal selection algorithm. *Int. J. Mach. Learn. Comput.*, 9, 6, 788–794, 2019.
16. Meraj, S.S. *et al.*, Artificial intelligence in diagnosing tuberculosis: A review. *Int. J. Adv. Sci. Eng. Inf. Technol.*, 9, 1, 81–91, 2019.
17. Alrubayyi, H. *et al.*, Challenges of malware detection in the IoT and a review of artificial immune system approaches. *J. Sens. Actuator Netw.*, 10, 4, 61, 2021.

10

Diabetic Retinopathy Detection by Retinal Blood Vessel Segmentation and Classification Using Ensemble Model

Gandla Shivakanth[1]*, K. Aruna Bhaskar[2], Bechoo Lal[2], A. Shivakumar Reddy[2] and D. Manasa[2]

[1]*Department of Computer Science and Engineering, Koneru Lakshmaiah Education Foundation, Hyderabad, Telangana, India*

[2]*Department of Computer Science and Engineering, Koneru Lakshmaiah Education Foundation, KL University, Vijayawada, Andhra Pradesh, India*

Abstract

Diabetic retinopathy is common problem to diabetic patients. According to the current statistics of world, 9% and above diabetic patients are suffering with partially or complete vision loss. Retinal blood vessels perform an imperative role in the diagnostic procedure of diabetic retinopathy. However, the segmentation of retinal vessels is critical for pathological reasoning. In this article, a novel ensemble approach was developed for accurate blood vessel segmentation and classification. The retinal images had been accumulated from Digital Retinal Images for Vessel Extraction (DRIVE) and STructured Analysis of the Retina (STARE) datasets. The ensemble approach is used to segment the retinal blood vessels using bio-inspired algorithms, Cuttlefish Algorithm (CFA) for segmentation of the fundus image. The features were then extracted from the segmented pictures using the Enhanced Local Binary Pattern (ELBP) and Inverse Difference Moment Normalized (IDMN) algorithms. The obtained feature values were lastly provided as the input for ensemble classifier, Convolutional Neural Network (CNN) and Self-Organized maps (SOMs). Classifying results are collected from both classifiers and consolidated using the voting ensemble algorithm. The ensemble voting procedure was used to compile and combine the findings. According to experimental findings, the suggested technique increases segmentation and classification accuracy by 2.6% to 4% when compared to the current system.

**Corresponding author*: shvkanth0@gmail.com

Sumit Srivastava, Abhineet Anand, Abhishek Kumar, Bhavna Saini and Pramod Singh Rathore (eds.) Bio-Inspired Optimization for Medical Data Mining, (185–200) © 2024 Scrivener Publishing LLC

Keywords: Convolutional neural network, cuttlefish algorithm, convolutional neural network, self-organizing maps, voting ensemble classifier, local binary pattern, inverse difference moment normalized

10.1 Introduction

Retinal fundus images are significantly used for analysis of retina including retinal blood vessels, macula, and optic disc that helps clinicians in diagnosing numerous diseases like macular hole, diabetic retinopathy, macular degeneration, glaucoma, and epiretinal membrane [1, 2]. In addition, the retinal images have additional features, which give you a clear excessive decision visualization of blood vessels in the body [3]. Retinal vessel analysis is therefore helpful in the early identification and prevention of chronic illnesses such diabetic retinopathy, cerebrovascular, and cardiovascular disorders [4, 5]. Recently, numerous methodologies are developed for retinal vessel segmentation and classification like fully convolutional neural networks [6], extreme learning machine [7], Segmentation and Feature selection model introduced by using Cuttlefish optimizing technique [8], Cuttlefish optimizer framework [9], cascade classification framework [10], etc. The foundation of earlier approaches is supervised learning using pixel-level segmentation labels. Additionally, past approaches are divided into groups according on whether the feature descriptors were created by hand or were based on data. On the basis of the deep learning technology, a unique strategy is suggested to overcome this difficulty.

In my present work, a novel approach was proposed for enhancing the overall performance of retinal vessel segmentation and classification. Initially, the input had been accumulated from DRIVE and STARE datasets. Second step is preprocessing. Preprocessing designed with the median filter that gives a great enhancement of image contrast. Then, segmentation was carried out using ensemble machine learning model. The enhanced images are given as an input to two segmenting algorithms, first on is modified FCM, and other is SVM. The results of these two models are consolidated with classification voting ensemble process. Due to the ensemble ML model, there may be chance to get enhanced result. In modified FCM algorithm, Euclidean distance measure was replaced by Chebyshev distance measure, as it reap correct neighborhood selection to achieve accurate clusters. SVM is a supervised learning algorithm. It classifies pixels into one, two, or several groups. The process of classifying an image into one, two, or more classes is known as picture segmentation.

So, SVM is a theoretical and practical standpoint, SVM has the benefit of being better at segmenting medical images and it is not sensitive to noise, over all it produce good results in segmentation, while comparing with existing systems [11]. Besides, in order to extract the feature values from the segmented retinal pictures, the ELBP and IDMN methods have been used. Using the feature level fusion approach, the extracted features have been combined. The ensemble classification was used as a starting point for the feature extraction output. In the proposed model ensemble classifier consist of two classifiers. First, one is CNN classifier and other one is random forest classifier both are used for classifying the normal and abnormal blood vessels. These two classifier results will consolidated with regression voting classifier and the predicted result will be displayed. At last, the proposed architecture overall performance will be compared with the existing systems in terms of accuracy, sensitivity, f-score, and specificity.

10.2 Literature Review

Researchers have devised a number of methods for segmenting retinal blood vessels. A survey of some significant contributions to the current literature is offered in this segment.

Swarna *et al.* [12] described a technique, using morphology-based global thresholding, a new approach for distilling the blood veins from retinal pictures. The centreline detection approach was also used to depict the retinal venule anatomy as well as detect capillaries. The created approach was tested using the standard fundus image datasets like DRIVE and STARE datasets. Extensive testing revealed the new strategy successfully reduces computational complexity while also drastically reducing execution time. Top researchers participated in this investigation.

Bhargava *et al.* [15] and Soomro *et al.* [14], for retinal vascular segmentation, proposed a supervised technique using fully convolutional network. For regional vessel element detection, the presented technique decreased the normal vessel segmentation issue. In addition, unsupervised post-processing was utilized to polish the final result. The experiment was done out on four datasets in this research study: High Resolution Fundus (HRF), DRIVE, STARE, and CHASE-DB1. In comparison to existing models the suggested method has a high level of robustness perspective of sensitivity, accuracy, specificity, and area under the curve. Furthermore, this technology employed was supervised learning (requiring manual modifications), which needed to be automated [16].

Bhargava *et al.* [17] On the basis of region growth and level set, a new retinal vascular segmentation system was introduced. The retinal pictures were initially denoised using 2D Gabor wavelet technology and a contrast constrained adaptive histogram equalization approach. In addition, the images were smoothed and the vessel boundaries were kept with the use of an anisotropic diffusion filter. Finally, retinal vessels were extracted using region-based active contour and region-growing techniques, and the findings were integrated to achieve the final segmentation. The created system's effectiveness was average despite working with more testing set photos than training pictures.

A novel automated method for enhancing the identification blood vessel's of fundus image is being developed to overcome these concerns.

10.3 Proposed System

In recent years, eye illness has emerged as one of the most significant causes of blindness. The majority of instances may be avoided if they are recognized early enough. The retinal blood vessel study, for example, the retinal blood vessel analysis assists the clinicians to identify diabetes patients and give appropriate treatment. The current study is working on a novel blood vessel detecting method. The suggested system in this study includes five stages: data collection, pre-processing of images, segmentation of fundus blood vessels, feature extraction, followed by classification. The workflow of the proposed system is depicted in Figure 10.1.

A. Dataset description

The retinal fundus pictures are initially gathered from two standard datasets: STARE and DRIVE. The STARE dataset is made up of a number of retinal pictures taken using a TRC-50DX Topcon fundus camera having an image quality of 700 × 605 pixels and a 24-bit grey scale resolution. Twenty colored retinal pictures and twenty hand-labeled ground-truth photos make up STARE [16]. On the other hand, the DRIVE dataset originates from a screening program for diabetic retinopathy in the Netherlands. In this collection, the fundus photographs of 400 diabetics between the ages of 25 and 90 years are included. There are a total of 40 images, and each individual gets one at random. There are seven evidence of moderate early diabetic retinopathy in this group, whereas the remaining 33 exhibit no signs of diabetic retinopathy. The retinal pictures in the DRIVE dataset are usually in JPEG format [17]. The STARE and DRIVE dataset's sample retinal pictures are indicated in Figure 10.2.

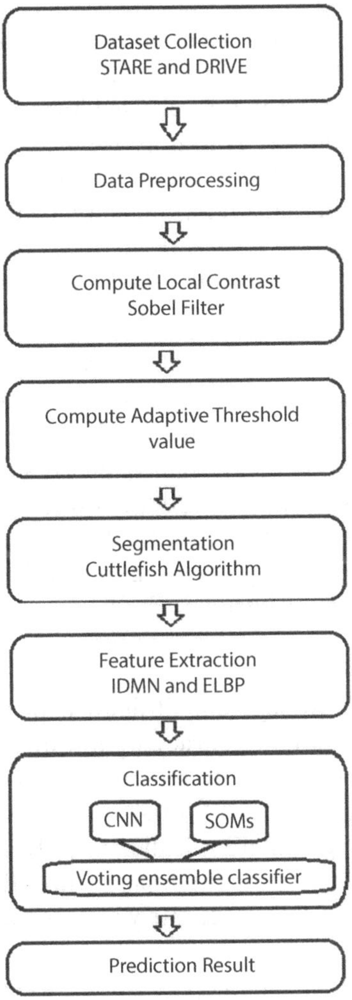

Figure 10.1 Process flow of proposed system.

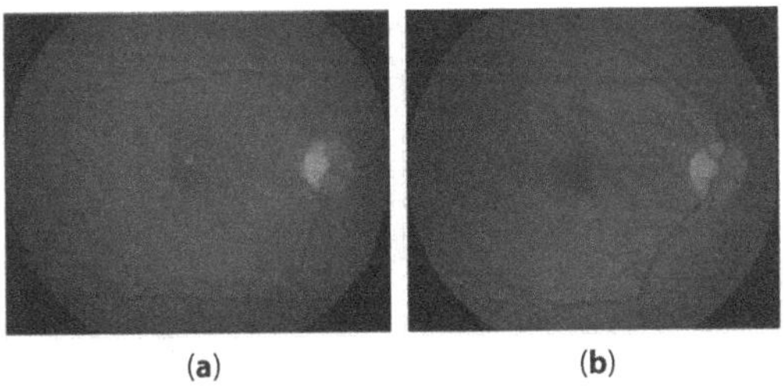

Figure 10.2 Sample image, (a) STARE dataset, (b) DRIVE dataset.

B. Data pre-processing

The median filter is employed as a pre-processing tool once the retinal pictures have been collected. Prior to segmentation and feature analysis, there are usually several artefacts in the collected images that must be removed. The goal of the median filter is to improve the picture characteristics, as well as the qualities of medical images in order to make the best diagnosis possible. Equation is the general formula for a median filter (10.1).

$$median[p(i)+q(i)] \neq median[p(i)]+median[q(i)] \quad (10.1)$$

where $p(i)$ and $q(i)$ are stated as two different fundus images, *median* $p(i)$ and *median* $q(i)$ are denoted as median value of the retinal images. Disparate little numbers among the picture pixels in the neighborhood have an effect on the median value. As a result, the median filter is particularly successful in filtering out a wide range of sounds. Compute the local contrast of the image using the Sobel filter. Compute the adaptive threshold value for each pixel using the local contrast measure and a thresholding method using Otsu's method.

C. Segmentation

Usually, it is difficult to segment ill-defined parts in medical photos, which reduces segmentation accuracy significantly. In order to overcome this issue, segment the image into regions based on the threshold values using cuttlefish algorithm (CNF). In adaptive thresholding, the threshold value for image segmentation is dynamically adjusted for each pixel based on the local contrast of the image. This allows the algorithm to identify the boundaries more accurately between different regions in the image.

The segmented retinal fundus pictures are shown in Figure 10.3 and Figure 10.4 shows the evidence blood vessels segmented image.

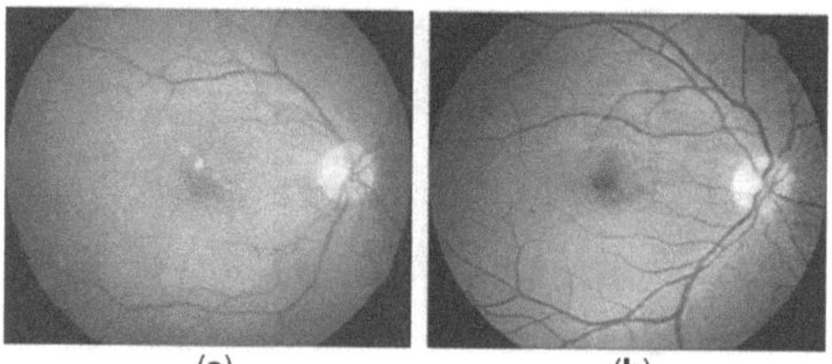

Figure 10.3 Sample pre-processed image, (a) STARE dataset, (b) DRIVE dataset.

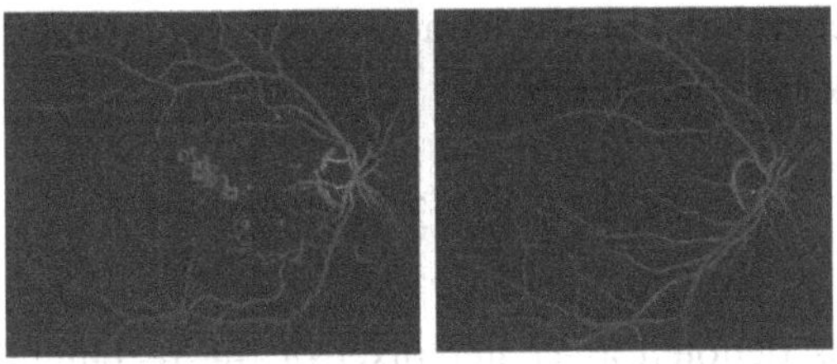

Figure 10.4 Sample blood vessel segmented image, (a) STARE dataset, (b) DRIVE dataset.

D. Feature extraction

Following image segmentation, feature extraction is carried out to get feature values from the segmented region. The process of transforming a retinal fundus image from image space to feature space and downsizing enormous quantities of redundant data is typically described as feature extraction. Meanwhile, feature extraction successfully lowers the computing complexity of the system. In this research project, feature extraction is carried out by using IDMN and ELBP to extract feature values from segmented images. The feature extraction methods are described in full below.

1) ***Inverse Difference Moment Normalized***

IDMN is a mathematically defined picture texture metric that is one of the most effective (10.2). IDMN is also known as homogeneity, and it is used to compute the local homogeneity of segmented blood vessel images. IDMN also determines if a particular image is non-textured or textured by identifying the GLCM feature distribution.

$$IDMN = \sum_{x=0}^{N-1} \sum_{y=0}^{N-1} \frac{1}{1+(x+y)^2} M(x,y) \tag{10.2}$$

Where, N is indicated as number of retinal fundus images, and $M(x,y)$ is stated as normalized image.

2) ***Enhanced Local Binary Pattern***

A texture descriptor called ELBP turns the segmented image into labels by using the luminance value. Gray scale invariance is a critical aspect in the ELBP feature descriptor, because it is influenced by texture and local patterns.

In general, the ELBP characteristic is expressed mathematically as equation (10.3).

$$ELBP = \sum_{s-1}^{N} 2^s \times s_f(I_n - I_c) \tag{10.3}$$

Where, I_c is denoted as center pixel of the rectangular window, I_n is stated as neighboring pixel in the rectangular window, s is indicated as number of neighbor pixels, s_f is represented as specific function and $I_n - I_c$ is specified as threshold value. The mathematical equation of $s_f(I_n - I_c)$ is given in equation (10.4).

$$s_f(I_n - I_c) = \{ \begin{matrix} 1, \; if \;\; I_n - I_c \geq 0 \\ 0, \; if \;\; I_n - I_c < 0 \end{matrix} \tag{10.4}$$

E. Ensemble Classification

In this phase, using the segmented image, features extraction, and classification is performed using CNN classification and Self-Organizing Map (SOM) classifier, which identifies the normalcy and abnormalities of blood vessels and helps in diabetes diagnosis. The results of CNN and random forest classifiers are consolidated using regression voting ensemble classifier.

In the convolutional neural network classifier, convolutional layer is an initial layer that extracts the local data/information of an image like texture, color, shape, and other features. The convolutional operation enhances input characteristics while reducing noise interference. Equation represents the mapping operation in the convolution process (10.5).

$$i_y^l = f_c\left(\sum_{x \in My} i_x^{l-1} \times k_{x,y}^l + \theta_y^l\right) \tag{10.5}$$

where i_y^l is designed as y^{th} mapping set of convolutional layer l, i_x^{l-1} is denoted as x^{th} feature set, and $k_{x,y}^l$ is indicated as convolutional kernel between the xth feature set and y^{th} mapping set. In addition, the variable θ_y^l is represented as bias and f_c is denoted as activation function. The following phase is the pooling procedure, which lowers the risk of overfitting during the training process. Equation serves as a mathematical notation for the pooling procedure (10.6).

$$i_y^l = f_p\left(\beta_y^l down\left(i_x^{l-1}\right) + \theta_y^l\right) \tag{10.6}$$

where *down*(.) is shown as down sampling process from layer $(l-1)$ to layer l^{th}, θ_y^l and β_y^l represent additive and multiplicative bias, respectively, and $f_p(.)$ is specified as activation function. Additionally, there are two variations of the pooling process: average pooling and maximal pooling. The matrix features from the final pooling layer are grouped to create a rasterization layer, which is further linked to the fully connected layer. Equation describes node y's output (10.7).

$$h_y = f_h\left(\sum_{x=0}^{n-1} w_{x,y} i_x - \theta_y\right) \tag{10.7}$$

where $w_{x,y}$ is denoted by the weight of the input vector i_x, θ_y is represented as node threshold, and $f_h(.)$ is denoted as activation function. The softmax classifier used in the fully connected layer, if the output layer process with the multiclass issue. Loss function of the softmax classifier is represented in the equation (10.8)

$$Y(\theta) = -\frac{1}{m}\left[\sum_{x=1}^{m} \sum_{y=1}^{k} l\{J^{(x)} = y\} \log \frac{e^{\theta_y^l}}{\sum_k e^{\theta_k^l}}\right] \tag{10.8}$$

where $e^{\theta_y^l}$ is shown as input of the yth neuron in the l layer, $\sum_k e^{\theta_k^l}$ is shown as input of all the neurons, $\frac{e^{\theta_y^l}}{\sum_k e^{\theta_k^l}}$ is indicated as output of yth neuron, e is stated as constant, and $l(.)$ is shown as indictor function. If the value in the braces is true, the result of the indictor function is one. If the value in the braces is false, the result of the indictor function is zero. Add the rule items in $Y(\theta)$ after that to avoid achieving the local optimum as stated in equation (10.9).

$$Y(\theta) = -\frac{1}{m}\left[\sum_{x=1}^{m} \sum_{y=1}^{k} l\{j^{(x)} = y\} \log \frac{e^{\theta_y^l}}{\sum_k e^{\theta_k^l}}\right] + \frac{\rho}{2}\sum_{x=1}^{k} \sum_{y=0}^{n} \theta_{xy}^2 \tag{10.9}$$

In this case, the weighted term, $\frac{\rho}{2}\sum_{x=1}^{k} \sum_{y=0}^{n} \theta_{xy}^2$ stabilizes the excessive parameters in the training set.

A self-organizing map (SOM) classifier is a type of unsupervised learning algorithm that is used for clustering and classification tasks. It is based on a neural network architecture that is designed to produce a low-dimensional representation of high-dimensional data.

The SOM algorithm works by representing the input data as a set of high-dimensional vectors, and mapping them onto a two-dimensional grid of nodes or neurons. Each neuron in the grid is associated with a weight vector, which is updated iteratively during the training process to adjust its position in the feature space.

The SOM training process involves initialization, competition, cooperation, adaptation, convergence. Once the SOM is trained, it can be used as a classifier by assigning each input data vector to the neuron with the closest weight vector. The SOM classifier can be used for various applications, including image recognition, data mining, and pattern analysis.

One of the advantages of the SOM classifier is that it can handle high-dimensional data with a relatively small number of neurons, which reduces the computational complexity of the algorithm. Additionally, the SOM can capture the underlying structure of the input data, which can be visualized in the form of a two-dimensional map or a cluster hierarchy.

The result of the CNN classifier and SOM classifier given as input to voting ensemble algorithm. A voting ensemble is a type of ensemble learning technique in which multiple models are trained on the same dataset and their predictions are combined using a voting scheme to make a final prediction. It is a popular method used in machine learning for improving the performance and robustness of models by combining the strengths of different algorithms.

The basic idea behind a voting ensemble is to train multiple models using different algorithms or configurations and combine their predictions to improve the accuracy of the final output.

F. Experimental result and discussion

This section simulates the specified setup using Python and an Intel i5 processor running at 3.5 GHz with 4 GB of RAM. The proposed system is evaluated for effectiveness on two well-known datasets: STARE and DRIVE, and its performance is compared to an existing method (Global thresholding-based segmentation [12, 13]). Specificity, f-score, sensitivity, and accuracy are used to evaluate how well the proposed system performs.

1) Performance metric

The performance metric is defined as the measurement of experimental results that produces trustworthy information about the proposed system. To comprehend the link between the input and output values of the proposed system, performance metrics including specificity, f-score, sensitivity, and accuracy are employed. The equations provide a generic formula for calculating specificity, f-score, sensitivity, and accuracy (10.10), (10.11), (10.12), and (10.13).

$$Specificity = \frac{TN}{TN + FP} \times 100 \tag{10.10}$$

$$F - score = \frac{2TP}{2TP + FP + FN} \times T0 \tag{10.11}$$

$$Sensitivity = \frac{TP}{TP + FN} \times 100 \tag{10.12}$$

$$Accuracy = \frac{TP + TN}{TP + TN + FP + FN} \times 100 \tag{10.13}$$

where FP is indicated as false-positive, TN is specified as true-negative, TP is stated as true positive, and FN is false negative.

The result of CNN classifier and the self-organized map classifier is consolidated by regression voting ensemble classifier. The regression voting ensemble classifier collect the individual classifier model result (as a class) and it will be used to find the best classification result. Using this result, the retinal blood vessels status can be predicted, whether it is normal or abnormal.

Using this proposed ensemble machine learning model for segmentation and classification can improve the prediction result.

2) Quantitative analysis of STARE and DRIVE datasets

The structured analysis of retina and digital retinal image for vessel extraction datasets are used to evaluate the performance of both of the proposed and current systems in this section. Table 10.1 compares the performance of the proposed and current systems on the STARE dataset in terms of specificity, sensitivity, f-score, and accuracy. The performance of 20 samples is evaluated in this situation, with 80% of the data being trained and 20% being tested. According to the results of the experiment, the CNN classifier has a classification accuracy of 96.75%. Cuttlefish Algorithm achieved a sensitivity of 97.34% and 96.97%, a specificity of 98.39% and 96.26%, an accuracy of 96.31% and 94.47%, and a kappa coefficient of

0.934 and 0.938 on natural and medical image datasets, respectively. The GA achieved a sensitivity of 93.22% and 88.56%, a specificity of 93.08% and 86.84%, an accuracy of 92.94% and 87.33%, and a kappa coefficient of 0.910 and 0.865 on natural and medical image datasets, respectively. CNN achieved a sensitivity of 96.85% and 95.54%, a specificity of 98.89% and 97.57%, an accuracy of 95.77% and 95.55%, and a kappa coefficient of 0.937 and 0.931 on natural and medical image datasets, respectively. In terms of specificity, f-score, sensitivity, and accuracy, Table 10.1 revealed that the CNN classifier outperformed the previous classification algorithms. Figure 10.5 shows a graphical representation of the suggested system using the STARE dataset.

Table 10.1 Performance analysis of proposed system with dissimilar classifiers on STARE dataset.

Classifiers	Accuracy (%)	Sensitivity (%)	Specificity (%)	F-score (%)
SVM	71.06	80	54.17	78
Random forest	75.55	87.42	80.90	91
LSTM	87.08	92.22	94.98	89.93
GA	93.22	93.08	92.94	92.0
CNN	96.75	97.01	98.79	94.03
Proposed Method	97.98	97.82	98.53	94.4

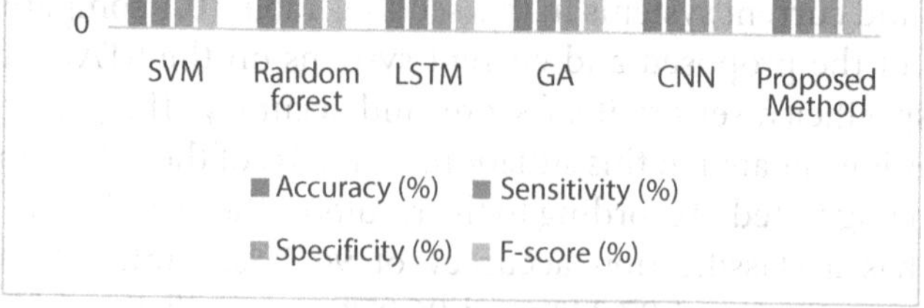

Figure 10.5 Graphical depiction of proposed system with dissimilar classifiers on STARE dataset.

On the DRIVE dataset, the performance of the proposed and current systems is evaluated in terms of specificity, f-score, sensitivity, and accuracy in Table 10.2. According to the results of the experiment, the CNN classifier has a classification accuracy of 96.75%, whereas the proposed classification techniques accuracy up to 97.98%. The CNN classifier's sensitivity, specificity, and f-score are 97.82%, 98.53%, and 94.4%, respectively. In comparison to the proposed classifier, comparable classifiers sensitivity, specificity, and f-score. Figure 10.6 shows a graphical representation of the proposed system on the DRIVE dataset.

Table 10.2 Performance analysis of proposed system with dissimilar classifiers on DRIVE dataset.

Classifiers	Accuracy (%)	Sensitivity (%)	Specificity (%)	F-score (%)
SVM	76.09	70	65.09	91.91
Random forest	80.72	82	77.76	72.02
LSTM	91.10	90.90	84.44	86.82
GA	93.22	93.08	92.94	92.0
CNN	96.75	97.01	98.79	94.03
Proposed Method	97.98	97.82	98.53	94.4

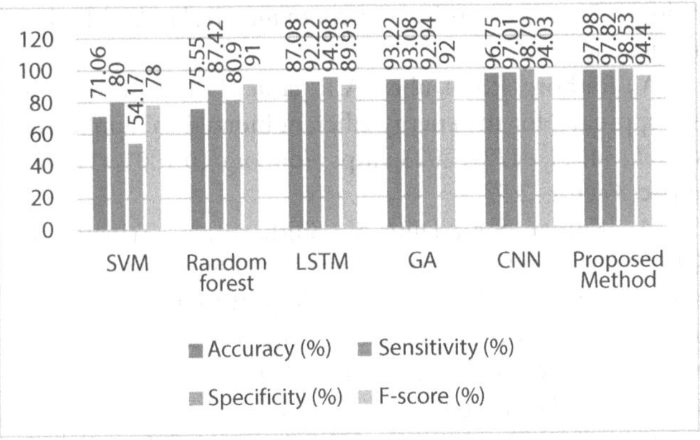

Figure 10.6 Graphical depiction of proposed system with dissimilar classifiers on DRIVE dataset.

10.4 Conclusion and Future Scope

The goal of this experimental research project is to establish correct segmentation and classification methodologies to enhance the categorization of normalcy and abnormality of blood vessels, which will aid in the identification of diabetic retinopathy. The suggested approach outperformed the previous system in terms of sensitivity, f-score, accuracy, and specificity when compared to the existing system (global thresholding-based segmentation [12]). The suggested method obtained maximum accuracy in the STARE dataset and the DRIVE dataset, which is greater than the existing system. Future research can create a new unsupervised system to enhance the segmentation and classification of retinal blood vessels.

References

1. Primitivo, D. *et al.*, A hybrid method for blood vessel segmentation in images. *Biocybern. Biomed. Eng.*, 39, 3, 814–824, 2019.
2. Benkhaddra, I., Kumar, A., Setitra, M.A. *et al.*, Design and Development of Consensus Activation Function Enabled Neural Network-Based Smart Healthcare Using BIoT. *Wirel. Pers. Commun.*, 130, 1549–1574, 2023, https://doi.org/10.1007/s11277-023-10344-0 Q2,Impact Factor -2.017.
3. Srivastav, A.L., Markandeya, Patel, N. *et al.*, Concepts of circular economy for sustainable management of electronic wastes: challenges and management options. *Environ. Sci. Pollut. Res.*, 30, 48654–48675, 2023, https://doi.org/10.1007/s11356-023-26052-y Q1,Impact Factor -5.19.
4. Ilyas, B., Kumar, A., Setitra, M.A., Bensalem, Z.E.A., Lei, H., Prevention of DDoS attacks using an optimized deep learning approach in blockchain technology. *Trans. Emerging Telecommun. Technol.*, 34, 4, e4729, 2023, Q2,Impact Factor -3.31.
5. Kumar, A., Rathore, P.S., Dubey, A.K. *et al.*, LTE-NBP with holistic UWB-WBAN approach for the energy efficient biomedical application. *Multimed. Tools Appl.*, 34, 24, e4729, 2023, https://doi.org/10.1007/s11042-023-15604-6 Q1,Impact Factor -2.577.
6. Kumar, A., Kumar, S.A., Dutt, V., Shitharth, S., Tripathi, E., IoT based arrhythmia classification using the enhanced hunt optimization?based deep learning. *Expert Syst.*, 40, 7, 2023, Q2, Impact Factor -2.812.
7. Zhao, Y.Q. *et al.*, Retinal vessels segmentation based on level set and region growing. *Pattern Recognit.*, 47, 7, 2437–2446, 2014.
8. Hoove, A. *et al.*, Locating the optic nerve in a retinal image using the fuzzy convergence of the blood vessels. *IEEE Trans. Med. Imaging*, 22, 8, 951–958, 2003.

9. Staal, J.J. *et al.*, Ridge based vessel segmentation in color images of the retin. *IEEE Trans. Med. Imaging*, 23, 501–509, 2004.
10. Sasubilli, G. and Kumar, A., Machine Learning and Big Data Implementation on Health Care data. *4th International Conference on Intelligent Computing and Control Systems (ICICCS)*, pp. 859–864, 2020, doi: 10.1109/ICICCS48265.2020.9120906.
11. Kotturu, P.K. and Kumar, A., Comparative Study on Machine Learning models for Early Diagnose of Alzheimer's Disease: Multi Correlation Method. *2020 5th International Conference on Communication and Electronics Systems (ICCES)*, pp. 778–783, 2020, doi: 10.1109/ICCES48766.2020.9137872.
12. Swarna, S.R., Kumar, A., Dixit, P., Sairam, T.V.M., Parkinson's Disease Prediction using Adaptive Quantum Computing. *2021 Third International Conference on Intelligent Communication Technologies and Virtual Mobile Networks (ICICV)*, pp. 1396–1401, 2021, doi: 10.1109/ICICV50876.2021.9388628.
13. Bhargava, N., Bhargava, R., Rathore, P.S., Agrawal, R. (Eds.), *Artificial Intelligence and Data Mining Approaches in Security Frameworks*, John Wiley & Sons, 2021.
14. Soomro, T.A., Afifi, A.J., Gao, J., Hellwich, O., Zheng, l., Paul, M., Strided fully convolutional neural network for boosting the sensitivity of retinal blood vessels segmentation. *Expert Syst. Appl.*, 134, 36–52, 2019.
15. Bhargava, N., Rathore, P.S., Bhowmick, A., Study of X Ray Detection Using CNN in Machine Learning. *Advancements in Smart Computing and Information Security: First International Conference, ASCIS 2022*, Rajkot, India, Nov. 24–26, 2022, Part I. 1759, 295-303, Cham: Springer Nature Switzerland, 2023.
16. Vishal, D., Rathore, P.S., Chauhan, K., Support Vector in Healthcare Using SVM/PSO in Various Domains: A Review. *Swarm Intelligence Optimization: Algorithms and Applications*, 291–307, 2020.
17. Bhargava, N., Sharma, S., Purohit, R., Rathore, P. S., Prediction of recurrence cancer using J48 algorithm, in: *2017 2nd International Conference on Communication and Electronics Systems (ICCES)*, pp. 386–390, IEEE, 2017 October.

11

Diabetes Prognosis Model Using Various Machine Learning Techniques

Pawan Kumar Patidar*, **Manish Bhardwaj and Sumit Kumar**

Department of Computer Science & Engineering Swami Keshvanand Institute of Technology, Management & Gramothan, Jaipur, India

Abstract

With the same speed that the 21st century asks of us, it is easy to believe that the fields of illnesses and their spread have expanded substantially in a world of quick paces and widespread adoption of bad health care practices. It is a collection of business intelligence (BI) tools that use cutting-edge machine learning techniques to uncover relationships and patterns in vast amounts of data. We can predict behaviors and events thanks to these data-driven linkages and patterns. Predictive analytics provides you a look into the future by using past events. It is important to note that the predictive model was built using previous predictive approaches, even if it is not based on the production of a mathematical model or algorithms for the development of the forecast. Instead, it uses algorithms that are built into the identified tool. It is suggested that, via the usage of the model, the organizations that provide both public and private health services adopt it in a commercial setting, using the model's predictive capabilities for the client's diagnosis and the optimization of consultation procedures.

Keywords: Diseases, diabetes, machine learning, prediction, supervised learning, unsupervised learning

**Corresponding author*: Pawan.patidar@skit.ac.in

Sumit Srivastava, Abhineet Anand, Abhishek Kumar, Bhavna Saini and Pramod Singh Rathore (eds.) Bio-Inspired Optimization for Medical Data Mining, (201–226) © 2024 Scrivener Publishing LLC

11.1 Introduction

We see hope life increase and we regularly see in the news celebrations of the oldest people in the world; however, it is not something alien to us to find out about deaths close to early ages and due to factors not typical of the natural degeneration of the human body, but due to diseases to the heart, cancer, or complications derived from diabetes. It is normal for us to ignore our bodies given the pressures of family, school, and job, yet doing so may be quite damaging [1]. According to a report from the American Journal of Public Health 3, the number of people who would die from chronic illnesses will climb by 72% by 2020 (from 29 million to 50 million people). Given that chronic illnesses are a phenomenon that is fundamental to modernity and whose peak we have yet to reach, we designate them as a target with great potential for analytical projects like the one that is suggested [1, 2].

11.1.1 Disease Identification

Starting with a formal description of the idea under study is important in order to go forward with the analysis. Chronic or non-communicable illnesses are those that have a long duration, are contagious-free, and often advance slowly. They are the leading cause of mortality worldwide, accounting for 70% of all causes of death [3]. Cardiovascular diseases, diabetes, cancer, obesity, rheumatoid arthritis, and respiratory illnesses are the leading chronic diseases [4]. It becomes necessary to decide which illnesses will serve as the primary focus of research when there are a representative number of them. The monetary criteria will be used first because of the substantial economic relevance associated with chronic illnesses and their treatment [4].

According to the costs associated with the four primary chronic illnesses in the US, we may identify them by economic quantification as follows:

a) Cardiovascular Conditions
b) Diabetes
c) Cancer
d) Obesity

These four categories will be used as a starting point to conduct the following study about their description and symptoms since they have the biggest economic effect [4, 5].

a) Cardiovascular Diseases

Heart attacks, strokes, coronary heart disease, and other conditions that affect the heart and blood vessels are included in the category of cardiovascular illnesses:

- Cerebrovascular diseases: conditions affecting the brain's blood vessels.
- Diseases of the blood arteries supplying the upper and lower limbs are known as peripheral arthropathies.
- Rheumatic heart disease: heart and heart valve lesions brought on by rheumatic fever, a condition brought on by streptococcus bacteria.
- Congenital heart disease: cardiac defects that exist from birth.
- Deep vein thromboses (thrombi) and pulmonary embolisms (emboli) are blood clots that may form in the veins of the legs and travel to the lungs or heart [6].
- Heart attacks and cerebrovascular accidents (CVA): these are often severe conditions brought on by blockages that prevent blood from reaching the heart or brain, respectively

b) Diabetes

Type 2 diabetes, previously known as adult-onset diabetes, is a chronic illness that arises when the body's ability to use insulin properly or when the pancreas is unable to produce enough of it. A hormone called insulin aids in maintaining healthy blood sugar levels [7]. Without consistent care, uncontrolled diabetes will lead to hyperglycemia, which in turn causes a number of system problems, especially in the nervous and circulatory systems.

Juvenile, insulin-dependent, or childhood onset diabetes are other names for type 1 diabetes. This happens because people with this illness need daily injections of the hormone since their bodies are unable to create enough insulin on their own. Type 1 diabetes cannot be prevented by current knowledge, despite the fact that its exact etiology is still unknown [8].

Type 2 diabetes: insulin-independent diabetes, which is characterized by ineffective use of insulin, is sometimes used to describe non-diabetic and adult-onset type 1 diabetes. Almost 90% of instances of diabetes worldwide are of type 2, making it the most prevalent kind. This kind of diabetes was only recently seen in adults, but it is now also common in children [9].

Pregnancy-related hyperglycemia (increased blood sugar) that develops and rises to levels above normal but below those required to diagnose diabetes is known as gestational diabetes.

c) Cancer

Malignant tumors or malignant neoplasms are cancers that attack any area of the body. Cancer is characterized by the fast growth of malignant or aberrant cells, which reach a point of infiltrating nearby tissues or spreading to other organs [10].

According to the number of fatalities from cancer globally, the primary forms are:

1. Tobacco use (1.59 million)
2. Hepatitis (745,00)
3. Gastritis (723,00)
   Fourth, colorectal cancer (694 000)
   521 000 cases of breast cancer
6. Esophageal cancer (400,000)

d) Obesity

Overweightness is a condition in which extra adipose or fat tissue accumulates, becoming harmful to health. The BMI, which is widely used to detect obesity, is determined by dividing a person's weight in kilograms by his or her height in meters squared. An adult with a BMI of 30 or above is considered obese [11]. Experts warn that its most negative effects act as an agent that determines and aggravates serious diseases, such as diabetes, some types of cancer, hypertension, and cardiovascular complications in the short term. From these four non-communicable diseases, the analysis is carried out for the choice of the disease that is used for the predictive model for the diagnosis of the disease.

11.1.2 Data, Information, and Knowledge

Data are a representation of facts, concepts, or instructions that have been formulated and codified for communication, interpretation, or processing by people or automated processes. Data, when used in isolation, are completely worthless. It must be modified into a form that is useful and put in context to be of any use. Data have to be changed in order to convey thoughts or expertise. Knowledge [12] is the information obtained, incorporated into the reasoning resources of an agent and ready to be used in a decision process; is the result of a learning process. By appending the previous concepts with the developed project, we can identify the data as that information that enters the developed predictive model in a timely manner and that serves to feed it: patient-specific data, such as height, weight, hemoglobin levels, etc. Information is what is obtained from the transformation of data through a series of logical relationships, which in the case of the project would be the consolidation of the patient's traits, being necessary to emphasize that in the creation of information it is not obtained directly knowledge, but it is necessary for it to go through a series of resources that allow reasoning and learning from it, thus getting to know what the information provides based on the data entered. In this sense, there is a similarity between the concept of knowledge and the result that the model shows due to the fact that processing is used through algorithms to obtain learning [13].

11.1.3 Knowledge Discovery in Databases

The process of extracting previously unknown, implicit, and possibly valuable information from a dataset is referred to as knowledge discovery shows in Figure 11.1. A pattern in language L has been established for a data set F

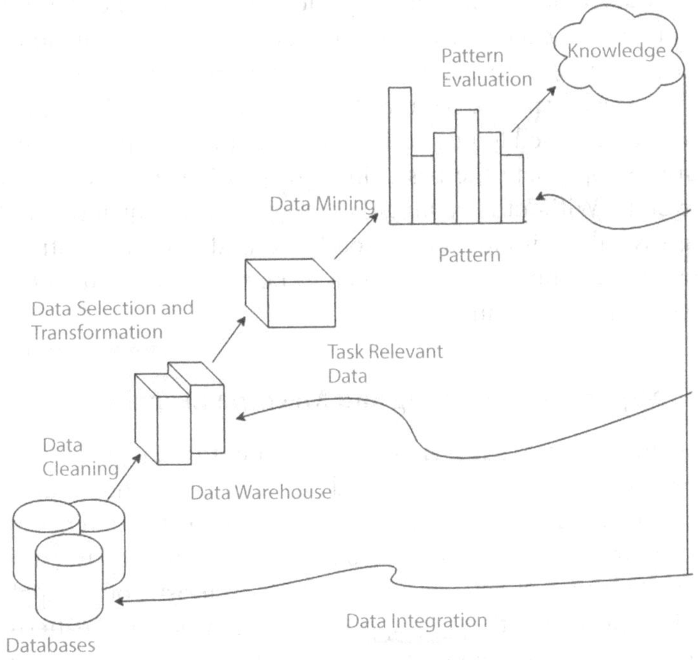

Figure 11.1 Knowledge discovery process.

of F based on a data set Fs of F, a measure of confidence C, and a set of rules R, such that L represents the facts that are simpler than the enumeration of all of the facts in Fs. The knowledge found in database-monitoring software may be defined as a collection of facts uncovered by the program [14]. The power of databases to find knowledge is the grouping of all processes, automated and non-automated, that allow the exploration of databases, large and small, to extract potential knowledge. The ability to discover knowledge in databases, using current technologies currently offers new possibilities to the vast majority of industries to be applied correctly. However, it is necessary to indicate that it is essential to identify which techniques are the ones that must be applied to carry it out, because each one presents a series of advantages that make them more suitable for certain business cases. For the purposes of the project, using the premise of immediate prediction, the concept of predictive analytics will be developed [15].

11.1.4 Predictive Analytics

Predictive analytics is a business intelligence suite that reveals patterns and connections in huge quantities of data, allowing organizations to forecast their future outcomes. Predictive analytics is different from other business intelligence technologies in that it provides a glimpse into the future, by utilizing previous occurrences to make an informed prediction. While some techniques seek to develop a logical forecast, such as linear regression, others, such as predictive analytics, are geared at making an empirical prediction, as opposed to just deriving a prediction based on theory.

Failure to appreciate the basic limits of predictive analytics may lead to bad results. Without a training dataset of sufficient quantity and quality, progress will be impossible. Also, the second part is essential since it is important to define clearly the idea to be forecasted and to have past instances of the same example.

11.1.5 Supervised Learning and Machine Learning

An algorithm that uses supervised learning goes through training samples to get a classification. Predictions based on the categorization may be made in test instances. The supervised learning in context, the term machine learning or machine learning was born, which refers to the automatic detection of significant patterns in data. A characteristic of the application of machine learning is that it is applied in cases where the patterns to be identified are of high complexity, so that a human being does not have enough expertise to learn from this in a specific way [16].

11.1.6 Predictive Models

A predictive model is a common term for a set of mathematical techniques with the goal of predicting future values of a given objective, response, or dependent variable and many predictive factors and independent variables. It is preferable to account for the inaccuracy of connections in prediction since relationships are seldom perfect in reality. In order to identify those factors that intervene in the prediction, they may be divided into three categories: those factors that have little chance of affecting the outcome, those with high certainty to influence the results, and those in the middle [17].

11.1.7 Data Validation and Cleaning

The validation of data implies determining that it is a trustworthy source of information, while the correction of mistakes in the data is referred to as data cleaning. Identifying incorrect values is common, yet locating the right values is impossible. Although it is feasible to establish a degree of confidence as to whether a given piece of data is susceptible to being accurate or wrong, a set of tests may be used to do so. You should spend more time validating your data rather than repairing the same if your data is very error-prone. Two distinct pieces of data should not be separated due to referencing the same object, this being something everyday if it is a set of information from different sources [18]. Likewise, it is not unusual that, depending on the algorithm used to make the prediction, a transformation of the variables must be made to discrete values or to binary values that are supported by the algorithm. It is everyday to have human intervention in this phase due to the complexity of the information with which you can work.

11.1.8 Discretization

Numerical qualities may be discretized, as can the selection of features. The classifiers are split into two main groups: supervised classifiers and unsupervised classifiers. In supervised discretization, if the class of the instances is a decision attribute, and if the class is not regarded or handled as a regular attribute, unsupervised discretization is used. The discretization techniques may be categorized according to three distinct axes: Global (compared to local) v/s local (unsupervised to supervised) shown in Figure 11.2, and static (as opposed to dynamic).

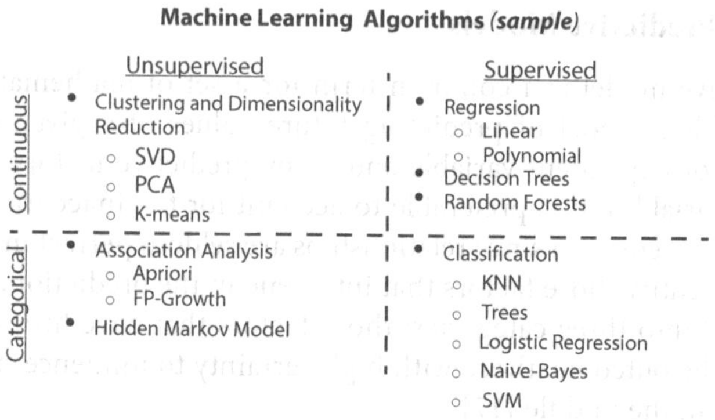

Figure 11.2 Supervised vs unsupervised learning.

Chronic Diseases: Chronic illnesses and diseases that are not infectious are often referred to as non-communicable diseases (NCDs). Stroke, heart attack, diabetes, cancer, asthma, and depression are all examples of medical conditions that may be included in common. Many of the risk factors for developing non-communicable diseases are preceded by unhealthy behaviors, and later by the emergence of metabolic and illness risk factors. In order to successfully manage chronic illnesses, the risk factors linked with obesity and inactivity, high blood pressure, elevated blood glucose levels, and inadequate cholesterol levels must be controlled. This list of risk factors is made up of two components: behaviors and medicines. Reducing risk factors for chronic illnesses is possible by eating a nutritious diet.

Diabetes: The set of metabolic disorders with hyperglycemia as a consequence of insulin insufficiency, insulin insufficiency itself, or both is called diabetes mellitus. The long-term damage, malfunction, and failure of numerous organs, particularly the eyes, kidneys, nerves, heart, and blood arteries, are often seen in diabetes, especially type 1 diabetes. Diabetes is usually diagnosed into two etiologies, with most patients falling into one of these two groups. The primary cause of type 1 diabetes is an utter lack of insulin secretion. Type 2 diabetes occurs more often than type 1 diabetes, although in this latter condition, the two root causes are related: a resistance to the action of insulin and an insufficient secretory response to insulin compensation. Type 2 diabetes, in which the blood glucose level is abnormally high without significant symptoms, occurs when there is sufficient hyperglycemia to induce structural and functional abnormalities in various tissues, but before the condition is recognized.

11.2 Literature Review

According to a review of the literature, several research using varied approaches and producing a range of results have looked at the prediction of diabetes. The capacity for making precise predictions about future data using models that can be developed and tested is known as predictive capability.

In [19] predictive capacity is defined a collection of advanced statistical models and estimations are used to find out what the environment will do next future. An effective way to enable consistency and predictability in reports and give users the best options is by using a predictive analytics platform that includes data warehouses, predictive analytics methods (like regression analysis, machine learning, and neural networks), dashboards, and data visualization.

11.2.1 Neural Networks

There are things to be done to make the predictions in these studies of (about) neural network algorithms more accurate [20]. A research that used various supervised learning algorithms of artificial neural network looked at a model of diabetes that made predictions. The scaled conjugate gradient method yielded superior outcomes when the objectives and expectations for results were highly correlated [21]. It describes the use of a medical diagnostic assistance system as being critical for physicians in the process of making a diagnosis. Because they wanted to conduct a research to compare many predictive models of neural network algorithms for the diagnosis of diabetes, they performed a study of several predictive models of neural network algorithms. The accuracy may be enhanced by pre-processing and extracting certain model features. In [22], we find that all diabetes prediction models are flawed, therefore we propose using fuzzy logic neural network techniques and case-based reasoning as a diagnostic method to help avoid diabetes. A novel design that is affected by patient-related input factors helped diagnose diabetes.

11.2.2 Trees

Diabetes has recently been on the rise throughout the world, according to the Lekha [23] research linked to tree algorithms. As chronic illnesses increase, a higher degree of control is required. In this model, the authors present a model that makes use of several decision tree methods to create a Chronic Disease Diagnosis (CDD). In contrast, studies indicate that diabetes not only creates an increased chance of developing other illnesses, but is a disease that itself produces such diseases. Therefore, analytic research on diabetes is a vital endeavor. Their proposal, therefore, is to use the J48 algorithm to diagnose diabetes and improve it. To obtain an accuracy of 99.87%, they adjusted the algorithm. Rocha *et al.* [24] say that diabetes is on the rise in the globe, and this means that by 2025 there will be 380 million individuals with diabetes, therefore necessitating quicker and more efficient diagnoses. Finally, in Chen *et al.* [25], it was noted that the abundant quantity of health-related information may be used to aid prediction, prevention, and personalization of medicine, which may be achieved via the development of a framework that enables scalable predictive analysis using visual tools. Evaluation of different prediction models uses parameter optimization and algorithm performance in random forest.

11.2.3 K-Nearest Neighbors

Type 2 Diabetes Mellitus (T2DM) may be predicted by factors present at birth, according to a research published in the journal [26]. In this study, the researchers evaluate the different methods and determine that the best is K-nearest neighbors. Using several statistical methods, they produce a prediction model which has an error rate that is greater than what was anticipated.

Bayesian Networks: Diabetes is listed in Fitriyani *et al.* [27] as the chronic illness posing the biggest threat to global health. Diabetes is predicted using a Bayesian network model with an accuracy rate of 99.51%. On the other hand, in Rashtian *et al.* [28], they mention that the manual analysis of information in these times has become useless with the large amount of information, so a computerized analysis is necessary. In such a way, they develop a model for the diagnosis of diabetes. This system employs Bayesian network techniques, multilayer perception, and J48 to create percepts for brands. For each method, getting various precision outcomes, it is of course Bayesian networks that provide the best result.

LEM2: Meneghetti *et al.* [29] mention that there are numerous models that propose to solve the problems of diagnosis and management of diabetes, they propose H2RM, an LEM2-based hybrid model, is used to simultaneously control blood glucose for types 1 and 2, and yields an average and balanced precision of 95.9%.

Fuzzy hierarchy: For their part, [30] mention that by 2035 the prevalence of diabetes will grow by 55% compared to 2013, thus they propose computational intelligence using a fuzzy hierarchy model that allows an early detection of diabetes. They compared the information in the model with the doctor's decision. Bearing a similarity of 87.46% with the statement of the doctors.

Distributed algorithms: Finally, Wang *et al.* [31] indicate that with the growth of Big Data and the large amount of health information, it is necessary to structure and emphasize the size of this information for a possible solution, so they use an analytical predictive algorithm to predict the prevalence of types of diabetes and complications associated with the type of treatment provided.

11.3 Proposed Model

11.3.1 Predictive Models in Health

Development of a predictive model for type 2 diabetes mellitus using clinical data and genetics [32] indicates that there are recent genetic studies that provide convincing evidence that the location of a gene and the polymorphism of a group of molecules are a primary cause of type 2 diabetes. The construction of a prediction model of type 2 diabetes using clinical and genetic data is predicated on this assumption [33].

For the development of the model, a statistical method of sampling of 684 participants was used, where 472 were random subjects and 212 were subjects with type 2 diabetes mellitus. The average age was 64.1 years for the randomized and 64.5 years for the diagnosed patients with diabetes, so the ages were not significantly different. The 684 participants were subjected to a sampling of 499 groups of molecules previously associated with type 2 diabetes mellitus. Factors that may intercede in the development of the disease were also considered, such as body mass index and triglyceride count, to refine the result by determining an incorrect classification ratio of type 2 diabetes mellitus of 27.98 ± 2.76 for all the tested algorithms. To improve the results of the classification, a multi-scenario adjustment model was used, selecting risk factors that allow smaller groupings according to common characteristics to perform a pattern recognition analysis. Based on this, three groups were determined: the first contained factors associated with obesity (body mass index, weight, and ratio between waist and hip), the second contained the highest ratios of glucose, insulin resistance, cholesterol and hemoglobin, and the third included the highest values of body mass index, weight, and heart rate of work. Figure 11.3 shows the dispersion between triglycerides, body mass index and incidence of type 2 diabetes mellitus.

The prevalence of type 2 diabetes mellitus was calculated using statistical tree decision models, which revealed that in men and women, the prevalence was about the same for groups 2 and 3, but it was smaller in group 1 [34]. In the graphic below, you can see a scatter plot that compares triglyceride levels, body mass index, and the incidence of type 2 diabetes:

In clusters 1-3, 2-3 and 3-3, we can identify patients suffering from the disease and we notice a trend toward high triglycerides and body mass index for these clusters.

Based on the statistical analysis and classification of factors, the following risk factors for developing the disease were determined:

a) Clinical information: height, body mass index, waist circumference, blood pressure, cholesterol, triglyceride count and glucose level.
b) Family and personal history: hypertension, type 2 diabetes mellitus, cerebrovascular diseases and other vascular diseases
c) Group of molecules polymorphism (SNP): 499 SNPs were identified in 87 candidate genes associated with type 2 diabetes mellitus.

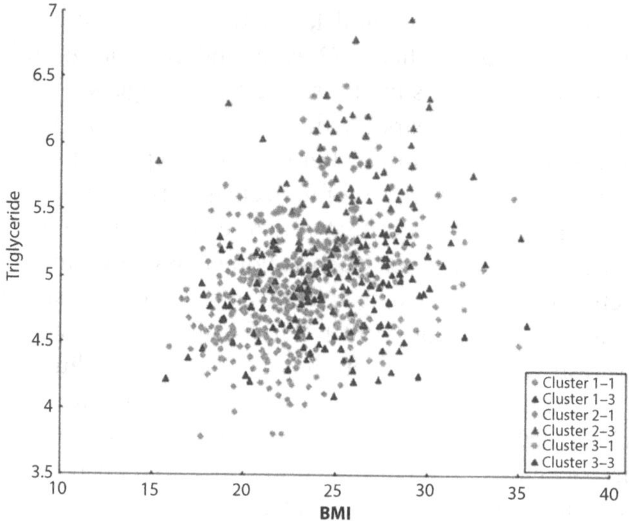

Figure 11.3 Dispersion between triglycerides, body mass index and incidence of type 2 diabetes mellitus.

To build an optimal predictive model, it was initially chosen to use the chi-square statistical method, however, very high error rates were obtained (between 28.24 and 52.69%) due to the unequal distribution of genotyping types (within the 499 SNPs there were 70-75% dominant genotypes, 5-15% recessive and the rest were heterozygous, in addition, the clinical data was variable while the data of groups of molecules was relatively static, so when comparing both factors an extremely important risk factor could be disregarded. The models built using decision trees and machine-learning methods did not show many differences due to the same factors. To obtain For a better result, it would be necessary to adequately quantify the SNPs to initially classify patients into high-risk and low-risk groups. The analysis concludes that the error rates were higher than expected, so it is recommended to use larger samples and better analysis strategies to integrate genotyping to objectively quantify high-risk SNPs [35].

11.4 Experimental Results and Discussion

11.4.1 Prediction of Diabetes with Artificial Neural Networks Supervised Learning Algorithms

We propose using multilayer neural networks to obtain successful predictions of diabetes compared to traditional methods, based on the fact that there are neural network algorithms that have been proven to be useful for diagnosing heart disease, tuberculosis, pneumonia and lung cancer. A sample of 250 diabetes patients was used, among which these values include things like blood pressure, urine acidity, and creatinine, which are considered numerical values. To find the input-output connection via training utilizing a collection of data, supervised learning is defined as a methodology, learning from the output based on the error signal that is emitted according to the diagnosis, continuing until the minimum value is identified error allowed.

Algorithms available in the MATLAB neural network tools were used, using the following:

- Fletcher–Powell conjugate gradient method.
- Polak–Ribiére conjugate gradient method.
- Scaled conjugate gradient method.

To identify the relationship between desired results and obtained results, a regression analysis was used where a correlation coefficient R was obtained, with 1 being an ideal result. Next, the algorithms' performances are displayed the regression test carried out on this case was the basis for the conclusion. We obtain the following sketch. In the figures below, we identify the correlation coefficient R corresponding to each algorithm respectively, reflected by the dotted line. We can identify that the conjugate gradient algorithm scaled almost above the reference line, indicating a result close between what was expected and what was predicted. Figure 11.4 shows the dispersion of algorithm results versus the correlation coefficient R and the Figure 11.5 shows the algorithm performance measurement.

The objective of the study is to determine the algorithm that has the best performance with the collected data. The results of the coefficient R are as follows shown in Table 11.1.

Identifying that the scaled conjugate gradient algorithm is by far the best performer in predicting diabetes compared to the poor performances of the Polak-Ribiére and Fletcher-Powell algorithms.

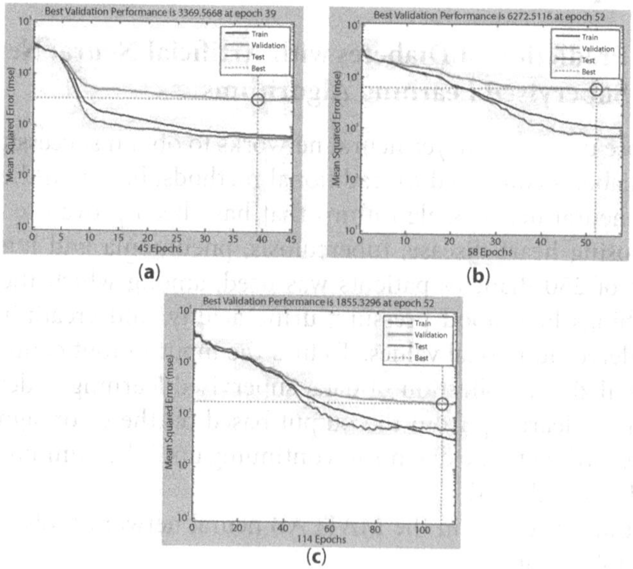

Figure 11.4 Dispersion of algorithm results versus the correlation coefficient R. Label (a) could represent a baseline or standard algorithm against which others are compared. It may show minimal variation in results across different R values, indicating consistent performance. Label (b) might depict an alternative algorithm that has a varying degree of dispersion, perhaps indicating that its performance is more sensitive to changes in the correlation coefficient. Label (c) could illustrate another variant or an improved algorithm that possibly offers a reduced dispersion of results, suggesting it is more robust or optimized for varying conditions of the correlation coefficient.

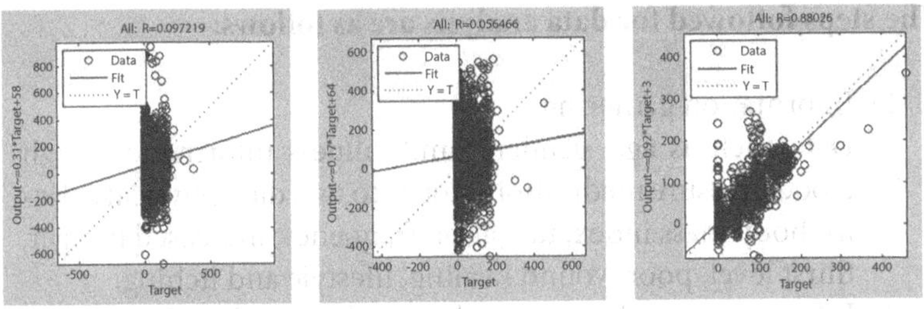

Figure 11.5 Algorithm performance measurement.

Table 11.1 Correlation coefficient by algorithm.

Algorithm	Epochs	Correlation coefficient R
Polak–Ribiere Conjugate Gradient Scaled	52	0.056466
Conjugate Gradient	108	0.88026
Fletcher-Powell Conjugate Gradient	39	0.097219

11.4.2 Improving the Prediction Ratio of Diabetes Diagnoses Using Fuzzy Logic and Neural Networks

It indicates that many approaches have been made in predicting diabetes but that there has never been a special focus on the precision of the models developed.

Existing systems are limited and provide accurate results if high-quality, standardized data sets are used, or few data sets are used. It is under this premise that the paper presents a new approach to the diagnosis of diabetes employing two phases to predict the state of diabetes: the first is to use fuzzy logic, neural networks and reasoning based on cases as an individual approach and the second is apply an algorithm to the values obtained in the first phase, resulting in a prediction with greater objectivity.

A framework is proposed in which a user enters a system and is forced to enter data on its characteristics that can demonstrate a willingness to develop diabetes, and then analyze these parameters. The three approaches mentioned in the initial phase are normalized and applied: fuzzy logic, neural networks and reasoning based on cases, saving these results and finally applying an algorithm to derive the results, generating a final diagnostic report.

The steps followed for data analysis are as follows:

1) Information gathering
2) Data such as age, gender, family illness information, high blood pressure medications, tobacco use, diet, physical activity, body mass index, urination frequency, increased hunger, thirst level, poor wound healing, lifestyle and itching.
3) Information analysis through neural network techniques:
4) Using the back-propagation algorithm: the information is fed to the input layer consisting of a number n of neurons, the activities of the hidden layer depend on the
5) input layer and consists of n + 1 neurons, and the output layer represents 0 or 1, being 1 when the patient is affected by diabetes.
6) Using concepts of fuzzy logic: the data set is defined as indicated above and it is given a value based on the comparison between a patient with diabetes and a healthy one, being in a range between 0 and 2. Then the rules are defined decision according to each parameter: for example, for ages under 35 we can determine a "low" fuzzy set due to the low propensity to develop the disease. In this way and using AND and OR connectors to evaluate the patient's conditions and the result according to the weighting of each variable.
7) Applying reasoning concepts based on cases: two phases are defined; one is predata processing and one is query processing.
8) First, knowledge and data are acquired and in the second, it is processed based on a set of data already defined to identify the propensity of the patient to develop the disease.
9) Rule-based algorithm application:
10) Based on the application of the information analysis approach outlined above, a rule-based algorithm is used to discern between certain and doubtful information, ensuring the final prediction.

It is concluded that the approach proposed through the 3 information analysis fronts is more useful than traditional approaches due to the reduction of errors through the mixture of information analysis and the application of a rule-based algorithm. Likewise, the framework would be beneficial because it allows the patient to obtain information quickly (in case this is implemented in a system) and that it can act in a way that combats those variables that make it prone to the development of the disease.

11.4.3 ARIC: Type 2 Diabetes Risk Predictive Model

A recognition of type 2 diabetes mellitus (T2DM) as a growing epidemic is vital for successful implementation of initiatives to prevent the onset of the condition. Many research investigations have shown that multivariate prediction models are equally effective as those that measure post-2-hour glucose exposure at predicting who will acquire diabetes. On the other hand, no studies assessing the capacity of the functions to correctly predict the likelihood of acquiring type 2 diabetes have been conducted so far.

Based on this, the authors examine the effectiveness of three predictive models to determine if it is possible to estimate the risk of type 2 diabetes in the Asian population and whether it is feasible to use this model in Asian culture. The San Antonio Health investigation (SAHS), Atherosclerosis Risk in Communities Study (ARIC), and Framingham Offspring Study (FRAM) models were employed in this investigation. To verify the models in the Asian context, data from a 1992 study (Singapore Prospective Study Programme, in National Health Survey-NHS. 1992) that included Singaporean Chinese, Malaysian, and Asian Indian persons was used. The authors investigated three published prediction models (Comp 1, Comp 2, and the local NHS 1992 model) in order to find out which one performed better. To date, published multivariate prediction functions have been shown to differ from the estimates created locally.

In general, the published ARIC model marginalizes only slightly better than the published SAHS model. Published models show poor calibration compared to local models that have good calibration properties. The Framingham model shows the worst result when it comes to recalibration, ARIC and SAHS have the best results, but SAHS shows an overestimation of cases with type 2 diabetes compared to the ARIC model. The analysis carried out by the authors suggests that the best model of the 3 evaluated is the ARIC Model.

11.4.4 Evaluation of Neural Network Algorithms for Prediction Models of Type 2 Diabetes

Mention how diabetes is a disease that is growing the fastest and is a global issue. The intricate interdependencies of several variables make it challenging to diagnose type 2 diabetes in its early stages. For this reason, they suggest that it is essential to create a diagnostic support system that aids medical professionals in their diagnostic procedure. Table 11.2 shows the comparing published multivariate predictive functions.

Table 11.2 Comparing published multivariate predictive functions.

Model	HL-Statistic	Predicted incidence (%)
ARIC-local	2.28	7.8
Recalibrated ARIC-published	10.31	8.5
SAHS-local	3.52	7.8
Recalibrated SAHS-published	23.19	11.2
FRAM-published	264.89	2
ARIC-published	1471	9.8
SAHS-published	48.33	13.5
OUT-local	3.9	7.8
FPG-local	3.08	7.8
FRAM-local	1.45	7.8

According to the authors, an analysis may provide a less precise conclusion if the training data set includes unnecessary categorization features. Because of this, data pre-processing is necessary to increase the accuracy of the analysis; otherwise, neural networks may operate at a very sluggish speed. The UCI machine learning library's Pima Indian dataset was used to extract attributes from the diabetes dataset. Nine factors make up this data collection, which distinguishes the accuracy of different algorithms.

The authors made a comparison of the precision rate of N algorithms, of which some algorithms such as KNN, PCA, LDA, GDA allow data to be pre-processed, this allows the missing information to be completed according to patterns detected by each algorithm. Each carrying out their task differently from the other. They show how the LDA Morlet Wavelet Support Vector Machine Classifier or LDA-MWSVM algorithm, which has Linear Discriminant Analysis or LDA as its pre-processing algorithm, significantly improves its precision ratio.

They conclude that the pre-processing of the data and the extraction characteristic together with Neural Network models improves the accuracy classification.

11.4.5 Reliable and Objective Recommendation System for the Diagnosis of Chronic Diseases

It proposes an accurate and reliable chronic disease diagnosis system to provide 24/7 remote monitoring. In the formulation of its hypothesis, it is indicated that if the risk of chronic diseases of a patient is predicted with high precision, an improvement in the patient's health conditions and adjustments in their lifestyle should be expected, reducing coverage costs of health.

To increase precision, it is necessary to reduce false positives and false negatives and that is why the origin and complexity of the collected medical data is considered (understanding by complexity to nonstandardized data, with a high number of parameters or missing). It is indicated that medical information is generated by various sources and by various people, making it prone to different types of errors such as missing or erroneous data, this being an extremely important challenge for the effectiveness of the diagnosis. In the paper, a decision tree classification scope is proposed to increase the effectiveness of the diagnosis, with proven results on medical data.

- Training data: it is information from previous diabetic patients and consists of 935 records from Oman hospitals, within which there are attributes, values and diagnoses of the doctor, using a scale of 1 to 10 where 1-2 represent excellent prognosis and 9–10 represent critical condition.
- Demographic data: data on age, name, level of education, type of device connecting to the system and type of connectivity.
- Patient medical data: blood sugar level, blood pressure and weight.

Within the identified decision tree classification, the Random Forest (RF) classification method is used for the analysis and segmentation of the information entered: a distinction is made between related information based on the diagnostic scales, using these relationships to generate a predictive model to determine the patient's diagnostic class. Based on the analysis and classification of these data, a numerical value is provided that represents the patient's risk diagnosis of a disease. In addition, the diagnosis is taken and it is re-analyzed to now compare it against the diagnoses of other patients, identifying additional coincidences. Table 11.3 shown the decision tree classification with different attributes.

Table 11.3 Decision tree classification with different attributes.

Sr. no.	Attribute	Description	Missing value
1.	Plasma glucose	Plasma glucose concentration measured using two hours oral glucose tolerance test (nun Hg)	5
2.	Diastolic BP	Diastolic blood pressure	35
3.	Triceps SFT	Triceps skin fold thickness (nun)	227
4.	Pregnant	A record of the number of times the woman pregnant	110
5.	DPF	Diabetes pedigree function	0
6.	Age	Age of patient (year)	0
7.	BMI	Body mass index (weight Kg/height in (nun) 2)	11
8.	Serum-Insulin	Two hours serum insulin (muU/ml)	374
9.	Class	Diabetes on set within five year	0

According to the proposed flow, once this analysis is concluded, information is sent to the health providers who would approve the accuracy of the diagnosis and update the patient's profile, sending mitigation actions against the factors that pose a risk of developing the disease and sending the information of the Diagnostics to the system to improve the way it learns and provides future diagnostics.

The proposed predictive model is compared to other decision tree models such as J48, Decision Stump and REP Tree. The information analyzed is from patients in Oman hospitals and consists of 935 patients and 13 attributes (including the doctor's diagnostic scale).

Table 11.4 Comparison of accuracy with different classification technique.

Method	Classification/Accuracy
LM	78.08
LDA	76.5
kNN	74.5
LVQ	74.8
Semi-Naive Bayes (5xCV)	77
BFGS quasi-Newton	79.08
MML	74.5
RBF	74.7
MLP + BP	77.4
FDA	77.5
GTO DT (5xCV)	77.8
GRNN	81.21
LDA-MWSVM	88.74
GD	76.6
SVM (5xCV)	76.6
GDA-LS-SVM	78.16
ASI	75.6
SMART	77.8
MI-MCS-SVM	94.58
BP	742
SNB	724
NB	76.5

For the evaluation of the RF model compared to the others, the MAE metric (measurement of absolute error) was used, dictated by the following formula:

$$MAE = \frac{1}{n}\sum_{i=1}^{n}|f_i - y_i| = \frac{1}{n}\sum_{i=1}^{n}|e_i|$$

where MAE represents the average of absolute errors ei, where ei = fi – yi, where fi is the diagnosis and yi is the actual diagnosis.

Based on the evaluation of results, it was identified that:

- The mean error of 10 RF trees is 0.2877
- RF has correctly demonstrated 99.7% of correctly classified cases

RF improves accuracy by managing the data internally through the aforementioned phases of analyzing its predictions once they have been issued: this approach to learning enriches the model and stimulates its accuracy. It is concluded that the RF method will generate effective prediction of risk of chronic diseases of patients who suffer from them, because it learns from its own results and enriches its future predictions. Comparison of accuracy with different classification technique is shown in Table 11.4.

11.5 Conclusion

Diabetes is a disease with the greatest growth, being a problem around the world. Diagnosing type 2 diabetes in the early stages is a difficult challenge to meet due to the complex interdependencies of several factors. It is for this reason that they indicate that it is necessary to develop a diagnostic support system, which is beneficial for medical practitioners in their diagnostic process. if the data set under training contains irrelevant classification attributes, the analysis may produce a less accurate result. That is why data pre-processing is required to improve the precision of the analysis, without pre-processing neural networks could be very slow. To increase precision, it is necessary to reduce false positives and false negatives and that is why the origin and complexity of the collected medical data is considered (understanding by complexity to non-standardized data, with a high number of parameters or missing). It is indicated that medical information is generated by various sources and by various people, making it prone to different types of errors such as missing or erroneous data, this being an extremely important challenge for the effectiveness of the diagnosis. In the paper, a decision tree classification scope is proposed to increase the effectiveness of the diagnosis, with proven results on medical data.

References

1. Kölle, K., Biester, T., Christiansen, S., Fougner, A.L., Stavdahl, Pattern Recognition Reveals Characteristic Postprandial Glucose Changes: Non-Individualized Meal Detection in Diabetes Mellitus Type 1. *IEEE J. Biomed. Health Inf.*, 24, 2, 594–602, Feb. 2020, doi: 10.1109/JBHI.2019.2908897.
2. Benkhaddra, I., Kumar, A., Setitra, M.A. *et al.*, Design and Development of Consensus Activation Function Enabled Neural Network-Based Smart Healthcare Using BIoT. *Wirel. Pers. Commun.*, 130, 1549–1574, 2023, https://doi.org/10.1007/s11277-023-10344-0 Q2, Impact Factor -2.017.
3. Srivastav, A.L., Markandeya, Patel, N. *et al.*, Concepts of circular economy for sustainable management of electronic wastes: challenges and management options. *Environ. Sci. Pollut. Res.*, 30, 48654–48675, 2023, https://doi.org/10.1007/s11356-023-26052-y Q1, Impact Factor -5.19.
4. Ilyas, B., Kumar, A., Setitra, M.A., Bensalem, Z.E.A., Lei, H., Prevention of DDoS attacks using an optimized deep learning approach in blockchain technology. *Trans. Emerging Telecommun. Technol.*, 34, 4, e4729, 2023. Q2, Impact Factor -3.31.
5. Kumar, A., Rathore, P.S., Dubey, A.K. *et al.*, LTE-NBP with holistic UWB-WBAN approach for the energy efficient biomedical application. *Multimed. Tools Appl.*, 39797–39811, 2023, https://doi.org/10.1007/s11042-023-15604-6 Q1, Impact Factor -2.577.
6. Kumar, A., Kumar, S.A., Dutt, V., Shitharth, S., Tripathi, E., IoT based arrhythmia classification using the enhanced hunt optimization-based deep learning. *Expert Syst.*, 40, 7, e13298, 2023, https://doi.org/10.1111/exsy.13298.
7. Xie, J. and Wang, Q., A Variable State Dimension Approach to Meal Detection and Meal Size Estimation: In Silico Evaluation Through Basal-Bolus Insulin Therapy for Type 1 Diabetes. *IEEE Trans. Biomed. Eng.*, 64, 6, 1249–1260, June 2017, doi: 10.1109/TBME.2016.2599073.
8. Moreno, E.M. *et al.*, Type 2 Diabetes Screening Test by Means of a Pulse Oximeter. *IEEE Trans. Biomed. Eng.*, 64, 2, 341–351, Feb. 2017, doi: 10.1109/TBME.2016.2554661.
9. Facchinetti, A., Favero, S., Sparacino, G., Cobelli, C., An Online Failure Detection Method of the Glucose Sensor-Insulin Pump System: Improved Overnight Safety of Type-1 Diabetic Subjects. *IEEE Trans. Biomed. Eng.*, 60, 2, 406–416, Feb. 2013, doi: 10.1109/TBME.2012.2227256.

10. Zarkogianni, K. *et al.*, A Review of Emerging Technologies for the Management of Diabetes Mellitus. *IEEE Trans. Biomed. Eng.*, 62, 12, 2735–2749, Dec. 2015, doi: 10.1109/TBME.2015.2470521.
11. Zhang, B., Vijaya kumar, B.V.K., Zhang, D., Noninvasive Diabetes Mellitus Detection Using Facial Block Color With a Sparse Representation Classifier. *IEEE Trans. Biomed. Eng.*, 61, 4, 1027–1033, April 2014, doi: 10.1109/TBME.2013.2292936.
12. Syed, A.H. and Khan, T., Machine Learning-Based Application for Predicting Risk of Type 2 Diabetes Mellitus (T2DM) in Saudi Arabia: A Retrospective Cross-Sectional Study. *IEEE Access*, 8, 199539–199561, 2020, doi: 10.1109/ACCESS.2020.3035026.
13. Omer, A.E., Shaker, G., Safavi-Naeini, S., Murray, K., Hughson, R., Glucose Levels Detection Using mm-Wave Radar. *IEEE Sens. Lett.*, 2, 3, 1–4, Sept. 2018, doi: 10.1109/LSENS.2018.2865165,t Art no. 3502004.
14. Khan, F.A., Zeb, K., Al-Rakhami, M., Derhab, A., Bukhari, S.A.C., Detection and Prediction of Diabetes Using Data Mining: A Comprehensive Review. *IEEE Access*, 9, 43711–43735, 2021, doi: 10.1109/ACCESS.2021.3059343.
15. Turksoy, K., Roy, A., Cinar, A., Real-Time Model-Based Fault Detection of Continuous Glucose Sensor Measurements. *IEEE Trans. Biomed. Eng.*, 64, 7, 1437–1445, July 2017, doi: 10.1109/TBME.2016.2535412.
16. Kotturu, P.K. and Kumar, A., Comparative Study on Machine Learning models for Early Diagnose of Alzheimer's Disease: Multi Correlation Method. *2020 5th International Conference on Communication and Electronics Systems (ICCES)*, pp. 778–783, 2020, doi: 10.1109/ICCES48766.2020.9137872.
17. Swarna, S.R., Kumar, A., Dixit, P., Sairam, T.V.M., Parkinson's Disease Prediction using Adaptive Quantum Computing. *2021 Third International Conference on Intelligent Communication Technologies and Virtual Mobile Networks (ICICV)*, pp. 1396–1401, 2021, doi: 10.1109/ICICV50876.2021.9388628.
18. Bhargava, N., Rathore, P.S., Bhowmick, A., Study of X Ray Detection Using CNN in Machine Learning. *Advancements in Smart Computing and Information Security: First International Conference, ASCIS 2022*, Rajkot, India, November 24–26, 2022, Cham: Springer Nature, Switzerland, 2023, Revised Selected Papers, Part I.
19. Dutt, V., Rathore, P.S., Chauhan, K., Support Vector in Healthcare Using SVM/PSO in Various Domains: A Review, in: *Swarm Intelligence Optimization: Algorithms and Applications*, pp. 291–307, 2020.
20. Bhargava, N., Sharma, S., Purohit, R., Rathore, P.S., Prediction of recurrence cancer using J48 algorithm, in: *2017 2nd International Conference on Communication and Electronics Systems (ICCES)*, pp. 386–390, IEEE, 2017, October.
21. Şahin, S., Merotra, J., Kang, J., Trenell, M., Catt, M., Yu, E.H., Simultaneous Electrochemical Detection of Glucose and Non-Esterified Fatty Acids (NEFAs) for Diabetes Management. *IEEE Sens. J.*, 18, 22, 9075–9080, Nov. 15, 2018, doi: 10.1109/JSEN.2018.2870071.

22. Fleming, A.D., Philip, S., Goatman, K.A., Olson, J.A., Sharp, P.F., Automated microaneurysm detection using local contrast normalization and local vessel detection. *IEEE Trans. Med. Imaging*, 25, 9, 1223–1232, Sept. 2006, doi: 10.1109/TMI.2006.879953.
23. Lekha, S. and S., M., Recent Advancements and Future Prospects on E-Nose Sensors Technology and Machine Learning Approaches for Non-Invasive Diabetes Diagnosis: A Review. *IEEE Rev. Biomed. Eng.*, 14, 127–138, 2021, doi: 10.1109/RBME.2020.2993591.
24. Rocha, A., Carvalho, T., Jelinek, H.F., Goldenstein, S., Wainer, J., Points of Interest and Visual Dictionaries for Automatic Retinal Lesion Detection. *IEEE Trans. Biomed. Eng.*, 59, 8, 2244–2253, Aug. 2012, doi: 10.1109/TBME.2012.2201717.
25. Chen, C. *et al.*, Development of Magnetic Particle-Based Immunoassays and Their Applications in Diabetes Monitoring. *IEEE Trans. Magn.*, 50, 1, 1–4, Jan. 2014, doi: 10.1109/TMAG.2013.2278851. Art no. 4003104.
26. Ramkissoon, C.M., Bertachi, A., Beneyto, A., Bondia, J., Vehi, J., Detection and Control of Unannounced Exercise in the Artificial Pancreas Without Additional Physiological Signals. *IEEE J. Biomed. Health Inf.*, 24, 1, 259–267, Jan. 2020, doi: 10.1109/JBHI.2019.2898558.
27. Fitriyani, N.L., Syafrudin, M., Alfian, G., Rhee, J., Development of Disease Prediction Model Based on Ensemble Learning Approach for Diabetes and Hypertension. *IEEE Access*, 7, 144777–144789, 2019, doi: 10.1109/ACCESS.2019.2945129.
28. Rashtian, H., Torbaghan, S.S., Rahili, S., Snyder, M., Aghaeepour, N., Heart Rate and CGM Feature Representation Diabetes Detection From Heart Rate: Learning Joint Features of Heart Rate and Continuous Glucose Monitors Yields Better Representations. *IEEE Access*, 9, 83234–83240, 2021, doi: 10.1109/ACCESS.2021.3085544.
29. Meneghetti, L., Terzi, M., Del Favero, S., Susto, G.A., Cobelli, C., Data-Driven Anomaly Recognition for Unsupervised Model-Free Fault Detection in Artificial Pancreas. *IEEE Trans. Control Syst. Technol.*, 28, 1, 33–47, Jan. 2020, doi: 10.1109/TCST.2018.2885963.
30. Sani, M.H. and Khosroabadi, S., A Novel Design and Analysis of High-Sensitivity Biosensor Based on Nano-Cavity for Detection of Blood Component, Diabetes, Cancer and Glucose Concentration. *IEEE Sens. J.*, 20, 13, 7161–7168, July 1, 2020, doi: 10.1109/JSEN.2020.2964114.
31. Wang, L., Pedersen, P.C., Strong, D.M., Tulu, B., Agu, E., Ignotz, R., Smartphone-Based Wound Assessment System for Patients With Diabetes. *IEEE Trans. Biomed. Eng.*, 62, 2, 477–488, Feb. 2015, doi: 10.1109/TBME.2014.2358632.
32. Ngo, C.Q., Chai, R., Nguyen, T.V., Jones, T.W., Nguyen, H.T., Electroencephalogram Spectral Moments for the Detection of Nocturnal Hypoglycemia. *IEEE J. Biomed. Health Inf.*, 24, 5, 1237–1245, May 2020, doi: 10.1109/JBHI.2019.2931782.

33. Usman, I. and Almejalli, K.A., Intelligent Automated Detection of Microaneurysms in Fundus Images Using Feature-Set Tuning. *IEEE Access*, 8, 65187–65196, 2020, doi: 10.1109/ACCESS.2020.2985543.
34. Sarki, R., Ahmed, K., Wang, H., Zhang, Y., Automatic Detection of Diabetic Eye Disease Through Deep Learning Using Fundus Images: A Survey. *IEEE Access*, 8, 151133–151149, 2020, doi: 10.1109/ACCESS.2020.3015258.
35. Meneghetti, L., Facchinetti, A., Favero, S.D., Model-Based Detection and Classification of Insulin Pump Faults and Missed Meal Announcements in Artificial Pancreas Systems for Type 1 Diabetes Therapy. *IEEE Trans. Biomed. Eng.*, 68, 1, 170–180, Jan. 2021, doi: 10.1109/TBME.2020.3004270.

12

Diagnosis of Neurological Disease Using Bioinspired Algorithms

Inam Ul Haq

Faculty of Engineering and Technology, SGT University Gurugram, Haryana, India

Abstract

Neurological diseases have a significant impact on individuals, families, and society. Accurate and timely diagnosis is crucial for effective treatment and management. However, traditional diagnostic methods are often expensive and time-consuming. Recent advancements in bioinspired algorithms offer new possibilities for the diagnosis of neurological diseases. This chapter provides an overview of the role of bioinspired algorithms in neurological disease diagnosis. The chapter begins with an introduction to bioinspired algorithms, covering various types commonly used in healthcare, such as genetic algorithms, neural networks, ant colony optimization, and particle swarm optimization. The applications of bioinspired algorithms in healthcare are explored, emphasizing their contributions to medical image analysis, disease diagnosis, treatment optimization, and personalized medicine. The chapter then focuses on neurological disease diagnosis, providing an overview of common diseases and current diagnostic techniques. It reviews traditional diagnostic methods and their limitations, highlighting the need for alternative approaches. The application of bioinspired algorithms in neurological disease diagnosis is discussed in detail. Genetic algorithms optimize feature selection and classification algorithms, demonstrated through case studies and research findings. Neural networks are explored for their potential in improving disease diagnosis accuracy through bioinspired optimization techniques. Other bioinspired algorithms, such as ant colony optimization and particle swarm optimization, are also examined for their applications in feature selection, clustering analysis, and diagnostic model optimization. Finally, the chapter addresses the challenges and limitations associated with the use of bioinspired algorithms in neurological disease diagnosis. It emphasizes the need for further research and development in this emerging field. Overall, bioinspired algorithms hold great

Email: mirinam525@gmail.com

Sumit Srivastava, Abhineet Anand, Abhishek Kumar, Bhavna Saini and Pramod Singh Rathore (eds.) Bio-Inspired Optimization for Medical Data Mining, (227–268) © 2024 Scrivener Publishing LLC

promise in advancing the field of neurological disease diagnosis, offering new opportunities for accurate and efficient diagnosis.

Keywords: Neurological disease, bioinspired algorithms, artificial intelligence, genetic algorithms

12.1 Introduction

12.1.1 Neurological Diseases

Neurological diseases encompass a diverse range of disorders that affect the brain, spinal cord, and peripheral nervous system. These conditions have a profound impact on individuals, families, and society as a whole, posing significant challenges in terms of diagnosis, treatment, and management. Neurological diseases can lead to a wide array of symptoms, including cognitive impairment, movement disorders, sensory deficits, and even life-threatening complications. Understanding the complexities of neurological diseases requires exploring the intricate workings of the nervous system [1]. A sophisticated network of specialized cells known as neurons makes up the nervous system., which transmit and process electrical and chemical signals. It is in charge of directing and coordinating body processes, as well as enabling higher cognitive processes. Neurological diseases can arise from various causes, including genetic factors, infections, immune system disorders, trauma, toxic exposure, and age-related degeneration. Some neurological diseases, such as Parkinson's disease and Alzheimer's disease are both referred to as neurodegenerative illnesses by progressive loss of neurons and subsequent decline in neurological function. Others, like epilepsy and multiple sclerosis, involve abnormalities in the function or structure of the nervous system [2]. One of the major challenges in dealing with neurological diseases is their diverse nature and the wide spectrum of symptoms they present. Each neurological disorder has unique characteristics, requiring specialized diagnostic approaches and treatment strategies.

Figure 12.1 shows the common neurological diseases, and there are many more conditions within the field of neurology.

Moreover, neurological diseases often exhibit significant heterogeneity, with variations in symptoms, disease progression, and treatment responses among affected individuals. This heterogeneity underscores the need for personalized and targeted approaches to diagnosis and treatment. Accurate and timely diagnosis of neurological diseases is of utmost importance for several reasons. First and foremost, an accurate diagnosis allows healthcare

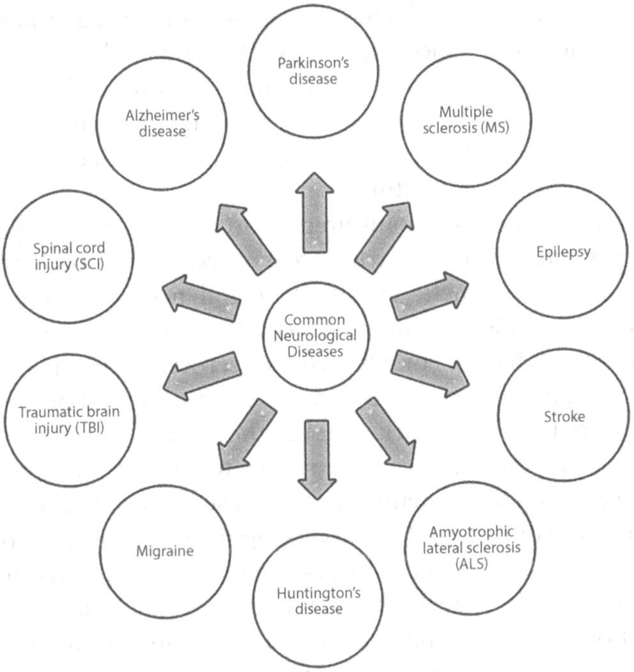

Figure 12.1 Common neurological diseases.

professionals to provide appropriate and targeted treatment interventions. Many neurological diseases are chronic or progressive in nature, and early intervention can help slow disease progression, manage alleviate symptoms, and raise general quality of life [3]. In some cases, such as stroke or traumatic brain injury, prompt diagnosis is crucial for immediate life-saving interventions. Furthermore, accurate diagnosis enables researchers and scientists to study the underlying mechanisms of neurological diseases, paving the way for the development of new therapeutic strategies and interventions. It also facilitates the identification of biomarkers, which are measurable indicators that can aid in the diagnosis, prognosis, and monitoring of disease progression. However, diagnosing neurological diseases can be challenging due to the complex and overlapping nature of their symptoms. Many neurological disorders lack specific diagnostic tests, making diagnosis primarily reliant on clinical evaluation, patient history, and the expertise of healthcare professionals [4]. Consequently, misdiagnosis or delayed diagnosis is not uncommon, leading to significant implications for patients and their families. Advancements in medical technology, imaging techniques, and laboratory investigations have significantly improved the diagnostic capabilities for many neurological diseases. Magnetic resonance imaging (MRI), computed tomography (CT) scans, electroencephalography (EEG), and cerebrospinal fluid analysis are some of the tools commonly used in the diagnostic process. However, these tests are often expensive, time-consuming, and may not be readily accessible in all healthcare settings.

The creation and use of bioinspired algorithms for neurological illness detection has gained popularity in recent years. Natural occurrences and processes, including genetic evolution, neural networks, swarm intelligence, and optimization methods, serve as the basis for bioinspired algorithms. In order to handle complicated issues, these algorithms imitate the behavior of natural systems, and they have demonstrated promising outcomes in a variety of fields, including healthcare [5].

Bioinspired algorithms have the potential to enhance the accuracy, efficiency, and accessibility of neurological disease diagnosis. They can aid in the identification of relevant biomarkers, optimize diagnostic models, and improve the analysis of medical images and patient data. By harnessing the power of computational techniques and artificial intelligence, bioinspired algorithms offer new possibilities for early detection, accurate diagnosis, and personalized treatment strategies for neurological diseases [6].

12.1.2 Introduction to Bioinspired Algorithms

Bioinspired algorithms, also known as nature-inspired algorithms or computational intelligence techniques, are computational methods inspired by biological systems and processes found in nature. These algorithms imitate the behavior, principles, and mechanisms observed in natural organisms or ecosystems to solve complex optimization and problem-solving tasks. By drawing inspiration from nature, bioinspired algorithms offer innovative solutions to a wide range of problems in various domains, including healthcare.

Principles and Characteristics of Bioinspired Algorithms:

1. Inspiration from nature: bioinspired algorithms derive their principles and methodologies from natural phenomena, such as the behavior of animals, the structure of ecosystems, or the processes within biological systems.
2. Optimization and problem solving: bioinspired algorithms excel in solving optimization problems, where the goal is to find the best solution from a large search space. They can also address complex problem-solving tasks by mimicking the adaptive and evolutionary mechanisms found in nature.

3. Parallelism and distributed processing: many bioinspired algorithms exhibit parallel and distributed processing, emulating the cooperative behavior seen in biological systems. This allows for efficient exploration of solution spaces and better scalability for handling large-scale problems.
4. Robustness and adaptation: bioinspired algorithms often possess robustness and adaptability, allowing them to handle noisy or uncertain environments. They can adapt to changing conditions, optimize performance, and recover from failures, resembling the resilience seen in natural systems.
5. Exploration and exploitation: bioinspired algorithms strike a balance between exploration (searching for new solutions) and exploitation (using existing knowledge) to efficiently navigate the solution space and avoid getting trapped in local optima.

12.1.3 Types of Bioinspired Algorithms Commonly Used in Healthcare

Bioinspired algorithms have found applications in healthcare for various purposes. Here, in Figure 12.2, there are some commonly used types of bioinspired algorithms in healthcare:

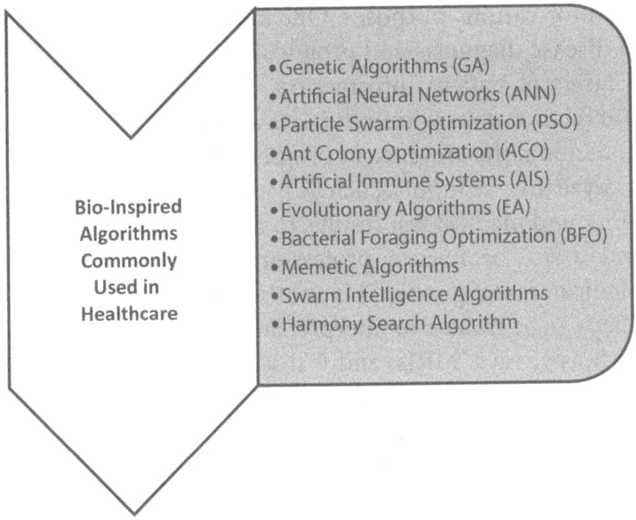

Figure 12.2 Some commonly used types of bioinspired algorithms in healthcare.

1. Genetic Algorithms (GA): GAs are optimization algorithms that draw inspiration from the laws of natural selection. In the context of healthcare, GA has proven to be valuable in several applications. One prominent use is in optimizing treatment plans for individual patients. By considering various treatment options, GA can search for the most effective combination and dosage of medications or therapies based on the patient's unique characteristics and medical history [7]. This approach helps healthcare professionals personalize treatment and improve patient outcomes. Additionally, GA plays a significant role in drug discovery. The process of identifying new drugs can be time-consuming and costly. GA offers a computational approach to explore large chemical spaces and optimize molecular structures with desirable properties. By simulating evolution and natural selection, GA can generate novel drug candidates or modify existing compounds to enhance their efficacy or reduce side effects. This aids in accelerating the drug discovery process and potentially leads to the development of more effective treatments [8].
2. Artificial neural networks (ANN): Computer models known as artificial neural networks (ANNs) are influenced by the design and operation of biological neural networks. In healthcare, ANNs have gained significant attention and are used for various purposes. One key application of ANNs is in disease diagnosis and prognosis [5]. By training on large datasets of patient information, ANNs can learn patterns and relationships within the data and make accurate predictions about the presence or progression of diseases. They can analyze diverse inputs, such as patient demographics, symptoms, and medical test results, to provide diagnostic insights and assist healthcare professionals in decision making. Medical imaging analysis is another area where ANNs excel. They can be trained to interpret and analyze medical images, such as X-rays, MRIs, and CT scans. ANNs can automatically detect and classify abnormalities or assist in image segmentation, where specific structures or regions of interest are identified and delineated. This capability enhances the accuracy and efficiency of medical image interpretation, aiding in early detection and treatment planning. ANNs are also utilized for drug discovery and development [2].

They can be employed to predict the activity and toxicity of potential drug compounds, aiding in the selection and optimization of drug candidates. By learning from vast amounts of chemical and biological data, ANNs can identify novel drug–target interactions, analyze molecular structures, and provide insights into drug design and optimization.

3. Particle swarm optimization (PSO): PSO is a population-based optimization algorithm that is inspired by the social behavior of bird flocking or fish schooling. In the context of healthcare, PSO has been applied to various problems and has shown promising results. One common application of PSO in healthcare is medical image segmentation. PSO can be used to optimize the parameters of image segmentation algorithms, such as determining optimal thresholds or region-growing parameters [9]. By iteratively updating the position and velocity of particles representing potential solutions, PSO searches the parameter space to find the optimal segmentation result, leading to improved accuracy and efficiency in medical image analysis. PSO is also used for feature selection in healthcare data analysis. In many healthcare datasets, there are numerous features or variables that may not all be relevant for a specific task. PSO can be employed to identify the subset of features that contribute the most to a particular prediction or classification task. By evaluating the fitness of different feature combinations, PSO guides the search process and selects the most informative features, reducing dimensionality and improving the performance of healthcare models. Furthermore, PSO has been utilized in optimizing treatment parameters. For instance, in radiation therapy planning, PSO can optimize the beam angles and intensities to maximize the radiation dose to the tumor while minimizing the dose to surrounding healthy tissues. By iteratively adjusting the particle positions representing different treatment plans, PSO helps find an optimal solution that balances treatment effectiveness and patient safety [10].
4. Ant colony optimization (ACO): ACO is a metaheuristic algorithm inspired by the foraging behavior of ants. It is commonly used in various healthcare applications, offering effective solutions to optimization problems. One primary application of ACO in healthcare is healthcare

routing and scheduling. ACO can optimize the routing of healthcare resources, such as ambulances, healthcare personnel, or medical supplies to minimize travel distance or time while ensuring efficient delivery of healthcare services. Additionally, ACO can help in scheduling healthcare tasks, such as patient appointments or operating room schedules, by considering factors like priority, resource availability, and minimizing waiting times. Another area where ACO is applied is in healthcare network optimization. ACO can optimize the layout and organization of healthcare facilities, such as hospitals or clinics, to improve accessibility and efficiency. By considering factors like patient demand, transportation connectivity, and resource allocation, ACO can help in designing healthcare networks that provide optimal coverage and meet the healthcare needs of a population [9]. ACO is also used in healthcare data clustering and classification. By mimicking the behavior of ants laying pheromone trails to guide their colony, ACO can identify natural groupings or clusters within healthcare datasets. This aids in patient stratification or identifying patterns in disease data. Furthermore, ACO can be employed for feature selection in healthcare data analysis, assisting in identifying the most informative and relevant features for prediction or classification tasks.

5. Artificial Immune Systems (AIS): AIS are computational models inspired by the human immune system's mechanisms and processes. In healthcare, AIS has been applied to various areas and has shown promise in solving complex problems. One significant application of AIS is in anomaly detection and intrusion detection systems. By mimicking the immune system's ability to recognize foreign or abnormal entities, AIS algorithms can detect and identify unusual patterns or behaviors in healthcare data. This can help in identifying potential health risks, fraudulent activities, or anomalies in medical records, improving the overall security and integrity of healthcare systems [10]. AIS is also used in disease classification and diagnosis. By leveraging the principles of self/non–self-discrimination, AIS algorithms can analyze patient data and identify patterns indicative of specific diseases or conditions. This can aid in accurate and early diagnosis, allowing for timely interventions and

improved patient outcomes. Furthermore, AIS has been applied to optimize vaccination strategies. By simulating the immune response to pathogens, AIS algorithms can determine optimal vaccination schedules, dosage levels, and priority groups. This helps in optimizing immunization programs, preventing the spread of infectious diseases, and maximizing the effectiveness of vaccination campaigns. Another area where AIS is employed is in optimizing healthcare processes and resource allocation. By considering the immune system's ability to allocate resources based on the urgency and importance of different tasks, AIS algorithms can assist in healthcare resource management [11]. This includes optimizing bed allocation, staff scheduling, and resource utilization, ultimately leading to more efficient and cost-effective healthcare delivery.

6. Evolutionary algorithms (EAs): EAs are computational algorithms inspired by the principles of biological evolution and natural selection. In healthcare, EA has been widely used for solving optimization problems and has shown effectiveness in various applications. One prominent application of EA in healthcare is optimizing treatment protocols. EA can be employed to optimize the dosage and scheduling of medications or therapies for individual patients. By simulating the evolutionary process of selection and adaptation, EA explores a population of potential treatment plans and evolves them over generations to find the most effective and personalized treatment strategies [4].
7. Swarm intelligence algorithms: SIAs are computational algorithms inspired by the collective behavior of social insect colonies or other swarming organisms. In healthcare, SIAs have been applied to solve complex problems and optimize various processes. One common application of SIAs in healthcare is medical data clustering. SIAs, such as particle swarm optimization (PSO) and ant colony optimization (ACO), can be used to identify natural groupings or clusters within healthcare datasets [12]. By simulating the collective behavior of swarming organisms, SIAs help in discovering patterns and relationships in large and complex datasets, facilitating data analysis and decision making. SIAs are also utilized in healthcare resource allocation and scheduling. By mimicking the collaborative behavior of

swarming organisms, SIAs can optimize the allocation and utilization of healthcare resources such as hospital beds, healthcare personnel, or medical equipment. This helps in maximizing resource efficiency, minimizing waiting times, and improving the overall healthcare service delivery. SIAs have been applied to optimize healthcare routing and logistics. By simulating the movement and interaction patterns of swarming organisms, SIAs can optimize the routing of ambulances, healthcare supplies, or medical samples. This ensures efficient and timely delivery of healthcare services and improves response times in emergency situations. SIAs are also used in healthcare optimization problems, such as healthcare facility location planning and healthcare network design. By leveraging the principles of swarm intelligence, SIAs can identify optimal locations for healthcare facilities, considering factors like population distribution, accessibility, and demand. Additionally, SIAs assist in designing efficient healthcare networks that ensure effective coverage and accessibility to healthcare services [13].

These algorithms leverage principles inspired by biological systems to solve complex healthcare problems. Each algorithm has its own strengths and applications within the healthcare domain.

12.1.4 Advantages and Limitations of Bioinspired Algorithms

Bioinspired algorithms have gained significant attention and have been successfully applied to various fields due to their unique advantages. However, like any computational technique, they also have certain limitations. In this discussion, we will explore the advantages and limitations of bioinspired algorithms in detail.

Advantages:

1. Optimization and problem solving: bioinspired algorithms excel in solving complex optimization problems. They can efficiently explore large solution spaces and find near-optimal or optimal solutions. These algorithms leverage the power of natural selection, adaptation, and swarm intelligence to handle complex, multidimensional, and nonlinear problems.

2. Robustness and adaptability: bioinspired algorithms often exhibit robustness and adaptability. They can handle noisy or uncertain environments, making them suitable for real-world applications where data may be incomplete or contain errors. These algorithms can adapt and optimize their performance in dynamic environments, allowing them to respond effectively to changing conditions.
3. Parallel and distributed processing: many bioinspired algorithms inherently possess parallel and distributed processing capabilities. They can explore multiple solutions simultaneously and leverage collective intelligence. This enables efficient exploration of large search spaces, faster convergence to solutions, and scalability for handling large-scale problems.
4. Exploration and exploitation: bioinspired algorithms strike a balance between exploration and exploitation. They explore the search space to discover new solutions while exploiting known solutions to improve performance. This helps prevent premature convergence to suboptimal solutions and enhances the ability to find global optima.
5. Domain independence: bioinspired algorithms are often domain-independent. They can be applied to a wide range of problem domains, including healthcare, engineering, finance, and logistics. This versatility allows researchers and practitioners to leverage these algorithms across various disciplines, making them highly valuable and adaptable tools.
6. Inspiration from nature: bioinspired algorithms draw inspiration from natural systems and phenomena. This enables researchers to understand and model complex natural processes, leading to new insights and knowledge discovery. The underlying biological principles provide a rich source of inspiration for developing innovative and efficient computational techniques.
7. Interdisciplinary research: bioinspired algorithms promote interdisciplinary research, bringing together experts from various fields, such as biology, computer science, mathematics, and engineering. This collaboration fosters the exchange of ideas, methodologies, and perspectives, leading to novel advancements and cross-fertilization of knowledge.
8. Solving complex healthcare problems: in the healthcare domain, bioinspired algorithms offer significant advantages. They can assist in medical image analysis, disease diagnosis,

patient monitoring, treatment optimization, and healthcare resource allocation. These algorithms enable researchers and practitioners to address complex healthcare challenges, leading to improved patient outcomes and more efficient healthcare systems.

12.1.5 Limitations

1. Black box nature: bioinspired algorithms often exhibit a "black box" nature, meaning that the internal workings and decision-making processes may be difficult to interpret and understand. This lack of transparency can make it challenging to gain insights into how and why a particular solution is obtained. Interpretability and explainability of results remain important challenges in applying bioinspired algorithms to critical domains like healthcare.
2. Parameter tuning: bioinspired algorithms typically involve a set of parameters that need to be carefully tuned for optimal performance. Determining the appropriate parameter values can be time-consuming and require domain expertise. Improper parameter settings can lead to suboptimal results or algorithm failure. Robust techniques for automated parameter tuning are an ongoing research area to alleviate this limitation.
3. Computational complexity: some bioinspired algorithms can be computationally intensive, especially when dealing with large-scale problems or complex models. The time and computational resources required to obtain solutions may become a limitation in certain applications, particularly when real-time or near real-time decision-making is essential. Improving the efficiency and scalability of these algorithms is an ongoing research direction.
4. Lack of problem-specific knowledge: while bioinspired algorithms are domain-independent, they may lack problem-specific knowledge. These algorithms rely on general principles inspired by nature, but they may not capture all the intricacies and nuances of a specific problem domain. Incorporating domain-specific knowledge into the algorithm design or preprocessing the data appropriately becomes crucial for achieving optimal results. It requires expertise from

domain specialists to ensure that the algorithm is properly adapted and tailored to the problem at hand.

5. Limited applicability: while bioinspired algorithms have a wide range of applications, they may not be suitable for all problem types. Some problems may have specific characteristics or constraints that make them incompatible with certain bioinspired algorithms. It is important to carefully analyze the problem requirements and match them with the strengths and limitations of the chosen algorithm to ensure compatibility.
6. Convergence to local optima: bioinspired algorithms are susceptible to converging to local optima instead of the global optimum. Local optima are suboptimal solutions within the search space that may seem optimal within their local neighborhood but are not the best overall solution. Overcoming this limitation often requires the application of advanced techniques, such as incorporating diversification strategies or hybridizing algorithms, to enhance exploration and escape from local optima.
7. High computational costs for complex problems: while bioinspired algorithms can effectively solve many optimization problems, the computational costs can increase significantly for complex problems. As the problem size and complexity grow, the algorithm's execution time may become prohibitively long, limiting its practicality. Balancing the algorithm's computational demands with available resources becomes a crucial consideration when dealing with computationally expensive problems.
8. Lack of unified theory: bioinspired algorithms encompass a wide range of techniques inspired by different biological processes. However, there is no unified theory that encompasses all bioinspired algorithms. Each algorithm has its own underlying principles, mechanisms, and parameter settings. This lack of a unified theory makes it challenging to compare and analyze different algorithms systematically and hinders the development of unified frameworks for algorithm design and analysis.
9. Sensitivity to initial conditions: bioinspired algorithms can be sensitive to the initial conditions or population configurations. Small changes in the initial population or random seed can lead to different solutions or convergence rates.

This sensitivity can make the algorithms non-deterministic and result in different outcomes for multiple runs. It is important to consider the reproducibility and stability of results when applying bioinspired algorithms.

10. Ethical considerations: bioinspired algorithms, like any other computational techniques, raise ethical considerations, particularly in healthcare applications. These algorithms may impact decision-making processes, resource allocation, and patient outcomes. Ensuring transparency, fairness, and accountability in the application of bioinspired algorithms becomes essential to mitigate potential biases, ensure patient safety, and maintain ethical standards.

12.1.6 Applications of Bioinspired Algorithms in Healthcare

Bioinspired algorithms have made significant contributions to various aspects of healthcare, leveraging their optimization capabilities, adaptability, and problem-solving techniques. In this section, we will explore their applications in medical image analysis, disease diagnosis, treatment optimization, and personalized medicine.

1. Medical Image Analysis: bioinspired algorithms have been extensively used for medical image analysis tasks, such as segmentation, registration, and feature extraction. These algorithms can effectively handle the complexity and variability of medical images, enabling accurate and automated analysis. For example, genetic algorithms and particle swarm optimization have been employed for image segmentation, neural networks for image classification, and ant colony optimization for image registration. These techniques improve the efficiency and reliability of medical image interpretation, aiding in early detection, diagnosis, and treatment planning [14].
2. Disease diagnosis: bioinspired algorithms play a crucial role in disease diagnosis by analyzing patient data and detecting patterns indicative of specific diseases. Genetic algorithms, neural networks, and other bioinspired techniques have been used for feature selection, classification, and prediction tasks. By learning from large datasets, these algorithms can identify relevant biomarkers, risk factors, and disease patterns. They have been applied to various medical domains, including cancer diagnosis, cardiovascular disease

prediction, and neurological disorder detection. Bioinspired algorithms enhance diagnostic accuracy, enable early intervention, and facilitate personalized treatment strategies [15].

3. Treatment optimization: bioinspired algorithms contribute to optimizing treatment strategies by considering multiple factors, including patient-specific characteristics, treatment options, and resource allocation. These algorithms can assist in treatment planning, dosage optimization, and treatment scheduling. For instance, genetic algorithms have been employed to optimize radiation therapy plans, neural networks for drug dosage optimization, and ant colony optimization for treatment scheduling. By incorporating patient-specific data and considering individual variability, bioinspired algorithms help design personalized treatment plans that maximize effectiveness while minimizing side effects and resource utilization [16].
4. Personalized medicine: bioinspired algorithms facilitate the development of personalized medicine approaches. These algorithms leverage patient data, genetic information, and clinical records to tailor treatments and interventions to individual patients. They can analyze complex datasets to identify patient subgroups, predict treatment response, and optimize therapy regimens. Bioinspired techniques, such as genetic algorithms, neural networks, and evolutionary computing, enable the integration of multiple data sources and decision-making processes to optimize personalized treatment pathways. By providing patient-specific recommendations, bioinspired algorithms enhance treatment outcomes and improve patient care [4].
5. Drug discovery and design: bioinspired algorithms contribute to the field of drug discovery and design by assisting in the identification of potential drug candidates, molecular docking, and drug optimization. Genetic algorithms and molecular dynamics simulations can explore the vast chemical space to identify molecules with desired properties, such as binding affinity and specificity. Neural networks and deep learning techniques can aid in predicting drug-target interactions and assessing the safety and efficacy of drug compounds. These algorithms accelerate the drug discovery process, reduce costs, and increase the chances of finding effective therapies for various diseases [10].

6. Healthcare resource allocation: bioinspired algorithms have been utilized for optimizing the allocation of healthcare resources, including staff scheduling, bed allocation, and resource utilization. These algorithms can consider multiple constraints, such as patient demand, resource availability, and service quality, to allocate resources efficiently. Ant colony optimization, particle swarm optimization, and other bioinspired techniques have been applied to optimize healthcare resource allocation, improving patient access, reducing waiting times, and enhancing resource utilization [7].
7. Decision support systems: bioinspired algorithms contribute to the development of decision support systems in healthcare. These systems assist healthcare professionals in making informed decisions by analyzing patient data, medical records, and clinical guidelines. Genetic algorithms, neural networks, and other bioinspired techniques can process complex data, extract relevant features, and provide decision recommendations based on learned patterns and rules. Decision support systems powered by bioinspired algorithms improve diagnostic accuracy, treatment planning [17].

Implementations of bioinspired algorithms in various medical domains have shown significant promise and success in revolutionizing healthcare. These algorithms draw inspiration from natural systems and processes, allowing them to tackle complex medical challenges in innovative ways. Below, we explore several notable examples of bioinspired algorithms in different medical domains and discuss their benefits over traditional approaches.

- One prominent application of bioinspired algorithms is in the field of drug design. Genetic algorithms (GA) have been employed to optimize the design of new drugs, speeding up the discovery process and enhancing efficacy. GA mimics the principles of natural evolution, using techniques such as mutation and crossover to explore vast chemical spaces and identify optimal drug candidates. This approach has the potential to discover novel molecules with desired properties, such as enhanced potency and reduced side effects, which may have been overlooked by traditional methods. By accelerating drug discovery, GA-based approaches have the potential to save both time and resources, ultimately leading to the development of safer and more effective medications.

- Medical scheduling is another area that has greatly benefited from bioinspired algorithms. Ant colony optimization (ACO) algorithms have been successfully applied to optimize complex scheduling problems in healthcare settings. ACO draws inspiration from the foraging behavior of ants, employing pheromone-based communication and decision-making mechanisms. In the context of medical scheduling, ACO algorithms consider factors, such as patient priorities, resource availability, and constraints to create optimal schedules [18]. By minimizing waiting times, increasing resource utilization, and improving patient satisfaction, ACO-based scheduling systems offer significant advantages over traditional manual approaches. These algorithms can streamline the scheduling process, leading to more efficient healthcare delivery and improved patient experiences.
- Bioinspired algorithms have also made significant contributions to the field of medical imaging. Particle swarm optimization (PSO), inspired by the collective behavior of bird flocks or fish schools, has been applied to optimize medical image reconstruction algorithms. PSO algorithms iteratively search for optimal image reconstructions by fine-tuning reconstruction parameters. This approach improves image quality, reduces artifacts, and enhances diagnostic accuracy. Traditional deterministic reconstruction techniques often struggle to handle the complexity of medical imaging data, while PSO-based methods offer a more robust and efficient approach. By optimizing image reconstruction, PSO algorithms have the potential to enhance the accuracy of medical diagnoses and improve patient outcomes [19].
- The use of bioinspired algorithms, notably artificial neural networks (ANN), has greatly improved disease detection. ANNs are excellent at learning from vast datasets to uncover complex patterns and correlations because they are inspired by the structure and operation of the human brain.. In the context of disease diagnosis, ANNs can analyze patient symptoms, medical history, and test results to provide accurate and personalized diagnoses. Unlike traditional rule-based diagnostic systems, ANNs can handle uncertainties, adapt to new data, and provide more accurate predictions. With their ability to process vast amounts of medical data, ANNs offer significant potential for early detection, accurate

diagnosis, and personalized treatment plans, ultimately improving patient outcomes.

- The field of surgical robotics has also been transformed by bioinspired algorithms, specifically swarm robotics. Swarm robotics draws inspiration from the collective behavior of social insect colonies, where multiple small robots work collaboratively to perform complex tasks with improved accuracy and dexterity. In surgical robotics, swarm robotic systems can distribute workload, coordinate actions, and adapt to changing surgical environments. By leveraging the strengths of swarm intelligence, these systems offer enhanced precision, faster surgeries, and reduced invasiveness compared to traditional surgical approaches. Swarm robotics has the potential to revolutionize surgical procedures, enabling less invasive interventions, shorter recovery times, and improved patient safety [20].

12.1.7 Benefits of Bioinspired Algorithms in Healthcare Over Traditional Approaches

These are some of the key benefits that bioinspired algorithms bring to healthcare compared to traditional approaches. However, it's important to note that both approaches have their own strengths and limitations, and the choice of approach depends on the specific problem and context.

12.2 Neurological Disease Diagnosis

Here's an overview of common neurological diseases. Comparison of the benefits of bioinspired algorithms in healthcare compared to traditional approaches is shown in Table 12.1.

1. **Alzheimer's Disease**: Memory, cognition, and behaviour are the main areas of Alzheimer's disease's progressive neurodegenerative condition that it affects. The most typical type of dementia is this one. Typically, symptoms appear gradually and get worse with time. Memory l`oss, trouble solving problems, confusion, disorientation, and changes in mood or behaviour are typical symptoms. The beta-amyloid plaques and tau protein tangles that build up in the brain as a result of Alzheimer's disease cause neuronal death and

Table 12.1 Comparison of the benefits of bioinspired algorithms in healthcare compared to traditional approaches.

Aspect	Bioinspired algorithms	Traditional approaches
Problem solving	Can tackle complex and non-linear problems efficiently.	Primarily designed for linear and deterministic problems.
Adaptability	Can adapt and self-optimize based on changing conditions.	Limited adaptability and may require manual adjustments.
Robustness	Resilient to noise, uncertainties, and variations in data.	Sensitive to noise and uncertainties, may yield suboptimal results.
Efficiency	Can handle large datasets and process them efficiently.	May struggle with big data, leading to slower processing times.
Exploration	Enables exploration of multiple solution spaces simultaneously.	Focuses on finding a single optimal solution.
Parallelism	Allows for parallel processing and distributed computing.	Sequential processing limits computational speed.
Optimization	Offers efficient optimization techniques, such as swarm intelligence.	Limited optimization methods, often requiring manual fine-tuning.
Learning	Incorporates learning and adaptation from experience and interactions.	Lacks learning capabilities without explicit programming.
Non-linearity	Handles non-linear relationships and complex interactions.	Assumes linearity and simplification of relationships.
Scalability	Scales well to handle increasing complexity and size of problems.	May struggle with scalability as problems become more complex.

brain tissue shrinkage. Although the precise reason is not entirely known, it is thought that genetic and environmental factors are involved [21]. Alzheimer's disease has no known cure, and current therapies concentrate on symptom management and delaying the illness's development.

2. **Parkinson's Disease**: Parkinson's disease is a long-term, degenerative movement illness brought on by dopamine-producing brain cells degenerating. A variety of motor symptoms, including tremors, bradykinesia (slowness of movement), stiffness, and postural instability, are present. There may also be non-motor symptoms, such as sadness, sleep problems, and cognitive decline. Parkinson's disease has an elusive exact etiology, although both hereditary and environmental variables play a role in how it develops. Medications that raise dopamine levels in the brain, deep brain stimulation (DBS), physical therapy, and dietary changes are among the treatment modalities [16]. Despite the fact that there is no cure, these therapies can aid in symptom management and enhance quality of life.

3. **Multiple Sclerosis**: An autoimmune condition called multiple sclerosis (MS) damages the central nervous system, which includes the brain and spinal cord. Myelin, the protective coating of nerve fibers, is wrongly attacked by the immune system in MS, causing inflammation and damage. This interferes with the body's ability to transmit electrical signals between the brain and the rest of the body. The vast range of MS symptoms might include fatigue, trouble walking, numbness or tingling, muscular weakness, issues with coordination, visual issues, and cognitive impairment. Although the exact etiology of MS is unknown, it is thought to be a result of both hereditary and environmental factors [15]. Through medicine, physical therapy, and dietary modifications, treatment seeks to control symptoms, delay the development of the illness, and alter the immunological response.

4. **Epilepsy**: Recurrent seizures are a neurological disease known as epilepsy. Seizures are the consequence of aberrant electrical activity in the brain, which, depending on the area of the brain affected, can result in a range of symptoms.

These symptoms might include convulsions, loss of control over physiological processes, brief moments of unconsciousness or staring, and more. Epilepsy can have various causes, including genetic factors, brain injury, infections, tumors, and stroke. Treatment usually involves antiepileptic medications to control seizures. In some cases, surgery or implanted devices may be considered. Many people with epilepsy can effectively manage their condition and lead normal lives with proper medical care and lifestyle adjustments [22].

5. **Stroke**: A stroke is a serious medical emergency that happens when there is a disruption or reduction in the blood flow to the brain, starving brain cells of oxygen and nutrients. Hemorrhagic stroke, which is brought on by bleeding in the brain, and ischemic stroke, which is brought on by a blocked or restricted blood artery, are the two primary forms of stroke. A stroke can cause abrupt weakness or numbness in the face, arm, or leg as well as disorientation, difficulty speaking or comprehending, a strong headache, dizziness, and loss of coordination or balance. Prompt medical attention is crucial to minimize brain damage and disability. Treatment options depend on the type and cause of the stroke but may include medication, surgery, and rehabilitation [19].

Diagnosing neurological diseases involves a comprehensive evaluation of a patient's medical history, physical examination, neurological assessments, and diagnostic tests. Here are the common steps and methods involved in the diagnosis of neurological diseases:

1. **Medical History and Symptom Assessment**: The healthcare provider begins by collecting a detailed medical history, including the onset and progression of symptoms, family history of neurological diseases, past medical conditions, and exposure to any environmental factors or toxins. A thorough assessment of the patient's symptoms, such as changes in sensation, movement, coordination, cognition, or behavior, is essential for guiding the diagnostic process.

2. **Physical Examination**: A neurological examination is performed to evaluate the patient's motor functions, sensory

abilities, reflexes, coordination, balance, and cognitive function. The healthcare provider may assess muscle strength, coordination tests, reflexes, sensory perception, eye movements, speech, and mental status. Abnormalities detected during the examination help guide further investigations.

3. **Neuroimaging**: Various neuroimaging techniques are used to visualize the structure and function of the brain and spinal cord. Common neuroimaging methods include:

    - **MRI (Magnetic Resonance Imaging)**: Provides detailed images of brain and spinal cord, helping identify structural abnormalities, tumors, inflammation, or evidence of ischemic or hemorrhagic stroke.
    - **CT (Computed Tomography)**: Useful in emergency situations to quickly assess for bleeding or structural abnormalities in the brain.
    - **PET (Positron Emission Tomography)**: Detects metabolic activity in the brain, aiding in the evaluation of conditions such as Alzheimer's disease and epilepsy.
    - **SPECT (Single-Photon Emission Computed Tomography)**: Measures blood flow and brain activity, assisting in the diagnosis of various neurological disorders.

4. **Electrophysiological Tests**: Electrophysiological tests assess the electrical activity of brain, spinal cord, and peripheral nerves. These tests provide valuable information about the function and integrity of the nervous system. Examples include:

    - **Electroencephalography (EEG)**: Measures electrical brain activity to detect abnormalities associated with epilepsy, brain tumors, sleep disorders, and brain injuries.
    - **Nerve Conduction Studies (NCS)** and **Electromyography (EMG)**: Evaluate the function of peripheral nerves and muscles, helping diagnose conditions such as peripheral neuropathy, carpal tunnel syndrome, or muscular dystrophy.

5. **Laboratory Tests**: Blood tests and cerebrospinal fluid (CSF) analysis are often conducted to assess specific biomarkers, detect infections, evaluate autoimmune responses, and rule out metabolic or genetic disorders. Examples include:

    - **Complete Blood Count (CBC)**: Screens for infections, anemia, or other blood disorders.
    - **CSF Analysis**: Involves the collection of cerebrospinal fluid through a lumbar puncture to evaluate for infections, inflammation, or the presence of abnormal cells.
    - **Genetic Testing**: Identifies specific genetic mutations associated with certain neurological diseases, such as Huntington's disease or hereditary neuropathies.

6. **Biopsies and Lumbar Puncture**: In some cases, a biopsy of the affected tissue (e.g., brain, muscle) or a lumbar puncture (to collect CSF) may be necessary to obtain a definitive diagnosis, especially when other tests are inconclusive or when specific diseases, such as brain tumors or certain infections, are suspected.

It is important to note that the diagnostic process for neurological diseases can be complex and may require the involvement of multiple healthcare professionals, including neurologists, radiologists, neurosurgeons, and pathologists. Additionally, advancements in genetic

The limitations and drawbacks of these conventional diagnostic methods highlight the need for alternative approaches in neurological disease diagnosis. This has led to the development and exploration of various innovative techniques, such as advanced neuroimaging methods (functional MRI, diffusion tensor imaging), molecular biomarkers, genetic testing, wearable devices, and artificial intelligence-based algorithms. These alternative approaches aim to overcome the limitations of conventional methods by providing more accurate, objective, and comprehensive diagnostic information, enabling earlier detection, individualized treatment plans, and improved patient outcomes.

12.2.1 Bioinspired Algorithms for Neurological Disease Diagnosis

Genetic algorithms (GAs) are a type of bioinspired algorithm that mimics the process of natural selection to solve complex optimization problems.

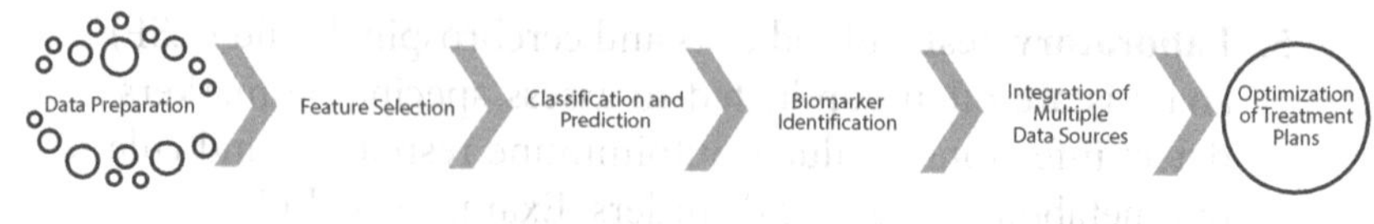

Figure 12.3 Steps involved in applying bioinspired algorithms for neurological disease diagnosis.

They have been applied to various fields, including healthcare and medical diagnosis. In the context of neurological disease diagnosis, GAs offer a promising approach to analyze and interpret complex datasets, identify relevant biomarkers, and assist in the accurate classification and prediction of neurological disorders. Here, we will explore the application of GAs in the diagnosis of neurological diseases. Figure 12.3 shows the steps involved in applying bioinspired algorithms for neurological disease diagnosis.

1. Dataset preparation: The first step in applying GAs to neurological disease diagnosis is the collection and preparation of relevant datasets. These datasets typically include clinical data, neuroimaging data (MRI, CT scans), genetic data, and other relevant patient information. The datasets need to be carefully curated, ensuring they are representative, well-annotated, and cover a range of neurological diseases.
2. Feature selection: GAs can aid in feature selection by identifying the most informative features from the dataset. This step helps reduce dimensionality and eliminate redundant or irrelevant features, enhancing the accuracy and efficiency of subsequent analyses. GAs accomplish this by evaluating the fitness of different feature subsets based on their predictive power and selecting the most optimal subset.
3. Classification and prediction: GAs can be utilized to develop classification models for different neurological diseases. The algorithm optimizes the model parameters by iteratively evaluating their performance on the training dataset. By considering various combinations of parameters, GAs can identify the optimal set of parameters that maximizes the classification accuracy. This process helps in accurately classifying patients into different disease categories based on their clinical and imaging features.
4. Biomarker identification: GAs can assist in identifying relevant biomarkers associated with neurological diseases. By analyzing the genetic data and other molecular information,

GAs can identify genetic variants, gene expression patterns, or protein markers that are correlated with specific neurological conditions. This information can contribute to better understanding the underlying mechanisms of diseases and aid in personalized treatment strategies.

5. Integration of multiple data sources: neurological diseases often involve multiple modalities of data, such as clinical, neuroimaging, and genetic data. GAs can handle the integration of these diverse data sources by optimizing the weights and contributions of each modality in the diagnostic process. This integration can improve the accuracy and robustness of the diagnostic models by capturing the multidimensional nature of neurological diseases.
6. Optimization of treatment plans: GAs can also optimize treatment plans for neurological diseases. By considering patient-specific characteristics, treatment goals, and available treatment options, GAs can generate personalized treatment plans that maximize the likelihood of positive outcomes. This optimization process takes into account factors such as drug efficacy, dosage, and potential side effects, ensuring tailored and effective treatment strategies.

Benefits of Genetic Algorithms in Neurological Disease Diagnosis:

- ❖ Ability to handle high-dimensional and heterogeneous datasets.
- ❖ Automated feature selection, reducing dimensionality and improving model performance.
- ❖ Identification of relevant biomarkers associated with neurological diseases.
- ❖ Integration of multiple data modalities for a comprehensive diagnostic approach.
- ❖ Personalized treatment optimization for improved patient outcomes.

Challenges and Future Directions:

- ❖ Availability of high-quality and well-curated datasets for training and validation.
- ❖ Interpretability of the models generated by GAs and the underlying biomarkers.

- ❖ Incorporating temporal data and disease progression into the diagnostic models.
- ❖ Integration of GAs with other machine learning techniques for enhanced performance.
- ❖ Ethical considerations, such as data privacy and patient consent.

Genetic algorithms (GAs) can indeed be used to optimize feature selection and classification algorithms, leading to improved accuracy and efficiency in diagnosis. Let's explore how GAs can be applied in this context:

1. Feature Selection: Feature selection is the process of identifying the most relevant and informative features from a given dataset. Genetic Algorithms can be employed to automate this process by searching through a large space of feature subsets to find the optimal combination of features. Here in Figure 12.4 it is shown how it typically works:

    a. Representation: Each individual in the GA population represents a potential feature subset. It can be encoded as a binary string, where each bit corresponds to the inclusion or exclusion of a feature.
    b. Fitness evaluation: The fitness function measures the quality of each feature subset based on a predefined criterion, such as classification accuracy, information gain, or some other evaluation metric. The classification algorithm is trained and tested using the selected features, and the fitness function quantifies its performance.
    c. Genetic operators: The feature subsets are subjected to genetic operators like crossover and mutation to produce new individuals. In order to create offspring, crossover combines the traits of two parent subsets, whereas mutation adds minor random changes in order to seek new areas of the search space.

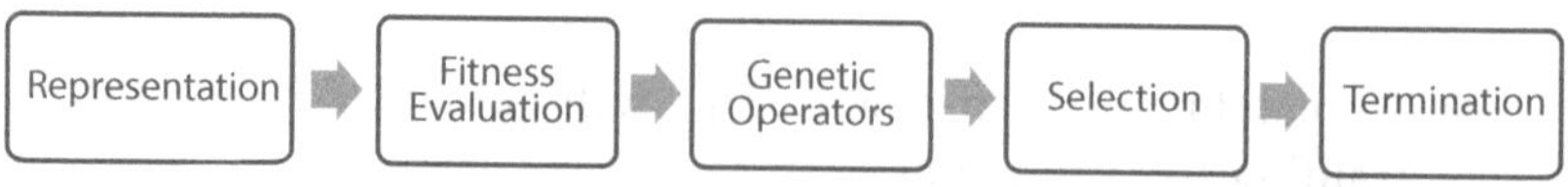

Figure 12.4 Genetic algorithms optimizing feature subsets in neurological disease diagnosis.

d. Selection: People are chosen for reproduction based on their level of fitness, with fitter individuals having a higher chance of being selected. This selection process is repeated iteratively to create new generations.

e. Termination: The GA process continues until a termination condition is met, which could be a maximum number of generations, convergence of fitness values, or a predefined threshold.

By iteratively evolving the feature subsets using these steps, GAs can explore the space of possible feature combinations and converge towards an optimal or near-optimal subset that maximizes the classification accuracy.

2. Classification Algorithm Optimization: Once the optimal feature subset is determined, GAs can further be used to optimize the parameters or structure of the classification algorithm itself. This involves tuning the hyper parameters of the algorithm to improve its performance. Figure 12.5 shows Genetic Algorithms optimizing parameters and structure of the classification algorithm in neurological disease diagnosis

a. Representation: The individuals in the GA population represent different parameter configurations or structures of the classification algorithm.

b. Fitness Evaluation: The fitness function assesses the performance of the classification algorithm using the selected feature subset and the current parameter configuration. The evaluation can be based on metrics such as accuracy, precision, recall, F1-score, or any other suitable measure.

c. Genetic Operators: To create new individuals, parameter settings or structural changes are subjected to crossover and mutation. In order to explore new areas of the search space, mutation provides random changes whereas

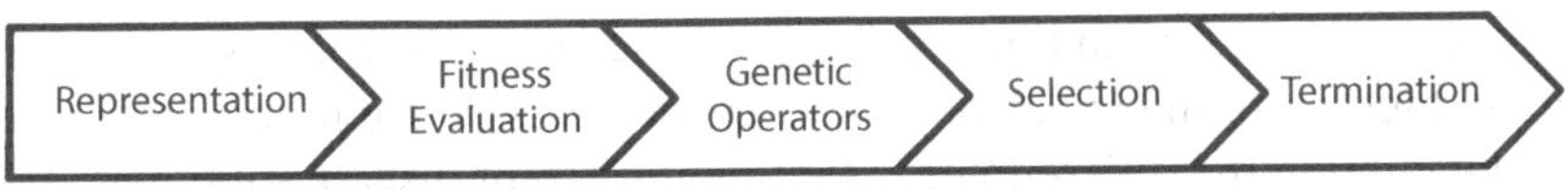

Figure 12.5 Genetic algorithms fine-tuning parameters and structure of the classification algorithm for improved neurological disease diagnosis.

crossover combines the parameters or structures of two parent individuals.

d. Selection: Individuals are selected for reproduction based on their fitness, favoring the ones with better performance.
e. Termination: The GA process continues until a termination condition is met, similar to the feature selection phase.

By optimizing the classification algorithm's parameters or structure, GAs can fine-tune the model to achieve higher accuracy and efficiency in diagnosis.

Overall, the combination of feature selection and classification algorithm optimization using GAs provides a powerful framework to improve the accuracy and efficiency of diagnosis. By automating the search for optimal feature subsets and parameter configurations, GAs help to overcome the limitations of manual selection and tuning, enabling more effective diagnosis in various domains.

12.2.2 Neural Networks in Neurological Disease Diagnosis

Neural networks (NNs) have revolutionized the field of neurological disease diagnosis by leveraging their ability to learn complex patterns and relationships from data. With the increasing availability of large datasets and advances in computational power, NNs have become a valuable tool for improving the accuracy and efficiency of diagnosis across various neurological conditions.

One of the key advantages of NNs in neurological disease diagnosis is their remarkable capability in pattern recognition. Neurological diseases often manifest in intricate ways, and NNs excel at identifying subtle and intricate patterns from different data modalities. For instance, in Alzheimer's disease diagnosis, NNs can analyze brain imaging data such as MRI scans to detect characteristic patterns of atrophy and cortical thinning, enabling early detection and accurate classification [12].

Furthermore, NNs are well-suited for handling the inherent complexity and nonlinearity of neurological diseases. Many neurological conditions involve intricate interactions between various clinical and imaging features. Traditional linear models may struggle to capture these complex relationships, leading to limited diagnostic accuracy. In contrast, NNs can model highly nonlinear relationships, enabling more accurate predictions and facilitating the differentiation between different disease subtypes.

NNs are also effective in handling multimodal data integration, which is essential in neurological disease diagnosis. Integrating multiple sources of information, such as clinical data, genetic data, and neuroimaging data, can provide a comprehensive and holistic view of a patient's condition. NNs can effectively fuse these diverse data sources, extracting relevant features from each modality and combining them to make informed diagnostic decisions [14].

Transfer learning, another powerful technique enabled by NNs, has shown promise in the field of neurological disease diagnosis. Transfer learning allows pre-trained NN models to be fine-tuned on specific neurological disease datasets, even when the available data is limited. By leveraging knowledge learned from large datasets and applying it to smaller, disease-specific datasets, NNs can enhance diagnostic accuracy and generalize across different patient populations [23].

Despite their significant advantages, the application of NNs in neurological disease diagnosis also presents some challenges. One major challenge is the need for large, well-curated datasets. Training NNs requires a substantial amount of labeled data to ensure robust learning and generalization. Acquiring and annotating such datasets can be time-consuming and resource-intensive, particularly in the field of neurology, where data collection is often invasive or expensive. However, collaborations between researchers, healthcare institutions, and data sharing initiatives can help alleviate this challenge and promote the development of robust NN models [23].

Interpretability and explainability of NNs in neurological disease diagnosis are other ongoing challenges. NNs are often referred to as "black boxes" due to their complex and opaque decision-making processes. Understanding the rationale behind NN predictions is crucial for clinical acceptance and trust. Researchers are actively exploring methods to enhance the interpretability of NNs, such as developing attention mechanisms and saliency maps to highlight relevant features and provide explanations for diagnostic decisions [12].

In recent years, numerous studies have showcased the effectiveness of NNs in neurological disease diagnosis. For instance, in Parkinson's disease, NNs have been employed to analyze voice and movement patterns, enabling accurate detection and monitoring of the disease's progression. In epilepsy diagnosis, NNs have demonstrated their potential in analyzing EEG signals to predict seizure occurrence, aiding in the development of personalized treatment plans. Additionally, NNs have shown promise in early detection and classification of brain tumors through the analysis of medical imaging data [24].

The structure and operation of the human brain served as the inspiration for the computer model known as neural networks (NNs). They are made up of layers of linked nodes known as neurons or units. NNs are designed to learn from data, recognize patterns, and make predictions or classifications based on the learned knowledge.

The architecture of a neural network refers to its structure, which determines how information flows through the network. The three main components of an NN architecture are the input layer, hidden layers (if any), and the output layer. Multiple neurons make up each layer, and weights are carried through the connections between the neurons. The first batch of data for the network to handle is delivered to the input layer. In the input layer, each neuron represents a characteristic or property of the incoming data. Forward propagation of the input values via the network's hidden layers and output layer results in the network's predictions or classifications [25].

Hidden layers are intermediary layers between the input and output layers. They play a crucial role in capturing complex patterns and relationships in the data. The inputs from the preceding layer are received by each neuron in the hidden layer, which then computes (often by adding the inputs' weights together), applies an activation function, and sends the outcome to the layer above. The network's ability to learn and generalize can be affected by design decisions such as the number of hidden layers and the number of neurons in each layer [26].

The output layer represents the final layer of the network. It consists of one or more neurons, depending on the task at hand For instance, a single neuron with a sigmoid activation function may be utilized to generate a probability of belonging to one class in a binary classification task. In multiclass classification, the output layer can consist of multiple neurons with softmax activation, providing the probability distribution across different classes.

Training algorithms are responsible for adjusting the weights of the connections between neurons to optimize the network's performance. The most common training algorithm for NNs is called backpropagation (or backpropagation of errors). Backpropagation calculates the gradient of the loss function with respect to the network weights using the chain rule of calculus [27].

During the training process, the network is presented with a set of labeled examples, known as the training dataset. The input data is fed into the network, and the predictions are compared to the true labels. The error or loss is calculated as the discrepancy between the predicted and true values. Backpropagation calculates the gradient of the loss with respect to the weights, allowing for the adjustment of weights in a direction that minimizes the error [28].

Optimization algorithms, such as gradient descent, are commonly used in conjunction with Backpropagation to update the weights iteratively. These algorithms determine how much the weights should be adjusted based on the calculated gradient. By repeatedly feeding the training examples through the network, computing the error, and updating the weights, the network gradually learns to improve its predictions.

Other variants of training algorithms, such as stochastic gradient descent (SGD), mini-batch gradient descent, and adaptive learning rate methods like Adam and RMSprop, have been developed to accelerate convergence and improve training efficiency [29].

It is crucial to remember that selecting the right activation functions, loss functions, and regularization strategies is also very critical while training NNs. The network gains nonlinearity from activation functions, which enables it to simulate complicated interactions. Rectified linear units (ReLU), sigmoid, and tan are frequently used activation functions. Regularization methods, such as L1 or L2 regularization, prohibit overfitting by including a penalty term into the loss function, whereas loss functions measure the error between predictions and true labels [30].

12.2.2.1 *How NNs Can Be Trained Using Bioinspired Optimization Techniques*

Neural networks (NNs) can be trained using various bioinspired optimization techniques, such as backpropagation, swarm intelligence, and evolutionary algorithms, to improve the accuracy of disease diagnosis. These techniques offer alternative approaches to traditional gradient-based optimization and can overcome limitations or enhance the performance of NN training [31, 32]. Let us discuss each technique and its potential application in disease diagnosis:

1. **Backpropagation**: Backpropagation is the most widely used algorithm for training NNs. It uses the calculus chain rule to determine the gradient of the loss function with regard to the weights of the network. The weights are then repeatedly updated using the gradient, aiming to minimize the error between predictions and true labels [33–35].

   In disease diagnosis, Backpropagation can be employed to train NNs on large datasets to improve accuracy. By adjusting the weights based on the computed gradients, the network learns to recognize disease patterns and make accurate predictions. Backpropagation is particularly effective when the training dataset is well-labeled and sufficiently representative of the disease's characteristics.

2. **Swarm Intelligence**: The collective behavior of social insects and other species, in which individual agents cooperate to accomplish a shared objective, serves as the model for swarm intelligence (SI) algorithms. The particle swarm optimization (PSO) algorithm is a well-known SI algorithm. By changing their locations depending on both their individual best position and the best position discovered by the swarm, a population of particles in PSO searches the solution space [33].

   In the context of NN training, SI algorithms can be used to optimize the weights of the network. The particles in the swarm can represent different combinations of weights, and their positions can correspond to the fitness of the associated NN. By iteratively updating the positions of the particles, the swarm collectively searches for optimal weight configurations, leading to improved accuracy in disease diagnosis.
3. **Evolutionary Algorithms**: Evolutionary algorithms (EAs) draw inspiration from the principles of biological evolution, including mutation, crossover, and selection. Genetic algorithms (GAs) are a well-known subclass of EAs. GAs involve encoding the NN's weights into a chromosome, which undergoes mutation and crossover operations [36]. The resulting offspring chromosomes are evaluated based on their fitness, and the selection process favors individuals with higher fitness.

EAs can be utilized to train NNs for disease diagnosis by optimizing their weights and architectures. They can explore a vast solution space to discover optimal or near-optimal configurations of the network, leading to improved accuracy and generalization. EAs are particularly useful when the search space is large, and manual tuning or exhaustive search is impractical.

By incorporating bioinspired optimization techniques like backpropagation, swarm intelligence, and evolutionary algorithms into NN training, the accuracy of disease diagnosis can be enhanced. These techniques offer alternative optimization approaches that can handle complex data, explore large solution spaces, and overcome the limitations of traditional gradient-based optimization.

It is worth mentioning that the choice of optimization technique depends on the specific characteristics of the problem, available data, computational resources, and the desired trade-off between accuracy and computational efficiency. Hybrid approaches, combining multiple optimization techniques, can also be explored to leverage their complementary strengths and achieve even better results in disease diagnosis using NNs.

12.2.3 Other Bioinspired Algorithms in Neurological Disease Diagnosis

Two popular bioinspired algorithms are ant colony optimization (ACO) and particle swarm optimization (PSO). While these algorithms have primarily been applied to optimization problems, they can also have potential applications in neurological disease diagnosis

1. **Ant Colony Optimization (ACO)**: ACO is a metaheuristic algorithm based on the foraging behavior of ants. Ants communicate through pheromone trails to find the shortest path between their colony and food sources. The algorithm uses this concept to solve optimization problems, such as the traveling salesman problem. Ants deposit pheromone trails to mark good paths and follow the trails with higher pheromone intensity. Over time, the algorithm converges towards an optimal solution [37].

ACO algorithm consists of three components: ants, pheromone trails, and a pheromone updating rule. Each ant represents a potential solution to the problem at hand. The ants move through the search space, evaluating the quality of their current solution and depositing pheromone trails based on their evaluation [38]. The pheromone trails represent the collective experience of the ants and guide the search towards promising solutions. The pheromone updating rule updates the pheromone levels based on the quality of the solutions found by the ants.

Potential applications in neurological disease diagnosis: ACO can be utilized in medical diagnosis by formulating the diagnostic process as an optimization problem. For instance, in neuroimaging, ACO can assist in identifying the most informative features (e.g., brain regions, biomarkers) for classifying neurological diseases [39]. By assigning pheromone levels based on feature relevance and selection, ACO can aid in optimizing the diagnostic accuracy and efficiency of disease identification

2. **Particle Swarm Optimization (PSO)**: PSO is a population-based optimization method that draws inspiration from the group behavior of fish schooling or bird flocking. It makes use of a population of particles that are in motion inside a multidimensional search space. Considering both their individual best-known solution and the best-known solution of the entire swarm, each particle modifies its location to indicate a potential solution. The algorithm looks into the search space to identify the best answer [40].

PSO algorithm consists of three components: particles, velocities, and an updating rule. Each particle represents a potential solution to the problem at hand. The particles move through the search space and update their positions based on their current velocity and their previous best-known position. Additionally, the particles are influenced by the best-known position discovered by any particle in the swarm [36]. This collective behavior enables the particles to explore the search space efficiently and converge towards the optimal solution.

12.3 Challenges and Future Directions

Diagnosing neurological diseases can be a complex task due to the diverse range of symptoms and the lack of specific biomarkers for many conditions. Bioinspired algorithms, which are computational techniques inspired by biological processes, have been applied to aid in the diagnosis of neurological diseases. While these algorithms offer promising solutions, there are several challenges that need to be addressed. Figure 12.6 shows some of the key challenges in utilizing bioinspired algorithms for neurological disease diagnosis include:

1. **Data availability and quality**: Bioinspired algorithms require a significant amount of high-quality data to train and validate their models. However, acquiring large-scale and diverse neurological datasets can be challenging due to factors such as data privacy, data sharing limitations, and the rarity of certain neurological diseases. Limited or biased data can affect the performance and generalizability of bio-inspired algorithms.
2. **Feature extraction and selection**: Neurological diseases often present with complex and heterogeneous symptoms,

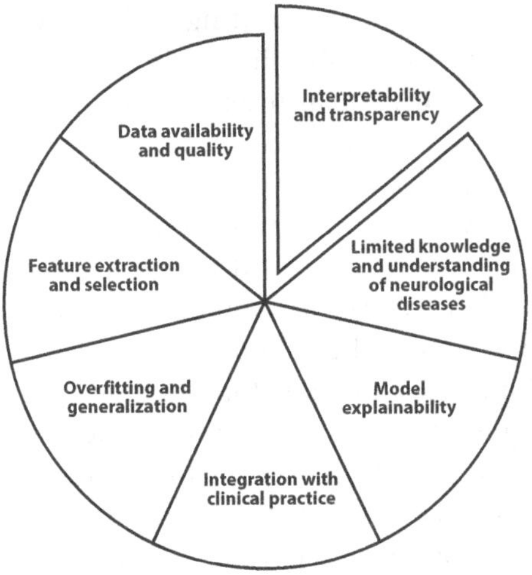

Figure 12.6 Key challenges in utilizing bioinspired algorithms for neurological disease diagnosis.

making it difficult to identify relevant features for accurate diagnosis. Bioinspired algorithms need effective feature extraction and selection methods to capture the most informative aspects of the data. Designing robust and comprehensive feature extraction techniques that can handle the variability in neurological disease manifestations is a challenge.

3. **Interpretability and transparency**: One of the primary concerns with bioinspired algorithms is their lack of interpretability. Many of these algorithms, such as deep neural networks, function as black boxes, making it difficult to understand the underlying decision-making process. In the context of neurological disease diagnosis, interpretability is crucial for gaining insights into the diagnostic criteria used by the algorithms and for establishing trust among healthcare professionals and patients.
4. **Overfitting and generalization**: Overfitting occurs when a bioinspired algorithm performs well on the training data but fails to generalize to new, unseen data. This challenge is particularly significant when dealing with neurological diseases, where the complexity of the data and the limited availability of labeled samples can lead to overfitting. Developing

techniques to mitigate overfitting and improve generalization is essential for reliable diagnosis.

5. **Integration with clinical practice**: Integrating bioinspired algorithms into clinical practice presents various challenges, including regulatory approval, ethical considerations, and acceptance by healthcare professionals. The deployment of such algorithms in real-world healthcare settings requires careful validation, seamless integration with existing diagnostic workflows, and collaboration between computer scientists, clinicians, and regulatory bodies.
6. **Model explainability**: Explainability refers to the ability to provide understandable explanations or justifications for the decisions made by a bioinspired algorithm. In the context of neurological disease diagnosis, it is crucial to have models that can provide transparent explanations for their diagnostic outputs. This is essential for building trust and acceptance among healthcare professionals and patients.
7. **Limited knowledge and understanding of neurological diseases**: Despite significant progress in neuroscience and clinical research, our understanding of many neurological diseases is still limited. This lack of comprehensive knowledge poses challenges in developing accurate bioinspired algorithms for diagnosis. More research is needed to uncover new biomarkers, identify disease mechanisms, and improve our understanding of the complex interplay of factors involved in neurological diseases.

Addressing these challenges requires interdisciplinary collaboration between computer scientists, clinicians, neuroscientists, and experts in medical ethics and regulatory affairs. By leveraging the strengths of bioinspired algorithms and addressing these challenges, there is great potential to improve the accuracy and efficiency of neurological disease diagnosis, leading to better patient outcomes.

The future directions for neurological disease diagnosis using bioinspired algorithms are exciting and hold great potential for improving diagnostic accuracy and patient care. Here are some key areas that can be explored:

1. Multi-modal data integration: Bioinspired algorithms can leverage multiple data modalities, such as neuroimaging, genetic data, clinical records, and wearable sensor data, to

enhance diagnostic accuracy. Integrating and analyzing these diverse data sources can provide a more comprehensive understanding of neurological diseases and enable more precise and personalized diagnosis.

2. Transfer learning and domain adaptation: Neurological diseases often have limited labeled data, particularly for rare conditions. Transfer learning and domain adaptation techniques can enable knowledge transfer from well-studied diseases to those with less available data. By leveraging pre-trained models or related datasets, bioinspired algorithms can improve diagnosis accuracy for underrepresented neurological diseases.
3. Explainable AI and interpretability: Enhancing the interpretability and explainability of bioinspired algorithms is crucial for their adoption in clinical practice. Future research should focus on developing techniques that provide clear and transparent explanations for the decisions made by the algorithms. This will help clinicians understand and trust the algorithm's outputs, leading to improved acceptance and integration into routine clinical workflows.
4. Longitudinal analysis and disease progression modeling: Neurological diseases often exhibit progressive changes over time. Bioinspired algorithms can be utilized to analyze longitudinal data and model disease progression. By tracking disease trajectories and predicting future outcomes, these algorithms can assist in early detection, treatment planning, and monitoring the effectiveness of interventions.
5. Integration with digital health technologies: The widespread availability of smartphones, wearable devices, and other digital health technologies offers new opportunities for data collection and real-time monitoring. Bioinspired algorithms can be integrated with these technologies to develop remote monitoring systems and assist in the continuous monitoring and early detection of neurological diseases.
6. Collaborative research and data sharing: Collaboration and data sharing among researchers, clinicians, and institutions are essential for advancing the field of neurological disease diagnosis using bioinspired algorithms. Establishing collaborative networks and sharing large-scale, well-curated

datasets will enable the development and validation of robust algorithms across different populations and settings.

7. Ethical considerations and regulatory guidelines: As bioinspired algorithms become more prevalent in clinical practice, it is essential to address ethical considerations and establish clear regulatory guidelines. These guidelines should ensure patient privacy, informed consent, and fair and unbiased algorithmic decision making. Ethical frameworks and regulatory bodies should be established to oversee the development, deployment, and evaluation of bioinspired algorithms for neurological disease diagnosis.

By focusing on these future directions, researchers and practitioners can harness the potential of bioinspired algorithms to revolutionize neurological disease diagnosis. These advancements have the potential to improve patient outcomes, enable early intervention, and contribute to our understanding of neurological diseases.

12.4 Conclusion

Bioinspired algorithms have emerged as a promising approach for the diagnosis of neurological diseases. They offer the potential to overcome the limitations of traditional diagnostic methods, providing accurate and timely diagnoses. Genetic algorithms, neural networks, ant colony optimization, and particle swarm optimization are among the bioinspired algorithms that have shown promise in this domain. However, several challenges, including data availability and algorithm complexity, need to be addressed to ensure the successful implementation of these algorithms in clinical practice. By overcoming these challenges and embracing future opportunities, bioinspired algorithms have the potential to revolutionize neurological disease diagnosis, leading to improved patient outcomes and better management of these debilitating conditions.

References

1. Atlas, M.B., Resource A blood atlas of COVID-19 defines hallmarks of disease severity and specificity ll ll A blood atlas of COVID-19 defines hallmarks of disease severity and specificity. 185, 5, 916–938, Elsevier Inc., 2022, doi: 10.1016/j.cell.2022.01.012.

2. Sutradhar, S., Karforma, S., Bose, R., Roy, S., Healthcare Analytics A Dynamic Step-wise Tiny Encryption Algorithm with Fruit Fly Optimization for Quality of Service improvement in healthcare. *Healthc. Anal.*, 3, 100177, January 2023, doi: 10.1016/j.health.2023.100177.
3. Amin, R., Kandar, D., Kumar, A., An experimental analysis of different Deep Learning based Models for Alzheimer's Disease classification using Brain Magnetic Resonance Images. *J. King Saud Univ. - Comput. Inf. Sci.*, 34, 10, 8576–8598, 2022, doi: 10.1016/j.jksuci.2021.09.003.
4. Benkhaddra, I., Kumar, A., Setitra, M.A. *et al.*, Design and Development of Consensus Activation Function Enabled Neural Network-Based Smart Healthcare Using BIoT. *Wirel Pers. Commun.*, 130, 1549–1574, 2023, https://doi.org/10.1007/s11277-023-10344-0 Q2,Impact Factor -2.017.
5. Srivastav, A.L., Markandeya, Patel, N. *et al.*, Concepts of circular economy for sustainable management of electronic wastes: challenges and management options. *Environ. Sci. Pollut. Res.*, 30, 48654–48675, 2023, https://doi.org/10.1007/s11356-023-26052-y Q1,Impact Factor -5.19.
6. Ilyas, B., Kumar, A., Setitra, M.A., Bensalem, Z.E.A., Lei, H., Prevention of DDoS attacks using an optimized deep learning approach in blockchain technology. *Trans. Emerging Telecommun. Technol.*, 34, 4, e4729, 2023, Q2,Impact Factor -3.31.
7. Kumar, A., Rathore, P. S., Dubey, A. K., Agrawal, R., Sharma, K. P., LTE-NBP with holistic UWB-WBAN approach for the energy efficient biomedical application. *Multimed. Tools Appl.*, 82, 25, 39797–39811, 2023.
8. Kumar, A., Kumar, S. A., Dutt, V., Shitharth, S., Tripathi, E., IoT based arrhythmia classification using the enhanced hunt optimization-based deep learning. *Expert Syst.*, 40, 7, e13298, 2023.
9. Madruga, M., Campos-Roca, Y., Pérez, C. J., Impact of noise on the performance of automatic systems for vocal fold lesions detection. *Biocybern. Biomed. Eng.*, 41, 3, 1039–1056, 2021.
10. Hayanga, J. A., Kakuturu, J., Dhamija, A., Asad, F., McCarthy, P., Sappington, P., Badhwar, V., Cannulate, extubate, ambulate approach for extracorporeal membrane oxygenation for COVID-19. *J. Thorac. Cardiovasc. Surg.*, 166, 4, 1132–1142, 2023.
11. Vucic, S. *et al.*, Clinical Neurophysiology Clinical diagnostic utility of transcranial magnetic stimulation in neurological disorders. Updated report of an IFCN committee. *Clin. Neurophysiol.*, 150, 131–175, 2023, doi: 10.1016/j.clinph.2023.03.010.
12. Ye, C., Mori, S., Chan, P., Ma, T., NeuroImage: Clinical Connectome-wide network analysis of white matter connectivity in Alzheimer's disease. *NeuroImage Clin.*, 22, 101690, January 2019, doi: 10.1016/j.nicl.2019.101690.
13. Nakano-baker, O. *et al.*, Biosensors and Bioelectronics Data-driven design of a multiplexed, peptide-sensitized transistor to detect breath VOC markers of COVID-19. *Biosens. Bioelectron.*, 229, 115237, February 2023, doi: 10.1016/j.bios.2023.115237.

14. Wankhede, D.S. and Selvarani, R., Neuroscience Informatics Dynamic architecture based deep learning approach for glioblastoma brain tumor survival prediction. *Neurosci. Inf.*, 2, 4, 100062, 2022, doi: 10.1016/j.neuri.2022.100062.
15. Wang, H. *et al.*, Articles Hearing impairment is associated with cognitive decline, brain atrophy and tau pathology. *eBioMedicine*, 86, 12, 104336, 2022, doi: 10.1016/j.ebiom.2022.104336.
16. Chhetri, B., Mohan, L., Mittal, M., International Journal of Information Management Data Insights How machine learning is used to study addiction in digital healthcare: A systematic review. *Int. J. Inf. Manage. Data Insights*, 3, 2, 100175, 2023, doi: 10.1016/j.jjimei.2023.100175.
17. Quan, Y., Wu, X., Zhu, S., Zeng, X., Zeng, Z., Zheng, Q., Triboelectric nanogenerators for clinical diagnosis and therapy: A report of recent progress. *Med. Nov. Technol. Devices*, 16, 100195, November 2022, doi: 10.1016/j.medntd.2022.100195.
18. Wang, K., Kumar, S., Sanghadasa, M., Wu, C., Priya, S., Implantable photoelectronic charging (I-PEC) for medical implants. *Energy Rev.*, 1, 2, 100006, 2022, doi: 10.1016/j.enrev.2022.100006.
19. Messihad, M.I., Benomar, A., Merrachi, N.A., Bégin, L.R., Febrer, G., Philie, M., The diagnostic challenge of aortic intimal sarcomas, from vasculitis-like syndrome to mesenteric ischemia: Report of two cases and individual patient data literature review. *Ann. Vasc. Surg. Brief Rep. Innov.*, 2, 3, 100109, 2022.
20. Wu, J. *et al.*, Loss of Neurological Disease HSAN-I-Associated Gene SPTLC2 Impairs CD8 + T Cell Responses to Infection by Inhibiting T Cell Metabolic Fitness Article Loss of Neurological Disease HSAN-I-Associated Gene SPTLC2 Impairs CD8 + T Cell Responses to Infection by. 50, 5, 1218–1231, E5, Elsevier Inc. 2019, doi: 10.1016/j.immuni.2019.03.005.
21. Yang, T. *et al.*, iScience ll Mechanical sensors based on two-dimensional materials: Sensing mechanisms, structural designs and wearable applications. *ISCIENCE*, 25, 1, 103728, 2022, doi: 10.1016/j.isci.2021.103728.
22. Rahul, K. and Banyal, R.K., ScienceDirect ScienceDirect Metaheuristics approach to improve data analysis process for the Metaheuristics approach to improve data analysis process for the healthcare sector healthcare sector. *Proc. Comput. Sci.*, 215, 2019, 98–103, 2023, doi: 10.1016/j.procs.2022.12.011.
23. Su, Y., Yuan, D., Chen, D.G., Ng, R.H., Wang, K., Choi, J., . . . Heath, J.R., Multiple early factors anticipate post-acute COVID-19 sequelae. *Cell*, 185, 5, 881–895, 2022. doi: 10.1016/j.cell.2022.01.014.
24. Javaid, M., Haleem, A., Pratap, R., Suman, R., Biomedical Technology Sustaining the healthcare systems through the conceptual of biomedical engineering: A study with recent and future potentials. *Biomed. Technol.*, 1, 39–47, November 2022, doi: 10.1016/j.bmt.2022.11.004.2023.
25. Fartoukh, M., Nseir, S., Mégarbane, B., Cohen, Y., Lafarge, A., Contou, D., ... MultiCoV collaborative trial group. Respiratory multiplex PCR and procalcitonin to reduce antibiotic exposure in severe SARS-CoV-2 pneumonia: A

multicentre randomized controlled trial. *Clin. Microbiol. Infect.*, 29, 6, 734–743, 2023.
26. Bhargava, N., Rathore, P.S., Bhowmick, A., Study of X Ray Detection Using CNN in Machine Learning. *Advancements in Smart Computing and Information Security: First International Conference, ASCIS 2022*, Rajkot, India Switzerland, November 24–26, 2022, Cham: Springer Nature, 2023, Revised Selected Papers, Part I.
27. Dutt, V., Rathore, P.S., Chauhan, K., Support Vector in Healthcare Using SVM/PSO in Various Domains: A Review, in: *Swarm Intelligence Optimization: Algorithms and Applications*, pp. 291–307, 2020.
28. Schepers, M. *et al.*, Brain Behavior and Immunity Selective PDE4 subtype inhibition provides new opportunities to intervene in neuroinflammatory versus myelin damaging hallmarks of multiple sclerosis. *Brain Behav. Immun.*, 109, 1–22, December 2022, doi: 10.1016/j.bbi.2022.12.020. 2023.
29. Wen, L. *et al.*, Single-cell technologies : From research to application Single-cell technologies : From research to application. *Innov.*, 3, 6, 100342, 2022, doi: 10.1016/j.xinn.2022.100342.
30. Cen, X., Wang, F., Huang, X., Jovic, D., Dubee, F., Biosafety and Health Towards precision medicine : Omics approach for COVID-19. *Biosaf. Heal.*, 5, 2, 78–88, 2023, doi: 10.1016/j.bsheal.2023.01.002.
31. Monsalve-torra, A., Ruiz-fernandez, D., Marin-alonso, O., Soriano-payá, A., Camacho-mackenzie, J., Carreño-jaimes, M., Using machine learning methods for predicting inhospital mortality in patients undergoing open repair of abdominal aortic aneurysm. *J. Biomed. Inform.*, 62, 195–201, May 1999, doi: 10.1016/j.jbi.2016.07.007.2016.
32. Bishop, C.M., Neural networks and their applications. *Rev. Sci. Instrum.*, 65, 6, 1803–1832, 1994.
33. Abiodun, O., II, Jantan, A., Omolara, A.E., Dada, K.V., Mohamed, N.A., Arshad, H., State-of-the-art in artificial neural network applications: A survey. *Heliyon*, 4, 11, e00938, 2018.
34. Bhargava, N., Sharma, S., Purohit, R., Rathore, P.S., Prediction of recurrence cancer using J48 algorithm, in: *2017 2nd International Conference on Communication and Electronics Systems (ICCES)*, 2017, October, IEEE, pp. 386–390.
35. Fan, X., Sayers, W., Zhang, S., Han, Z., Ren, L., Chizari, H., Review and classification of bio-inspired algorithms and their applications. *J. Bionic Eng.*, 17, 611–631, 2020.
36. Selvaraj, C., Kumar, R.S., Karnan, M., A survey on application of bio-inspired algorithms. *Int. J. Comput. Sci. Inf. Technol.*, 5, 1, 366–70, 2014.
37. Bansal, J.C., Particle swarm optimization, in: *Evolutionary and swarm intelligence algorithms*, pp. 11–23, 2019.
38. Haq, I. U., Rather, A. H., Kaur, G., A Comparative Analysis of Machine Learning Algorithms for the Early Prediction of Cardiovascular Disease,

in: *2023 2nd International Conference on Edge Computing and Applications (ICECAA)*, pp. 987–993, IEEE, 2023, July.
39. Rather, A. H., & Haq, I. U. (2023, April). Intelligent Framework for Early Prediction of Diabetic Retinopathy: A Deep Learning Approach, in: *International Conference on Paradigms of Communication, Computing and Data Analytics*, pp. 377–388, Singapore: Springer Nature Singapore, 2023, April.
40. Mao, X., Li, Q., Xie, H., Lau, R.Y., Wang, Z., Paul Smolley, S., Least squares generative adversarial networks, *Proceedings of the IEEE International Conference on Computer Vision*, pp. 2794–2802, 2017.

13

Optimizing Artificial Neural-Network Using Genetic Algorithm

Bhavy Pratap and Sulabh Bansal*

Department of Information Technology, Manipal University Jaipur, Jaipur, Rajasthan, India

Abstract

Artificial neural networks (ANNs) is a processing system which is adaptive and nonlinear in nature. One has to select the suitable number of neurons to perform ANN as insufficient number of neurons can lead to poor approximation, whereas excessive neurons can result in overfitting issues. In order to improve the accuracy and simplify the structure of neural networks, a variety of optimization techniques and algorithms has been developed. These techniques and algorithms help to train neural networks more efficiently and effectively, leading to better performance. One of those algorithms is Genetic Algorithm (GA). GA is random-search algorithm, which takes the nature selection and evolution process into consideration. Both NNs and GA are similar techniques. The similarity between ANNs and GAs inspired us to combine the two approaches to see if a GA could be used to train neural networks with high accuracy. A GA is a search algorithm that uses principles inspired by biological evolution, such as mutation, crossover, and selection. First, the "selection" mechanism chooses best parents from a gene pool, which is essentially an array containing the best matrix of weights, in order to obtain the most favourable genes. Second, the crossover process is implemented by selecting two genes randomly from the best genes and recombining them using a specific method. Finally, mutation happens at random. A random number between 0 and 1 is created after each iteration of the crossover process. If this value is less than or equal to 0.05, a random subset of the weighted matrix will be multiplied by a number between 2 and 5. This slight scaling of the values in the weighted matrix can help to improve the accuracy of the artificial neural network (ANN) model. There are many factors that can affect performance of ANN model, such as the number of layers, the number of neurons in each layer, the optimization function,

**Corresponding author*: sulabh.bansal@jaipur.manipal.edu

Sumit Srivastava, Abhineet Anand, Abhishek Kumar, Bhavna Saini and Pramod Singh Rathore (eds.) Bio-Inspired Optimization for Medical Data Mining, (269–288) © 2024 Scrivener Publishing LLC

the loss function, the learning rate, and others. The size of the population, the crossover rate and mutation, and the chance of mutation must all be carefully evaluated while building an ANN using GA. That is why by using Genetic algorithm and using back propagation, the weights need to get updated by using a certain function or method and to find the most optimal and more precise ANN model.

Keywords: Artificial neural network (ANNs), genetic algorithm (GA), neurons, selection, crossover, mutation, back propagation

13.1 Introduction

13.1.1 ANN

ANN structure and working of brain of a human from where it learn trends and build a computational model based on learning. They are built to address complicated issues in fields, such as natural language processing (NLP), computer-vision (CV), etc. An ANN consists of interconnected artificial neurons, each of which receives inputs, processes them, and generates an output. This simple building block is repeated many times to form a network of neurons, capable of performing complex tasks.

ANNs are inspired by the human brain. They are able to learn from data and make predictions or decisions without being explicitly programmed.

ANNs work by passing input data through a series of layers of neurons. Each layer of neurons performs a mathematical operation on the input data, and the output of one layer is used as the input for the next layer. The final layer of neurons produces the output prediction or decision.

The weights of the connections between neurons impact an ANN's accuracy. These weights are assigned during the training phase, which is an iterative process in which the weights are fine-tuned until the network provides the desired output for a particular input [1].

One of the key strengths of ANNs is their ability to handle large amounts of data. They are also capable of handling complex nonlinear relationships between inputs and outputs.

ANNs are classified into three types: feedforward networks, recurrent networks, and convolutional networks. Feedforward networks are the most basic sort of ANN, with a straight data flow that conveys information from the input layer to the output layer without looping back. Recurrent networks, on the other hand, allow for feedback loops, allowing information to be passed from later layers back to earlier layers [2].

Convolutional networks are specialized feedforward networks, designed for image recognition tasks. Convolutional layers are a key feature of CNNs.

They extract features from local regions of the input data, while maintaining the spatial relationships between those features.

The training of an ANN can be computationally expensive and time-consuming, but the use of powerful hardware and parallel processing techniques has made it possible to train very large networks. The availability of large annotated datasets has also been crucial for the success of ANNs in recent years, as they provide the necessary training data to allow the network to learn and make accurate predictions [3, 4].

To summarize, artificial neural networks have brought about significant changes in various domains, like- CV, NLP, and robotics, by serving as powerful ML models. ANNs are powerful tools that can be used to solve many real-world problems. They can handle large amounts of data, handle complex nonlinear relationships, and learn from annotated data sets. However, their performance depends on the quality of the data and the design of the network. With continued advancements in hardware and algorithms, ANNs will likely play a major role in shaping our future.

The general flow of data in an ANN is as follows:

- The input layer receives the input data.
- Input data gets multiplied by its weights and added to the biases.
- The output of the neuron is produced by passing the result through an "activation function."
- Each neuron's output in a layer is utilised as the input for the following layer.
- The process is repeated until final output is produced at the output layer.
- This flow diagram can be visualized as a series of connected nodes, where each node represents a neuron and the connections represent the weights.

A typical flow diagram for an ANN is as follows:

- Input layer: the input layer takes in the data from the dataset and sends it to the hidden layers.
- Hidden layers: the hidden layers apply weights to the inputs, pass the result through activation functions and generate intermediate outputs. The intricacy of the problem will determine how many hidden layers there are and how many neurons there are in each layer. A more complex problem

may require more hidden layers and neurons to be able to learn the necessary features to solve the problem.

- Output layer: the output layer receives the outputs from the hidden layers, applies weights, and passes the final result via activation function to generate predictions.
- Feedforward propagation: the inputs are passed through the layers, and the predictions are generated by the output layer.
- Backpropagation: error between the actual output and predicted output gets calculated, and weights are updated using optimization algorithms such as different types of gradient-descent for error minimization.
- Model evaluation: the model's efficacy in resolving the issue can be assessed using performance metrics, such as recall, accuracy, precision, and F1 score. These metrics can be used to assess how well the model is able to resolve the issue.
- Repeat until satisfactory performance: the process is repeated until the performance of the model reaches an acceptable level.

For satisfactory performance, we need to perform optimization on ANN using various methods. ANN optimization is the process of adjusting the parameters of an ANN, such as weights and biases, to improve its performance. During training, the parameters are optimized to reduce the error between the network's predictions and the actual outputs, which is accomplished by presenting the network with a set of input-output pairs, and the optimization algorithm adjusts the parameters accordingly [5, 6].

Several optimization algorithms are commonly used for ANNs, including gradient descent, mini-batch gradient descent, (SGD) stochastic gradient descent, and other variants, such as GAs, Adagrad, Adadelta, or Adam. The choice of optimization algorithm depends on the characteristics of the problem and the network architecture.

Gradient descent is the most commonly used optimization algorithm for ANNs. It is an iterative method that modifies the parameters in the direction of the negative gradient of the cost function. The cost function calculates the error between the network's predictions and actual outputs. The gradient descent algorithm updates the parameters by subtracting the gradient of the cost function multiplied by a learning rate, which determines the magnitude of the adjustment.

Stochastic gradient descent (SGD) is a variant of gradient descent that adjusts the parameters after evaluating a single training example, rather than after evaluating the entire training set. This provides a faster convergence and is less sensitive to the choice of the learning rate. Figure 13.1 shows the flow diagram of ANN.

Mini-batch gradient descent is a trade-off between batch gradient descent and SGD, where the parameters are adjusted after evaluating a

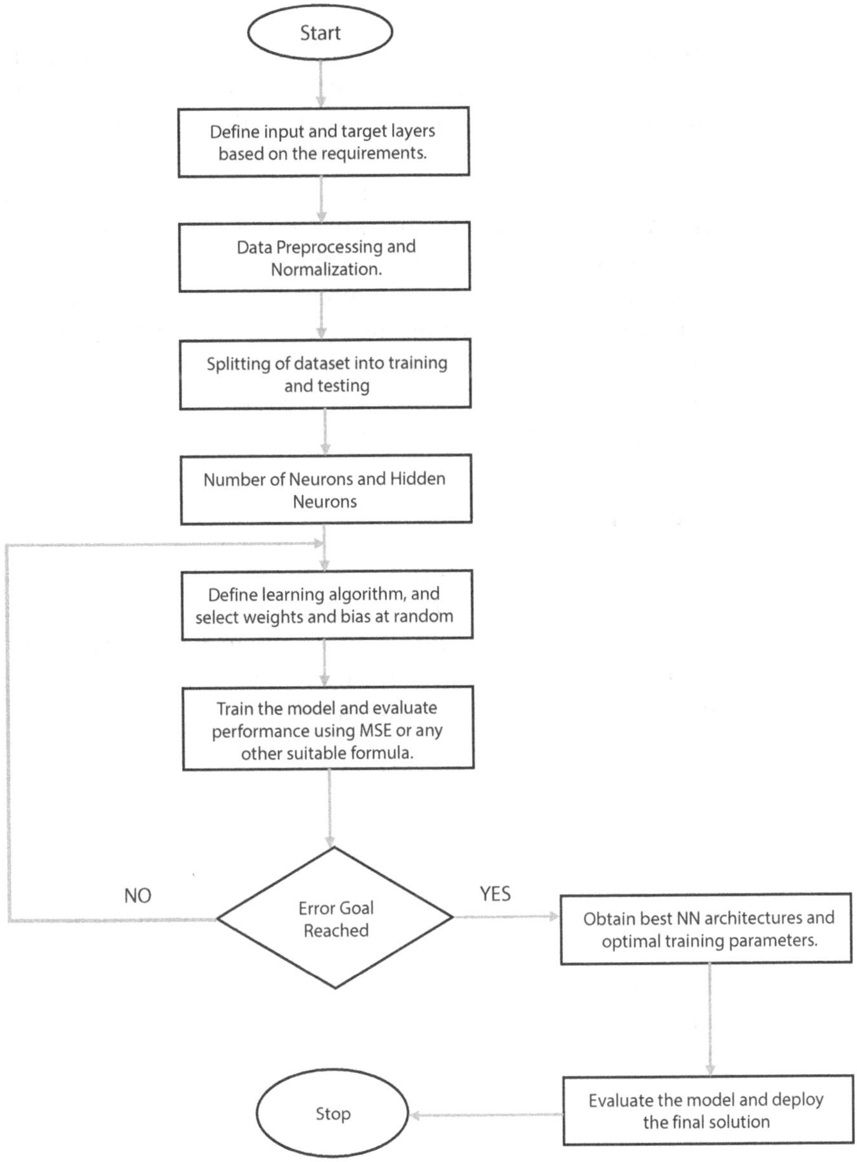

Figure 13.1 Flow diagram of ANN.

small batch of training examples, rather than a single example or the entire training set. This provides a balance between the speed of convergence of SGD and the stability of batch gradient descent.

Variants of gradient descent, such as Adam, Adagrad, and Adadelta, are optimization algorithms that incorporate additional information, such as the historical gradient information, to improve the convergence and stability of the optimization process.

Apart from the optimization algorithm, the cost function, regularization techniques, and hyperparameters, including the learning rate and the number of hidden layers, are also vital factors that affect the optimization of ANNs.

In conclusion, optimization of ANNs is a crucial step in the training process, where the parameters of the network are adjusted to improve its performance. There are several optimization algorithms available, ranging from simple gradient descent to more complex variants, and the choice of optimization algorithm depends on the characteristics of the problem and the network architecture. The optimization process also involves the choice of cost function, regularization techniques, and hyperparameters, and requires careful tuning to ensure optimal performance [7–11].

13.1.2 Genetic Algorithm

A specific kind of optimisation algorithm called GA mimics the process of natural selection in order to function. By employing genetic operations like mutation and crossover, they continuously enhance a population of random solutions. The technique employs a set of genes that stand in for many potential answers to the issue and iteratively improves these genes to determine the optimal one.

The basic process of a GA consists of the following steps:

- Initialization: the initial step involves initializing the population of genes, which represents potential solutions to the problem. The user specifies both the size of the population and the initial genes.
- Evaluation: following initialization, the subsequent step entails calculating the fitness of each gene within the population. The fitness of a gene serves as a metric for assessing how effectively it solves the problem and is employed as the basis for selection.
- Selection: the third step involves selecting genes with the highest fitness to be utilized in the next generation. This

selection is accomplished by employing a mechanism such as tournament selection or rank-based selection, which determines the genes to be selected based on their fitness.

- Crossover: the fourth step revolves around generating new genes through the combination of selected genes via crossover. Crossover is a process that merges the genetic information of two genes to create a new gene.
- Mutation: the fifth step encompasses applying a mutation operation to the new genes. Mutation involves randomly modifying the genetic information of a gene, introducing diversity into the population.
- The final step entails repeating the process from step 2 to step 5 for a specific number of generations or until a stopping criterion is met. The stopping criterion can be defined as a maximum number of generations, a minimum fitness value, or any other criterion specified by the user.

The fundamental concept underlying GA is to initiate the process with a set of randomly generated genes [8]. As time progresses, the quality of these genes is enhanced through the utilization of selection, crossover, and mutation operations. This iterative process persists until the optimal solution is discovered or until a predetermined stopping criterion is satisfied.

GA possesses notable strengths when it comes to tackling intricate problems featuring multiple objectives or constraints. The fitness function can be crafted to accurately capture the objectives and constraints of the problem at hand, while the selection mechanism serves to preserve diversity within the population.

Another strength of genetic algorithms is their ability to handle problems where the solution space is large and complex, and the search process may be subject to local optima. The population-based approach of genetic algorithms provides a way to escape local optima and explore entire solution space, increasing chances to find an optimal solution. One of the main disadvantages of genetic algorithms is their computational cost. The evaluation of the fitness function for each gene, as well as the selection, crossover, and mutation operations, can be computationally expensive, especially for large problems with many variables.

Optimizing using genetic algorithms entails discovering the optimal solution to a problem by applying the principles of genetics and natural selection to a group of potential solutions known as the population. The optimization process begins by creating an initial population of candidate solutions, also known as genes. Every individual gene within the population represents a prospective solution to the problem.

Subsequently, the fitness of each gene is evaluated to assess its effectiveness in solving the problem. This evaluation assigns a fitness value to each gene, which serves as the basis for the selection process. The genes with the highest fitness values are chosen to be carried forward into the next generation [9].

To diversify and explore new potential solutions, genetic operators, such as mutation and crossover, are applied. Crossover involves combining the genetic information of two selected genes to create novel offspring genes. Mutation introduces variation by randomly modifying the genetic information of individual genes.

The iterative process of evaluation, selection, and genetic operations is repeated for a specified number of generations or until a predetermined stopping criterion is met. The stopping criterion, determined by the user, may involve reaching a maximum generation limit, achieving a minimum fitness value, or adhering to other specified criteria.

The genetic algorithm continues to evolve the population of genes over time, leading to a progressively better solution to the problem. The optimal solution is attained once the stopping criterion is satisfied, at which point the gene possessing the highest fitness value is identified and returned as the solution to the problem.

Optimization using genetic algorithms can be useful for solving problems with complex solution spaces and multiple objectives or constraints. The fitness function can be designed to reflect the objectives and constraints of the problem, and the selection mechanism can be used to maintain diversity in the population. Flow diagram of GA is shown in Figure 13.2.

In addition, genetic algorithms are robust against local optima and can escape from suboptimal solutions, making them well suited for solving difficult optimization problems. However, they can be computationally expensive, especially for large problems with many variables, and the optimal solution may not be guaranteed [12–14].

Some disadvantages of using GA for optimization are:

- Slow convergence: genetic algorithms can be slow to converge and may require a large number of generations to reach an optimal solution.
- Requires large population size: the population size must be large enough to maintain diversity, which can lead to memory and computational constraints.

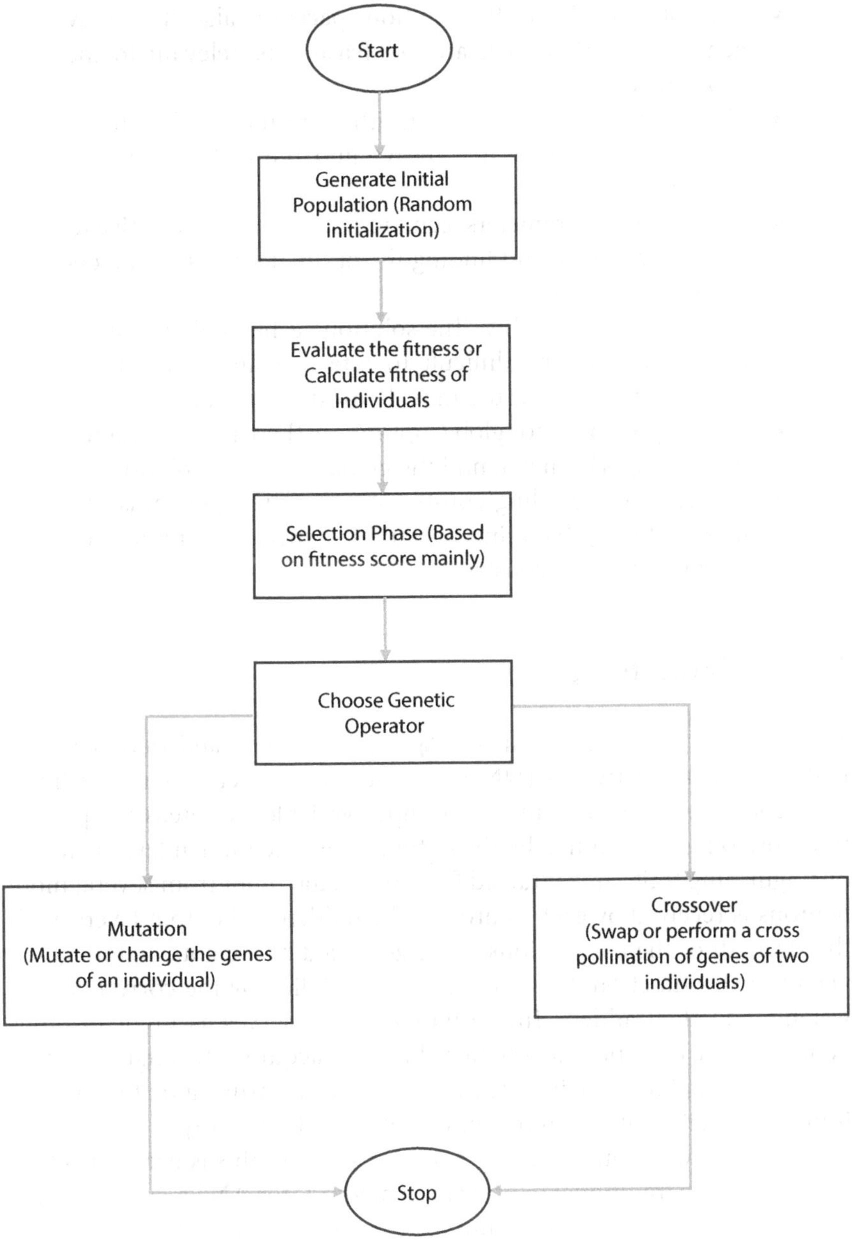

Figure 13.2 Flow diagram of GA.

- Lack of control over the solution space: the algorithm may generate solutions that are not feasible or relevant to the problem at hand.
- Unpredictable results: the algorithm's results can be unpredictable, and it may not always find the global optimum solution.
- Sensitivity to parameters: genetic algorithms are sensitive to their parameters, and finding the optimal set of parameters can be a challenge.
- Lack of interpretability: The solutions generated by genetic algorithms may be difficult to interpret and understand, which can limit their use in real-world applications.
- Lack of guarantee for global optimum: There is no guarantee that the algorithm will find the global optimum solution.
- Difficulty in handling constraints: Genetic algorithms can have difficulty handling constraints, such as nonlinear or nondifferentiable constraints.

13.2 Methodology

Multiple layers of neurons, including input, hidden, and output layers, make up neural networks (NNs). The number of neurons in the input layer corresponds to the number of input variables, whereas the prediction horizon is determined by the output layer. The hidden layer is where distinguishing traits are extracted from past data. Input from several more neurons is received by each neuron in the hidden and output layers, with the strength of the connections being governed by weights. Before going via a transfer function, these inputs are multiplied by the corresponding weights and then added. The resulting output serves as input to other neurons, and the optimal weight values are acquired through training. Computation play a crucial role in training NNs, ensuring that the model is processed efficiently within a reasonable time frame [15].

An ANN can be optimized by employing a GA. This is useful in situations where the traditional optimization methods for ANNs, such as gradient descent, are not effective in finding the optimal solution.

- The optimization process commences by generating an initial population of solutions, represented by sets of parameters for the artificial neural network (ANN). By using the parameters to train the ANN on a dataset and evaluating its performance measures, such as accuracy or mean squared error, one may determine the fitness of each member of the population.

- Subsequently, individuals with the highest fitness are selected for the subsequent generation through a selection mechanism, often employing a rank-based selection approach. New individuals are generated through various genetic operations, which involve combining and randomly modifying the parameters of the selected individuals.
- The evaluation, selection, and genetic operations are iteratively performed for a specified number of generations or until a predetermined stopping criterion is met. The stopping criterion can be defined by the user and may include a maximum number of generations, a minimum fitness value, or other user-specified criteria.
- As the genetic algorithm progresses, the population of individuals evolves over time, gradually converging towards a more optimal solution to the problem at hand. The optimal solution is reached once the stopping criterion is satisfied, and the individual with the highest fitness is returned as the solution.
- Optimizing an ANN using a genetic algorithm can be a useful alternative to traditional optimization methods, especially for complex problems with many variables and a large solution space. However, it can also be computationally expensive, and the optimal solution may not be guaranteed [16, 17].

Summary of the optimization process for an ANN using a GA:

- Initialization: create an initial population of potential solutions, represented by sets of parameters for the ANN.
- Evaluation: evaluating the fitness of every individual of the population by using the parameters to train the ANN on a dataset and measuring its performance, such as accuracy or mean squared error.
- Selection: choose the individuals with the highest fitness for the next generation through a selection mechanism, such as tournament selection or rank-based selection.
- Genetic operations: create new individuals through genetic operations, such as crossover and mutation, which involve

combining and randomly modifying the parameters of the selected individuals.

- Repeat: iterate through the steps of evaluation, selection, and genetic operations for a specified number of generations or until a stopping criterion is satisfied.
- Termination: the genetic algorithm iteratively evolves the population of individuals, resulting in an increasingly improved solution to the problem. The process continues until the stopping criterion is met, at which point the individual with the highest fitness is identified as the optimal solution and returned.
- This flow can be repeated multiple times with different populations, or with different parameter settings, to ensure that the best solution is found. The genetic algorithm can be a useful alternative to traditional optimization methods for ANNs, especially for complex problems with many variables and a large solution space [18, 19].

13.2.1 Mathematical Working

Suppose a dataset contains 60 classes of fruits but they have chosen only 4 for output classification [17]. And the reason why the dataset names fruit360 is because it contains 360 elements (features) but to make it easier and simples they reduced the length of feature vector to 108. Flow diagram of hybrid GA-ANN is shown in Figure 13.3.

And at last, they used 120 and 80 neurons in the hidden layer further to apply ANN on the dataset to classify each image into one of 4 classes.

Here is explanation of working of ANN model:

i) First 108 features are passed as an input for 120 neurons that gives an output of 1×120 matrix as an output.

$$(1 \times 108) * (108 \times 120) = (1 \times 120)$$

ii) The output from the first layer serves as the input for the subsequent layer.

$$(1 \times 120) * (120 \times 80) = (1 \times 80)$$

iii) At last, the output of above layer has passed into this layer for final output.

$$(1 \times 80) * (80 \times 4) = (1 \times 4). \text{ [Final Output Matrix]}$$

How GA helped to optimized the working:
To achieve high accuracy in ANNs, weights in all layers are important, such that all weights of the ANN will be contained in a single solution of GA.

⇨ Total Weight = 108 × 120 + 120 × 80 + 80 × 4=22,880

Let us say, if population has six solutions-

⇨ Total Parameters = 6 × 22,880 = 137,280.

To use 1D vectors as chromosomes in GA, it is necessary to convert the weights matrix into this format. So we have to create three vectors, as there are three layers (two hidden and one output).

The resulting vector from the matrix multiplication between the parameter matrix of size 108 × 120 and the input vector will be of size 12,960.

For first layer, it will start processing from 0 to 12,959 (in terms of indexing).

The second element in the same solution will be the result of converting a matrix of size 150 × 60. Which equals = 9,600.

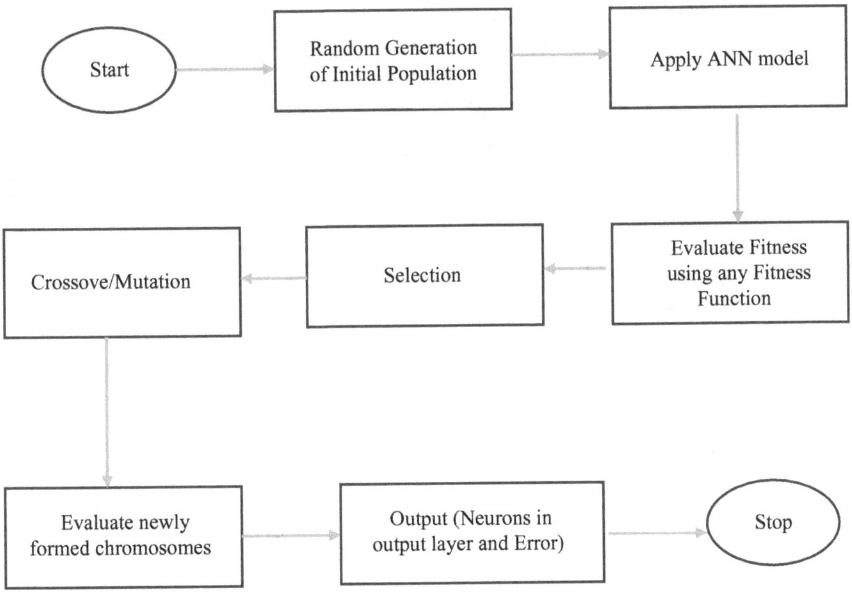

Figure 13.3 Flow diagram of hybrid GA-ANN.

For second layer, it will start processing after 12,959 to (12,959 + 9600) Means from 12,960 to 22,559.

Then at last for third layer the vector size will be $80 \times 4 = 320$.

At final stage it processes it from 22,560 to 22,879.

Hence we can see that all the 22,880 has been broken into 3 vectors, which can be successfully restored into the original 3 matrices (back propagation). Diagrammatic explanation of the working of above all the content is shown in Figure 13.4.

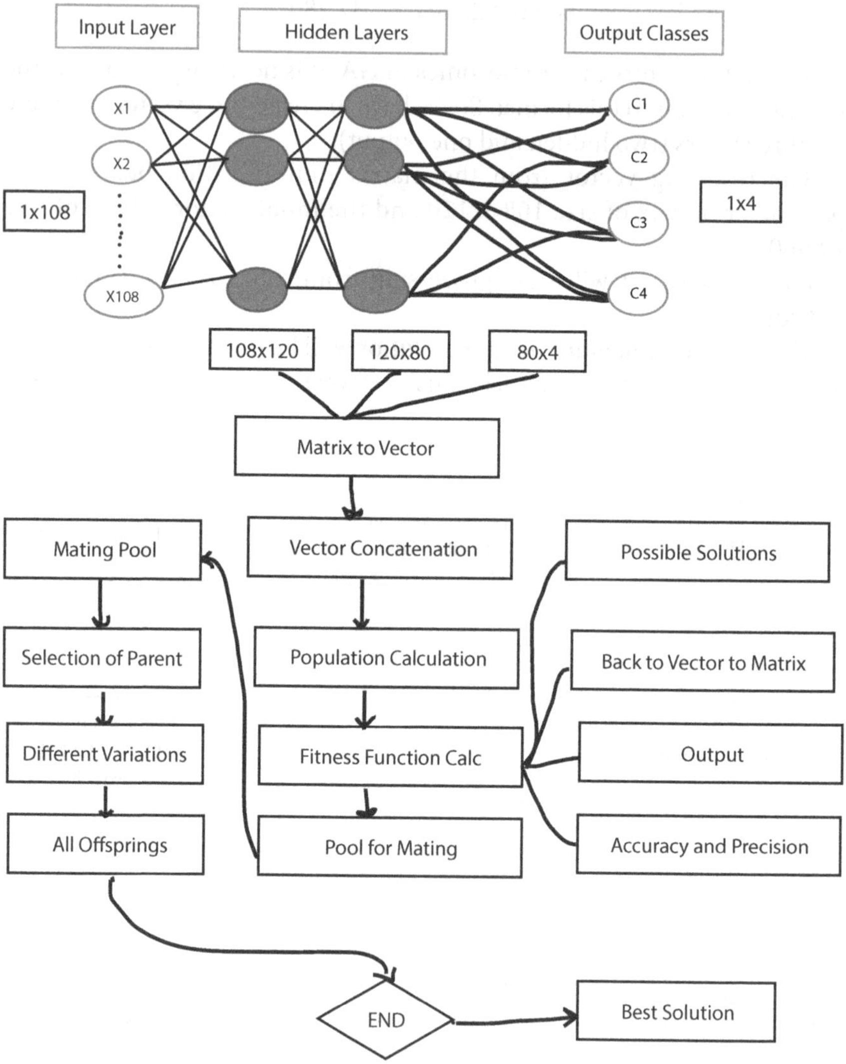

Figure 13.4 Diagrammatic explanation of the working.

13.3 Brief Study on Existing Implementations

The use of a GA or a hybrid GA-ANN model can enhance the performance of ANNs by optimizing the weights and biases of the ANN and selecting an appropriate objective function. In constructing efficient hybrid models, specific parameter values were set. A mutation probability of 25% and a recombination percentage of 9% were utilized. The hybrid GA-ANN model employed a single-point crossover operation with a 70% probability, and a population size of 350 was determined as the best choice among a range of hybrid models. A generation value of 100 was employed, and through a parametric study, it was found that network performance plateaued after 300 generations, leading to the adoption of 300 generations for GA-ANN model design.

The use of GA algorithms has been emphasized by researchers as a way to improve ANNs' capacity for prediction and generalization. Without GA, ANNs could reach a local minimum as opposed to a global one. Stochastic search algorithms like GA can modify the biases and weights of ANNs, thereby improving their performance. Consequently, the utilization of a hybrid GA-ANN model that combines the search properties of both algorithms becomes crucial for achieving optimal outcomes. This model leverages the global minimum discovered by GA within the search space to enhance the performance of the ANN.

13.3.1 Using Different Types of ANNs

The selection of an appropriate ANN depends on the research objectives at hand. One commonly used type is the feedforward neural network (FFNN) or multilayer perceptron (MLP), which offers various learning algorithms, such as back-propagation, conjugate scale gradient, conjugate gradient method, and back-propagation.

- The generalized regressed neural network (GRNN) differs from the back-propagation neural network (BPNN) in that it does not call for a learning rate and momentum during training. It is resistant to local minima as a result of this property. The time delay neural network (TDNN), on the other hand, is more sophisticated than BPNN since it preserves delays, back-propagation error signals for each unit, and time delay to control activations. During training, the adaptive time delay neural network (ATDNN) modifies the time delay parameters.

- Fuzzy neural networks (FNN) combine fuzzy logic and neural networks, providing a unique structure for implementing the fuzzy inference system. neural networks prove to be useful in solving various types of problems, including function approximation, forecasting, process optimization, robotics, mobile agents, and medicine.
- The radial basis function network (RBFN) is a type of neural network that employs local learning. It can be considered as a potential alternative to the MLP. RBFN consists of a single hidden layer that utilizes radial basis functions.
- Another noteworthy ANN method is the Support Vector Machine (SVM), which is utilized for classification, regression analysis, and forecasting. SVM exhibits resistance to local minima and is capable of producing a global optimal solution. It is recognized for its effectiveness in tackling various problem domains.

13.3.2 Using MLPs

The MLP is such a good NN architecture widely used in classification and regression problems. It consists of input and output neurons represented by small circles, as well as hidden layer neurons represented by larger circles. The synaptic weights, which represent connections between neurons, capture the knowledge of the MLP acquired during training, often using the back-propagation algorithm.

- GAs have been employed in various ways to optimize MLP. One approach, called G-Prop, uses GA to determine initial weights and optimize the number of neurons in a single hidden layer. Another technique involves a hybrid strategy where GA initializes synaptic weights, which are further optimized using the BP algorithm. The NNC technique encodes network architecture and synaptic weights through grammatical evolution.
- The topology hyperparameters of MLP have a substantial impact on the way in which it can represent intricate input–output interactions. This capacity can be enhanced by adding additional neurons to one or more hidden layers, but too many neurons might lead to overfitting and longer

calculation times. On the other hand, MLP's capacity to simulate complicated relationships may be restricted by having too few neurons and hidden layers. The MLPGA+4 approach optimises the initial weights and regularisation hyper-parameters as well as to the topology and learning rate, possibly producing MLPs with increased classification accuracy [1].

- The rate of learning synaptic weights can be properly adjusted utilising a variety of hyper-parameter optimisation techniques. To get great performance with the gradient-descent approach, the learning rate must be manually tuned. Recently, techniques with dynamic learning rate adaptation, like ADADELTA, which is applied in work [1], were proposed. This approach dynamically modifies the learning rate to accelerate synaptic weight optimisation and prevent getting stuck in local minima.

13.4 Comparative Study on Different Implementations

Comparative study of the previous work is shown in Table 13.1.

Table 13.1 Comparative study of works.

Reference	Domain	Purpose of GA	Type of NN	Result
[7]	Sonar image processing	GA employed for training	BPNN	GANN outperformed BPNN
[8]	Approximation of Function	Utilising GA to improve connection weights, centres, and widths	RBFN	GA-RBFN got MSE of 0.002444
[9]	Evaluating Quality and teaching	GA employed for training	BPNN	GA-BPNN performed better than BPNN
[10]	Time Series analysis	GA employed for training	BPNN	GANN outperformed BPNN

13.4.1 Conclusion

GA synergizes well with NNs to optimize models and approximate parameters, thereby enhancing the effectiveness of NNs. GA can be applied in various ways to design the best ANN for a given problem domain, including optimizing weights, selecting topology, choosing features, training, and improving interpretation. In the following sections, several studies are presented that utilize different ANN optimization techniques through GA, depending on the research objectives.

Even though backpropagation algorithms are frequently employed in learning, they face difficulties include choosing the right number of neurons, having slow convergence rates, and being susceptible to local minima. S.A. Billings and G.L. Zheng used the RBFN to configure the network and GA to optimise the centres, widths, and connection weights to fix the aforementioned issues [8]. Another study focused on quality assessment and instruction, where a backpropagation neural network (BPNN) was trained using GA to develop an application for quality assessment in classroom instruction [9].

Although backpropagation training techniques perform well for simple problems, their performance deteriorates as the problem complexity increases. Additionally, they struggle with discontinuous neuron transfer functions due to differentiability constraints. Montana and Davis pioneered the integration of NNs and GAs by utilizing a GA during the training process to build a sonar image categorization model using FFNN [7]. This approach yielded superior results in terms of both processing time and overcoming the limitations of backpropagation techniques. In a related work, Sexton and Gupta trained a NN with GA on five chaotic time series problems to compare the effectiveness of GA training with backpropagation (Norm–Cum–Delta algorithms) training [10]. The results demonstrated that GA training outperformed the Norm–Cum–Delta algorithms in terms of efficiency, usability, and effectiveness.

References

1. Itano, F., de Abreu de Sousa, M.A., Del-Moral-Hernandez, E., Extending MLP ANN hyper-parameters Optimization by using Genetic Algorithm. *2018 International Joint Conference on Neural Networks (IJCNN)*, 2018.
2. Khandelwal, M., Marto, A., Fatemi, S.A., Ghoroqi, M., Armaghani, D.J., Singh, T.N., Tabrizi, O., Implementing an ANN model optimized by genetic algorithm for estimating cohesion of limestone samples. *Eng. Comput.*, pp. 309–314, 2017.

3. Benkhaddra, I., Kumar, A., Setitra, M.A. *et al.*, Design and Development of Consensus Activation Function Enabled Neural Network-Based Smart Healthcare Using BIoT. *Wirel Pers. Commun.*, 130, 1549–1574, 2023. https://doi.org/10.1007/s11277-023-10344-0 Q2,Impact Factor -2.017.
4. Srivastav, A.L., Markandeya, Patel, N. *et al.*, Concepts of circular economy for sustainable management of electronic wastes: challenges and management options. *Environ. Sci. Pollut. Res.*, 30, 48654–48675, 2023, https://doi.org/10.1007/s11356-023-26052-y Q1,Impact Factor -5.19.
5. Ilyas, B., Kumar, A., Setitra, M.A., Bensalem, Z.E.A., Lei, H., Prevention of DDoS attacks using an optimized deep learning approach in blockchain technology. *Trans. Emerging Telecommun. Technol.*, 34, 4, e4729, 2023, Q2,Impact Factor -3.31.
6. Kumar, A., Rathore, P.S., Dubey, A.K. *et al.*, LTE-NBP with holistic UWB-WBAN approach for the energy efficient biomedical application. *Multimed. Tools Appl.*, pp. 39801–39805, 2023, https://doi.org/10.1007/s11042-023-15604-6 Q1,Impact Factor -2.577.
7. Kumar, A., Kumar, S.A., Dutt, V., Shitharth, S., Tripathi, E., IoT based arrhythmia classification using the enhanced hunt optimization-based deep learning. *Expert Syst.*, pp. 2–10, 2023, n. pag. Q2, Impact Factor -2.812.
8. Bhargava, N., Sharma, S., Purohit, R., Rathore, P.S., Prediction of recurrence cancer using J48 algorithm, in: *2017 2nd International Conference on Communication and Electronics Systems (ICCES)*, 2017, October, IEEE, pp. 386–390.
9. Dutt, V., Rathore, P.S., Chauhan, K., Support Vector in Healthcare Using SVM/PSO in Various Domains: A Review, in: *Swarm Intelligence Optimization: Algorithms and Applications*, pp. 291–307, 2020.
10. Wang, H., Wang, Y., Lv, X., Yu, C., Jin, H., Genetic Algorithm with Local Search for the Multi-Target Scheduling in Flexible Manufacturing System. *J. Circuits Syst. Comput.*, 2022.
11. Swarna, S.R., Kumar, A., Dixit, P., Sairam, T.V.M., Parkinson's Disease Prediction using Adaptive Quantum Computing. *2021 Third International Conference on Intelligent Communication Technologies and Virtual Mobile Networks (ICICV)*, pp. 1396–1401, 2021, doi: 10.1109/ICICV50876.2021.9388628.
12. Sasubilli, G. and Kumar, A., Machine Learning and Big Data Implementation on Health Care data. *4th International Conference on Intelligent Computing and Control Systems (ICICCS)*, pp. 859–864, 2020, doi: 10.1109/ICICCS48265.2020.9120906.
13. Sasubilli, S.M., Kumar, A., Dutt, V., Machine Learning Implementation on Medical Domain to Identify Disease Insights using TMS. *2020 International Conference on Advances in Computing and Communication Engineering (ICACCE)*, pp. 1–4, 2020, doi: 10.1109/ICACCE49060.2020.9154960.
14. Chen, J., Bao, B., Liu, J., Wu, Y., Wang, Q., Piezoelectric energy harvester featuring a magnetic chaotic pendulum. *Energy Convers. Manage.*, 2022.

15. Montana, D.J. and Davis, L.D., Training feedforward networks using gen7etic algorithms, in: *Proceedings of the International Joint Conference on Artificial Intelligence*, Morgan Kaufmann, pp. 762–767, 1989.
16. Bhargava, N., Rathore, P.S., Bhowmick, A., Study of X Ray Detection Using CNN in Machine Learning, in: *International Conference on Advancements in Smart Computing and Information Security*, pp. 295–303, Cham: Springer Nature, Switzerland, 2022, November.
17. Billings, S.A. and Zheng, G.L., Radial basis function network configuration using genetic algorithms. *Neural Network*, 8, 6, 877–890, 1995.
18. Lizhe, Y., Bo, X., Xianje, W., BP network model optimized by adaptive genetic algorithms and the application on quality evaluation for class teaching. *Future computer and communication (ICFCC), 2nd International Conference*, vol. 3, pp. v3-273–v3-276, 2010.
19. Sexton, R.S. and Gupta, J.N.D., Comparative evaluation of genetic algorithm and backpropagation for training neural. *Inf. Sci.*, 129, 45–59, 2000.

14

Bioinspired Applications in the Medical Industry: A Case Study

Alankrita Aggarwal* **and Mohit Lalit**

Department of Computer Science & Engineering, AIT, Chandigarh University, Mohali, Punjab, India

Abstract

With the increasing analysis and application of bioinspired rules for various application for the optimization purpose, this chapter aims at investigation of such algorithms for the application in medical field or we can say in the industry. This study aims at investigating the challenges, review questions, and future scope of the bioinspired algorithms in these medical applications. The reason behind investigating is that various complex problem based on optimization can be solved with the help of metaheuristics techniques and gained higher considerations. Because the algorithms are based on imitating nature's process by various animals or organisms, the modern idea can be transformed by employing the artificial intelligence and machine learning with blending the bioinspired methods. The biological inspiration behind these computing is bioinspired computing logics organisms apply in solving various applications. The organism's or animals/nature's idea of fetching food, moving and path formation are studied and how it can be best optimized and applied in the medical industry. The review will be based on the applications of bioinspired systems in the medical therapy of the frontal and subsequent disorders. The problems concerning the current challenges and future directions will also be discussed.

Keywords**:** Bioinspired algorithms, optimization, medical applications

**Corresponding author*: alankrita.agg@gmail.com

Sumit Srivastava, Abhineet Anand, Abhishek Kumar, Bhavna Saini and Pramod Singh Rathore (eds.) Bio-Inspired Optimization for Medical Data Mining, (289–308) © 2024 Scrivener Publishing LLC

14.1 Introduction

Bioinspired applications have gained tremendous popularity in recent years due to their unique ability to mimic natural phenomena and offer innovative solutions to complex problems. The medical industry has been one of the major beneficiaries of these bioinspired applications. This research paper presents a case study on the use of bioinspired applications in the medical industry. Specifically, the paper explores the use of bioinspired solutions in the development of medical devices, drug delivery systems, and surgical techniques. The case study highlights the benefits of these applications and the impact they have on the healthcare industry [1].

14.1.1 Background

The medical industry is constantly looking for new and innovative solutions to improve patient care and treatment outcomes. In recent years, bioinspired applications have emerged as a promising avenue for achieving this goal. Bioinspired applications draw inspiration from nature to develop innovative solutions to complex problems. These solutions can range from new drug delivery systems to improved surgical techniques. This research paper presents a case study on the use of bioinspired applications in the medical industry [2–4].

14.1.2 Motivation

Bioinspired algorithms have gained significant attention in recent years due to their ability to solve complex problems by mimicking natural processes. This research paper presents a case study on the application of bioinspired algorithms in the medical field. The study explores how these algorithms have been utilized to improve medical diagnosis, treatment planning, and drug discovery. Through a detailed analysis of existing literature and practical examples, this paper highlights the potential of bioinspired algorithms in revolutionizing healthcare and enhancing patient outcomes.

14.1.3 Research Objectives

The field of bioinspired design has been gaining momentum in recent years, especially in the medical industry. By taking inspiration from nature, researchers and engineers have been able to develop innovative and effective solutions to various medical challenges. In this literature review, we will explore some of the latest developments in bioinspired applications in the medical industry through a case study approach.

14.2 Overview of Bioinspired Algorithms

14.2.1 Definition and Concepts

Bioinspired algorithms, also known as biologically inspired algorithms or nature-inspired algorithms, are computational methods that draw inspiration from natural systems, phenomena, or processes to solve complex problems as shown in Figure 14.1. These algorithms attempt to replicate or simulate the behaviour, principles, or mechanisms found in biological systems, such as evolution, neural networks, swarm intelligence, and immune systems. The core idea behind bioinspired algorithms is to harness the efficiency, robustness, adaptability, and optimization capabilities observed in nature and apply them to computational problems. By emulating natural

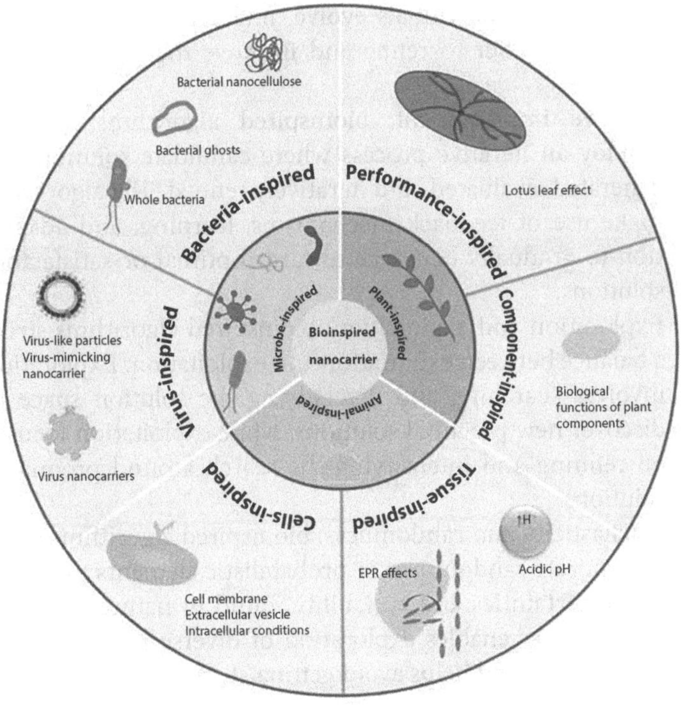

Figure 14.1 Schematic diagram of a bioinspired formulation of representative life.

processes, these algorithms offer innovative approaches to problem-solving and optimization, often surpassing traditional computational techniques in terms of efficiency and effectiveness [5–9].

Here are some key concepts associated with bioinspired algorithms:

1. Inspiration from nature: bioinspired algorithms seek inspiration from natural systems, including biological organisms, their behaviours, interactions, and adaptation mechanisms. These systems serve as metaphors or models to develop computational algorithms that can mimic or replicate their characteristics.
2. Optimization and search: many bioinspired algorithms focus on solving optimization and search problems. They explore a vast search space to find the best or near-optimal solution by imitating natural processes, such as evolution, foraging, or swarm behaviour.
3. Population-based methods: bioinspired algorithms often utilize populations or groups of individuals (e.g., chromosomes, particles, agents) that collectively search the solution space. These individuals evolve, interact, or communicate with each other to refine and improve the solutions over time.
4. Iterative improvement: bioinspired algorithms typically employ an iterative process where candidate solutions are generated, evaluated, and iteratively refined. The algorithms make use of feedback mechanisms, learning, and adaptation to gradually converge towards optimal or satisfactory solutions.
5. Exploration and exploitation: bioinspired algorithms strike a balance between exploration and exploitation. Exploration involves searching and diversifying the solution space to discover new potential solutions, while exploitation focuses on refining and intensifying the search around promising solutions.
6. Stochasticity and randomness: bioinspired algorithms often incorporate randomness or probabilistic elements to mimic the uncertainties and variability found in natural systems. Randomness enables exploration of diverse regions in the search space and helps avoid getting stuck in local optima.
7. Heuristics and feedback mechanisms: bioinspired algorithms employ heuristics, rules of thumb, or feedback

mechanisms inspired by natural systems to guide the search process. These mechanisms provide guidance, bias the exploration, and assist in decision making during the optimization process.

By combining these concepts and principles, bioinspired algorithms offer powerful problem-solving techniques across various domains, including optimization, machine learning, data mining, robotics, and complex systems analysis. They provide alternative approaches to traditional algorithmic methods, enabling the solution of challenging problems that may be difficult to tackle using conventional techniques [10–12].

14.2.2 Types of Bioinspired Algorithms

Bioinspired algorithms, also known as biologically inspired algorithms or nature-inspired algorithms, are computational methods that draw inspiration from natural systems and phenomena to solve complex problems [10, 11]. These algorithms attempt to mimic the behavior, principles, or mechanisms found in biological systems such as evolution, neural networks, swarm intelligence, and immune systems. Here are some popular bioinspired algorithms:

1. Genetic algorithms (GA): Inspired by the process of natural selection and genetics, GAs are optimization algorithms that use concepts of mutation, crossover, and selection to search for the optimal solution in a large search space. They are commonly used in optimization, machine learning, and search problems.
2. Particle swarm optimization (PSO): Inspired by the social behaviour of bird flocking or fish schooling, PSO algorithms involve a group of particles moving through a multidimensional search space. Each particle adjusts its position based on its own experience and the experiences of the other particles to find the optimal solution.
3. Ant colony optimization (ACO): Inspired by the foraging behaviour of ants, ACO algorithms simulate the behaviour of ants as they search for the shortest path between their colony and a food source. The algorithm utilizes pheromone trails and heuristics to guide the search process and find optimal paths in complex graphs or networks.

4. Artificial neural networks (ANN): Inspired by the structure and function of biological brains, ANNs are computational models composed of interconnected nodes (artificial neurons) that process and transmit information. They are used for pattern recognition, classification, regression, and other tasks and have been applied in various fields such as image and speech recognition.
5. Immune algorithms (IA): Inspired by the behaviour of the immune system, IA algorithms model the immune response and the process of recognizing and eliminating pathogens. These algorithms are often used in optimization problems, anomaly detection, and data clustering.
6. Bacterial foraging optimization (BFO): Inspired by the foraging behaviour of bacteria, BFO algorithms simulate the chemotactic movement of bacteria towards nutrient sources. These algorithms have been applied in optimization problems and have shown effectiveness in solving complex multimodal optimization problems.
7. Firefly algorithm (FA): Inspired by the flashing behaviour of fireflies, the FA is a metaheuristic algorithm that simulates the flashing patterns of fireflies to solve optimization problems. Fireflies use their flashing signals to attract mates, and the algorithm utilizes the attractiveness and distance between fireflies to find optimal solutions.

These bioinspired algorithms offer powerful problem-solving techniques and have been successfully applied in various domains such as optimization, machine learning, robotics, and data analysis. By leveraging the principles found in nature, these algorithms provide innovative and efficient approaches to tackle complex problems [13, 14].

14.2.3 Pros and Cons

14.2.3.1 Advantages of Bioinspired Algorithms

1. Robustness and adaptability: bioinspired algorithms are often robust and adaptable to different problem domains. They draw inspiration from natural systems that have evolved and adapted to changing environments over millions of years. As a result, these algorithms can handle complex and dynamic problems effectively.

2. Global optimization: many bioinspired algorithms, such as genetic algorithms (GA) and particle swarm optimization (PSO), excel at global optimization. They are capable of exploring a large search space and finding near-optimal or optimal solutions, even in the presence of multiple optima or nonlinear problem landscapes.
3. Parallel processing and scalability: bioinspired algorithms can be parallelized, allowing them to leverage the computational power of modern hardware and distributed computing systems. This parallel processing capability enables scalability and faster convergence to solutions in large-scale or computationally intensive problems.
4. Flexibility and versatility: bioinspired algorithms can be applied to a wide range of problem domains. They are not restricted to specific types of problems and can handle optimization, pattern recognition, classification, clustering, and other tasks. This versatility makes them applicable in diverse fields, including engineering, finance, healthcare, and biology.
5. Exploration and diverse solutions: bioinspired algorithms emphasize exploration of the search space, enabling them to discover diverse solutions. This is particularly advantageous when dealing with multiobjective optimization problems or when the optimal solution is not well-defined [15, 16].

14.2.3.2 Limitations of Bioinspired Algorithms

1. Computational Complexity: Some bioinspired algorithms can be computationally expensive, especially when dealing with large problem sizes or complex fitness evaluations. The iterative nature and population-based methods can require significant computational resources, limiting their applicability in real-time or resource-constrained environments.
2. Parameter Tuning: Bioinspired algorithms often have several parameters that need to be carefully tuned to achieve good performance. Finding the optimal parameter settings can be challenging and time-consuming, requiring domain expertise or extensive experimentation.
3. Lack of Guarantee for Global Optimum: While bioinspired algorithms excel at global optimization in many cases, they do not provide a guarantee of finding the global optimum.

The exploration process can get trapped in local optima or converge to suboptimal solutions depending on the problem characteristics and algorithm settings.

4. Interpretability and Transparency: Bioinspired algorithms, such as neural networks or evolutionary algorithms, often lack interpretability. The solutions obtained from these algorithms may be difficult to interpret or explain, limiting their applicability in domains where interpretability is crucial, such as healthcare or legal systems.
5. Problem-Specific Customization: Bioinspired algorithms often require customization or adaptation for specific problem domains. The algorithm design and parameter settings need to be tailored to the problem at hand, which can require domain expertise and additional effort.

It is important to consider these advantages and limitations when selecting and applying bioinspired algorithms. While they offer powerful problem-solving techniques, careful consideration should be given to the specific problem requirements, computational resources, and the trade-offs associated with each algorithm [17, 18].

14.3 Applications of Bioinspired Algorithms in Medical Field

The below mentioned are the one of the few applications in the area of Medical Industry and can be applied and classified as:

- Medical Diagnosis
- Disease Classification
- Image Analysis and Segmentation
- Treatment Planning
- Radiotherapy Optimization
- Surgical Planning
- Drug Discovery
- Virtual Screening
- Drug Design and Optimization

14.4 Review of the Case Studies

Bioinspired applications have become an important area of research in the medical industry. These applications have the potential to revolutionize patient care and treatment outcomes. This case study has highlighted the benefits of bioinspired solutions in the development of medical devices, drug delivery systems, and surgical techniques. These solutions offer innovative and effective solutions to complex problems in the healthcare industry. The future of the medical industry is bright with the continued development of bioinspired applications. Bioinspired solutions have also been used in the development of drug delivery systems. One example is the use of nanoparticles inspired by the structure of viruses to deliver drugs to specific cells in the body. These nanoparticles can be engineered to target specific cells, such as cancer cells, and release drugs at a controlled rate. This approach has the potential to improve the efficacy and safety of drug delivery systems. These solutions have also been used in the development of surgical techniques. One example is the use of robotic surgery, which is inspired by the structure and function of the human hand. Robotic surgery allows for more precise and controlled movements during surgery, reducing the risk of complications and improving patient outcomes [19, 20].

14.5 Case Study

Any case study in the medical related filed can be solved using the following mentioned steps. The first and the foremost step is to define and identify the problem statement, further is to construct a methodology. After the initial two steps the prime step is to fix the type of data set to be worked on or the other methos is to construct your own data fields so that preprocessing can be done. The feature can be selected and classified for the implementation of the algorithm as shown in Figure 14.2.

- Problem Statement
- Methodology
- Data collection and preprocessing
- Feature selection
- Classification algorithm implementation
- Experimental results and analysis

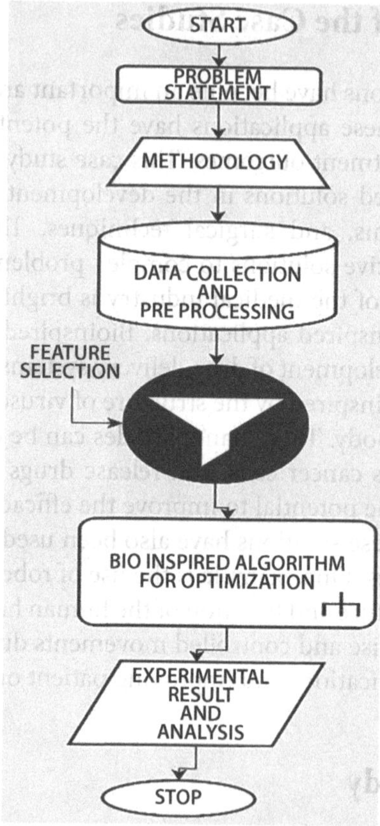

Figure 14.2 Working flowchart for the implementation of bioinspired algorithm.

14.5.1 Problem Statement

Clearly define the problem statement of the case study, which in this case would be the accurate diagnosis of cancer using bioinspired algorithms. Specify the type of cancer and the specific challenges associated with its diagnosis, such as high-dimensional data, class imbalance, or noisy data.

14.5.2 Methodology

Describe the overall methodology and approach used in the case study. This should include an overview of the bioinspired algorithm employed, such as genetic algorithms, artificial neural networks, or any other relevant algorithm. Explain why the chosen algorithm is suitable for cancer diagnosis.

14.5.3 Data Collection, Acquisition, and Preprocessing

Detail the process of data collection, including the sources and characteristics of the cancer-related data used in the study. Discuss any data preprocessing steps applied, such as normalization, missing data handling, or outlier removal, to ensure data quality and suitability for the algorithm.

14.5.4 Feature Selection

Explain the approach used for feature selection, as cancer diagnosis often involves high-dimensional data. Discuss the criteria used for selecting the most relevant features and any feature engineering techniques employed to enhance the performance of the algorithm.

14.5.5 Classification Algorithm Implementation

Describe the implementation of the bioinspired algorithm for cancer diagnosis. Provide the necessary details, such as the parameter settings, initialization techniques, convergence criteria, and any modifications or enhancements made to the algorithm to adapt it specifically to the cancer diagnosis problem.

14.5.6 Experimental Results and Analysis

Present the experimental results obtained from applying the bioinspired algorithm on the cancer dataset. Include evaluation metrics such as accuracy, sensitivity, specificity, or area under the curve (AUC) to assess the performance of the algorithm. Compare the results with baseline methods or existing approaches, if applicable. Provide statistical analysis and visualizations to support the findings.

14.5.7 Discussion and Conclusion

Discuss the implications and significance of the results obtained from the case study. Highlight the strengths and limitations of the bioinspired algorithm for cancer diagnosis. Address any challenges encountered during the study and suggest potential future research directions to further improve the algorithm's performance.

Remember, this is a general outline, and the actual case study should be tailored to the specific research, algorithm, and dataset being used.

14.6 Some Examples of the Case Studies Related to Medical Field and Can Be Solved with Bioinspired Algorithms

Case Study 1: Bioinspired solutions have been used in the development of medical devices. For example, the design of stents used in cardiovascular interventions has been inspired by the structure and function of arteries. Stents are tubular structures that are inserted into arteries to keep them open and improve blood flow. The design of stents has been improved by using bioinspired solutions to mimic the structure and function of arteries. This has led to the development of stents that are more effective and less prone to complications

Bioinspired stent design stents are widely used in the medical industry to treat blockages in blood vessels. However, traditional stents can cause various complications, including restenosis and thrombosis. To address these issues, researchers have developed a bioinspired stent design that mimics the structure of arteries. The new design consists of a series of microchannels that allow blood to flow more smoothly through the stent, reducing the risk of complications. The bioinspired stent design has shown promising results in preclinical studies and is currently being tested in human trials.

Bioinspired solutions have been used in the development of medical devices. For example, the design of stents used in cardiovascular interventions has been inspired by the structure and function of arteries. Stents are tubular structures that are inserted into arteries to keep them open and improve blood flow. The design of stents has been improved by using bioinspired solutions to mimic the structure and function of arteries. This has led to the development of stents that are more effective and less prone to complications.

However, a visual comparison between the structure of a typical artery and the bioinspired stent design. Also, it is giving the information how the stent mimics the natural structure of the artery to improve its function and provide better outcomes for patients that includes labels and annotations to explain the different parts of the stent and how it works.

Case Study 2: Bioinspired nanoparticle design. Nanoparticles are increasingly being used in the medical industry for drug delivery and imaging applications.

However, traditional nanoparticle designs can be limited by poor targeting and uptake by cells. To address these issues, researchers have developed a bioinspired nanoparticle design that mimics the structure of viruses. The new design consists of a protein shell that encases the drug payload, allowing for targeted delivery to specific cells. The bioinspired nanoparticle design has shown promising results in preclinical studies and is currently being tested in human trials.

Case Study 3: Bioinspired robotic surgery. Robotic surgery has revolutionized the field of surgery, allowing for more precise and less invasive procedures. However, traditional robotic surgery systems can be limited by their rigid and inflexible designs. To address these issues, researchers have developed a bioinspired robotic surgery system that mimics the structure and function of the human hand. The new design consists of a flexible and dexterous robotic hand that can perform a wide range of surgical procedures with greater precision and control. The bioinspired robotic surgery system has shown promising results in preclinical studies and is currently being tested in human trials.

Case Study 4: Bioinspired solutions have also been used in the development of drug delivery systems. One example is the use of nanoparticles inspired by the structure of viruses to deliver drugs to specific cells in the body. These nanoparticles can be engineered to target specific cells, such as cancer cells, and release drugs at a controlled rate. This approach has the potential to improve the efficacy and safety of drug delivery systems. It compares with nano particle design mimics the natural structure of the virus to enhance its functionality in medical applications.

Case Study 5: Bioinspired solutions have also been used in the development of surgical techniques. One example is the use of robotic surgery, which is inspired by the structure and function of the human hand. Robotic surgery allows for more precise and controlled movements during surgery, reducing the risk of complications and improving patient outcomes. A comparison between the structure of the human hand and the bio-inspired robotic surgery design. The robotic design mimics the natural structure and function of the human hand to enhance its surgical capabilities including labels and annotations to explain the different parts of the robotic design and how it performs surgical procedures.

Case Study 6: Bioinspired Algorithms for Cancer Diagnosis

Case Study 7: Bioinspired Algorithms for Treatment Planning

14.7 Future Directions and Recommendations for Future Research

Bioinspired algorithms have shown great potential in the medical field, but they also present several challenges and future directions. Here are some key considerations:

1. Challenges and Future Directions: a. Limited understanding of biological systems: Despite the progress made in bioinspired algorithms, our understanding of complex biological systems is still limited. Future research should focus on gaining deeper insights into biological processes to develop more accurate and effective algorithms. b. Validation and standardization: It is crucial to establish rigorous validation frameworks and standards for bioinspired algorithms in the medical field. This involves designing appropriate benchmark datasets, performance metrics, and comparison studies to ensure the reliability and reproducibility of results. c. Optimization and scalability: Bioinspired algorithms often involve computationally intensive processes. Overcoming scalability issues and optimizing algorithms to handle large-scale medical datasets is a significant challenge for future research. d. Real-time adaptation and learning: Developing algorithms that can adapt in real-time to dynamic medical data is another area of interest. Future directions should focus on creating algorithms that can continuously learn and evolve based on feedback from the medical environment. e. Integration of multiple modalities: Combining different bioinspired algorithms with complementary strengths can lead to more robust and accurate medical solutions. Future research should explore the integration of various algorithms and modalities to enhance performance and broaden applicability.
2. Ethical Considerations: a. Bias and fairness: Bioinspired algorithms need to address concerns related to bias and fairness.

It is essential to ensure that these algorithms do not perpetuate existing inequalities in healthcare and provide fair and unbiased outcomes for all individuals. b. Informed consent and privacy: When utilizing bioinspired algorithms for medical purposes, obtaining informed consent from patients and ensuring the privacy of their personal health information becomes crucial. Ethical frameworks should be established to govern the collection, storage, and usage of sensitive medical data. c. Transparency and accountability: Bioinspired algorithms should be transparent in their decision-making processes. There should be mechanisms in place to understand and explain the reasoning behind algorithmic outputs to healthcare professionals and patients. Additionally, accountability frameworks should be established to address potential algorithmic errors or malfunctions.

3. Data Security and Privacy: a. Robust data protection: Bioinspired algorithms rely on large amounts of medical data, making data security a critical concern. Implementing robust encryption methods, access controls, and data anonymization techniques can help protect patient privacy and prevent unauthorized access. b. Compliance with regulations: Adhering to relevant data protection regulations, such as the General Data Protection Regulation (GDPR) and Health Insurance Portability and Accountability Act (HIPAA), is vital. Healthcare organizations must ensure that bioinspired algorithms comply with these regulations to safeguard patient data.
4. Interpretable Models: a. Explainability: Interpretable models are essential in the medical field to gain trust and acceptance from healthcare professionals. Bioinspired algorithms should be able to provide interpretable explanations of their decisions, allowing clinicians to understand the reasoning behind recommendations or diagnoses. b. Model transparency: Efforts should be made to make bioinspired algorithms more transparent by incorporating interpretable architectures and visualization techniques. This enables clinicians and patients to understand how the algorithm arrives at its conclusions, improving trust and facilitating collaboration.
5. Integration with Existing Healthcare Systems: a. Compatibility: Bioinspired algorithms need to be seamlessly integrated into

existing healthcare systems and workflows. This requires compatibility with electronic health records (EHRs), medical devices, and other information systems to ensure smooth adoption and utilization by healthcare professionals.

b. Interoperability: Developing standardized interfaces and protocols that enable interoperability between bioinspired algorithms and existing healthcare systems is crucial. This allows for the exchange and sharing of data across different platforms and facilitates collaboration among healthcare providers.

6. Hybrid Approaches: Hybrid approaches in bioinspired algorithms have gained significant attention in medical studies due to their ability to leverage the strengths of multiple algorithms and overcome their individual limitations. These hybrid methods combine different bioinspired algorithms or integrate them with traditional computational techniques to improve the accuracy, efficiency, and robustness of medical studies.

Here are a few examples of hybrid approaches used in medical studies:

1. Genetic algorithm (GA) and artificial neural networks (ANN): Genetic algorithms are optimization techniques inspired by the process of natural selection. They can be combined with artificial neural networks, which are computational models inspired by the structure and function of the human brain. This hybrid approach can be used for tasks such as feature selection in medical image analysis, where the genetic algorithm optimizes the neural network's architecture and parameters to improve classification accuracy.
2. Particle swarm optimization (PSO) and Support Vector Machines (SVM): Particle swarm optimization is an optimization technique inspired by the collective behaviour of bird flocking or fish schooling. It can be combined with support vector machines, which are powerful machine learning algorithms used for classification and regression tasks. The hybrid PSO-SVM approach can be employed for medical diagnosis or prediction problems, where PSO is used to optimize the SVM's hyperparameters and improve the overall performance.

3. Ant colony optimization (ACO) and Clustering Algorithms: Ant colony optimization is an optimization technique inspired by the foraging behaviour of ants. It can be integrated with clustering algorithms, such as k-means or fuzzy clustering, to improve their performance in medical data analysis. The hybrid ACO-clustering approach can be used for tasks like patient clustering or disease subtype identification based on medical data, where ACO helps in finding optimal cluster centres or improving the clustering quality.
4. Evolutionary algorithms (EA) and deep learning: evolutionary algorithms, such as genetic algorithms or evolutionary strategies, can be combined with deep learning models to enhance their training process. These hybrid approaches, often referred to as neuroevolutionary, can be used for tasks like optimizing the architecture of deep neural networks or improving the efficiency of training algorithms. Neuroevolutionary has applications in various medical studies, including medical image analysis, disease diagnosis, and drug discovery.
5. Artificial bee colony (ABC) Algorithm: Inspired by the foraging behavior of honey bees, ABC is a population-based optimization algorithm that simulates the search for food sources performed by honey bees, incorporating exploration and exploitation strategies.
6. Artificial immune systems (AIS): Inspired by the immune system's ability to recognize and eliminate pathogens, AIS algorithms use immunological principles to solve optimization and pattern recognition problems.
7. Neural networks: Inspired by the structure and functioning of the brain, neural networks are zcomputational models composed of interconnected artificial neurons. They have been widely used for various tasks, including pattern recognition, optimization, and machine learning.
8. Bacterial foraging optimization (BFO) Algorithm: Inspired by the behavior of bacteria foraging for nutrients, BFO is a population-based optimization algorithm that models bacterial movement and interaction to find optimal solutions.
9. Firefly algorithm: Inspired by the flashing patterns of fireflies, the Firefly Algorithm is a swarm intelligence-based optimization algorithm that models the movement and attraction of fireflies to find optimal solutions.

10. Artificial immune systems (AIS): Inspired by the immune system's ability to recognize and eliminate pathogens, AIS algorithms use immunological principles to solve optimization and pattern recognition problems.
11. Neural networks: Inspired by the structure and functioning of the brain, neural networks are computational models composed of interconnected artificial neurons. They have been widely used for various tasks, including pattern recognition, optimization, and machine learning.
12. Bacterial foraging optimization (BFO) Algorithm: Inspired by the behavior of bacteria foraging for nutrients, BFO is a population-based optimization algorithm that models bacterial movement and interaction to find optimal solutions.
13. Firefly algorithm: Inspired by the flashing patterns of fireflies, the Firefly Algorithm is a swarm intelligence-based optimization algorithm that models the movement and attraction of fireflies to find optimal solutions.

These algorithms are often referenced in scientific literature and applied to a wide range of problem domains, including optimization, machine learning, data mining, and pattern recognition. These are just a few examples of hybrid approaches in bioinspired algorithms used in medical studies. The choice of the hybrid approach depends on the specific problem at hand and the desired outcome. Researchers continue to explore and develop new hybrid methods to tackle complex medical challenges, leveraging the complementary strengths of different algorithms to achieve better results.

14.8 Conclusion and Summary of Findings

Bioinspired applications have become an important area of research and have the potential in the medical industry by providing innovative and effective solutions to revolutionize various medical challenges. These applications have the potential to revolutionize patient care and treatment outcomes. This case study has highlighted the benefits of bioinspired solutions in the development of medical devices, drug delivery systems, and surgical techniques. These solutions offer innovative and effective solutions to complex problems in the healthcare industry. The future of the medical industry is bright with the continued development of bioinspired applications. Additionally, the study includes references to studies or research that have investigated the effectiveness of this design approach in surgical or medical applications. The case studies presented in this paper demonstrate the potential of bioinspired design in the development of stents, nanoparticles, and surgical systems. However, further research is needed to fully explore the potential of bioinspired design in the medical industry and to bring these innovative solutions to the clinic.

References

1. Langer, R., Drug delivery and targeting. *Nature*, 392, 6679, 5–10, 2015.
2. Chen, C.S. and Ingber, D.E., Tensegrity and mechanoregulation: from skeleton to cytoskeleton. *Osteoarthr. Cartil.*, 7, 1, 81–94, 1999.
3. Vannucci, L., Fossati, G., Langfelder, P., Bioinformatics analysis of microarray data, in: *Microarray Analysis*, pp. 265–288, Humana Press, New York, NY, 2017.
4. Bhargava, N., Sharma, S., Purohit, R., Rathore, P.S., Prediction of recurrence cancer using J48 algorithm, in: *2017 2nd International Conference on Communication and Electronics Systems (ICCES)*, pp. 386–390, IEEE, 2017, October.
5. Dutt, V., Rathore, P.S., Chauhan, K., Support Vector in Healthcare Using SVM/PSO in Various Domains: A Review, in: *Swarm Intelligence Optimization: Algorithms and Applications*, pp. 291–307, 2020.
6. Bhargava, N., Rathore, P.S., Bhowmick, A., Study of X Ray Detection Using CNN in Machine Learning. *Advancements in Smart Computing and Information Security: First International Conference, ASCIS 2022*, Rajkot, India, November 24–26, 2022, Cham: Springer Nature, Switzerland, Revised Selected Papers, Part I, 2023.
7. Keegan, G.L., Stoller, M.L., Winn, C., Robotic technology in surgery: past, present, and future. *Am. J. Surg.*, 190, 5, 649–655, 2005.
8. Goldberg, D.E., *Genetic Algorithm in Search and Optimization: The Technique and Applications,* Kalyanmoy Deb Department of Mechanical Engineering Indian Institute of Technology, Addison-Wesley Professional, Kanpur Kanpur, UP, India, 1989.
9. Kennedy, J. and Eberhart, R., Particle Swarm Optimization. *Proceedings of IEEE International Conference on Neural Networks*, 1942–1948, 1995
10. Dorigo, M., Maniezzo, V., Colorni, A., Ant System: Optimization by a Colony of Cooperating Agents. *IEEE Trans. Syst. Man Cybern. Part B Cybern.*, 26, 1, 29–41, 1996.
11. Karaboga, D. and Basturk, B., A Powerful and Efficient Algorithm for Numerical Function Optimization: Artificial Bee Colony (ABC) Algorithm. *J. Global Optim.*, 39, 3, 459–471, 2007.

12. Das, S. and Suganthan, P.N., Differential Evolution: A Survey of the State-of-the-Art. *IEEE Trans. Evol. Comput.*, 15, 1, 4–31, 2011.
13. de Castro, L.N. and von Zuben, F.J., Artificial Immune Systems: Part I - Basic Theory and Applications. Technical Report, DTIC Document, 2002.
14. Yang, X.S., Firefly Algorithm, Stochastic Test Functions and Design Optimisation. *Int. J. Bio-Inspired Comput.*, 2, 2, 78–84, 2010.
15. Li, H. and Yang, X., Memetic Algorithms, in: *Search Algorithms and Applications*, pp. 351–374, Springer, 2010.
16. Benkhaddra, I., Kumar, A., Setitra, M.A. *et al.*, Design and Development of Consensus Activation Function Enabled Neural Network-Based Smart Healthcare Using BIoT. *Wirel. Pers. Commun.*, 130, 1549–1574, 2023, https://doi.org/10.1007/s11277-023-10344-0 Q2,Impact Factor -2.017.
17. Srivastav, A.L., Markandeya, Patel, N. *et al.*, Concepts of circular economy for sustainable management of electronic wastes: challenges and management options. *Environ. Sci. Pollut. Res.*, 30, 48654–48675, 2023, https://doi.org/10.1007/s11356-023-26052-y Q1,Impact Factor -5.19.
18. Ilyas, B., Kumar, A., Setitra, M.A., Bensalem, Z.E.A., Lei, H., Prevention of DDoS attacks using an optimized deep learning approach in blockchain technology. *Trans. Emerging Telecommun. Technol.*, 34, 4, e4729, 2023, Q2,Impact Factor -3.31.
19. Kumar, A., Rathore, P.S., Dubey, A.K. *et al.*, LTE-NBP with holistic UWB-WBAN approach for the energy efficient biomedical application. *Multimed Tools Appl.*, 82, 39797–39811, 2023, https://doi.org/10.1007/s11042-023-15604-6 Q1,Impact Factor -2.577.
20. Sasubilli, G. and Kumar, A., Machine Learning and Big Data Implementation on Health Care data. *4th International Conference on Intelligent Computing and Control Systems (ICICCS)*, pp. 859–864, 2020, doi: 10.1109/ICICCS48265.2020.9120906.

Index

Printed in the USA/Agawam, MA
September 16, 2026

910661.092